Immunological Aspects of Infection in the Fetus and Newborn

The second of a series of occasional colloquia on aspects of infection which are of current concern to clinicians and scientists.

Medical Society of London
19th–21st September, 1979

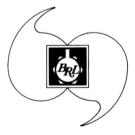

Immunological Aspects of Infection in the Fetus and Newborn

Editors

H. P. LAMBERT

Professor of Microbial Diseases
St. George's Hospital
London

C. B. S. WOOD

Professor of Child Health
Medical College of
St. Bartholomew and the
London Hospital and
Queen Elizabeth Hospital
for Children
London

1981

ACADEMIC PRESS

A Subsidiary of Harcourt Brace Jovanovich, Publishers

London New York Toronto Sydney San Francisco

ACADEMIC PRESS INC. (LONDON) LTD.
24/28 Oval Road,
London NW1

United States Edition published by
ACADEMIC PRESS INC.
111 Fifth Avenue
New York, New York 10003

British Library Cataloguing in Publication Data

Immunological aspects of infection in the fetus and new—born.
1. Fetus—Diseases—Immunological aspects—Congresses
2. Infants (Newborn)—Diseases—Immunological
aspects—Congresses   3. Infection in children—Congresses
I. Lambert, H. P.   II. Wood, C. B. S.
618.3'2   RG627   80-41978

ISBN 0–12–434660–X

Filmset by Willmer Brothers Limited
Birkenhead, Merseyside
and printed in Great Britain by
Whitstable Litho, Kent

Foreword

Immunology has of late begun to make enormous strides in its factual content and its concepts, which are far-reaching in their impact upon medicine and surgery. Yet when one looks at the new knowledge which has been gathered and asks of it questions concerning the immunological problems which surround birth, it is soon apparent that there are still very many mysteries particularly in relation to infection.

The care and protection bestowed by the mother on her offspring begins *in utero*, where the fetus is cocooned by the mother's immunological defence against infection, so that it is remarkably well cared for during nine months of sojourn. Relatively few organisms succeed in penetrating this defence, and in wrecking the fetus before it has had a chance to develop its own powers of resistance.

The moment of birth brings about a rude exposure to the environment in all its most ugly aspects. Perhaps we may ask three questions: why does such a small proportion of the environmental agents of infection succeed in disturbing the innocence of the newborn baby? How does the mother succeed in equipping the baby for the fight against infection in the early weeks of postnatal life? And how can we, as practising physicians and immunologists, help to bridge this immunological gap by buttressing the maternal umbrella of defence?

There is much to discuss in the development of the baby's own acquired resistance to infection, as it takes over the struggle from the mother, and it is perhaps here that we are beginning to realize the fragility of immunological mechanisms. Certainly the inability of immunizing materials to evoke an adequate response to parenteral innoculations has only become obvious comparatively recently with our failure with the newer polysaccharide materials.

Sir Charles Stuart-Harris
Chairman

v

Preface

The fetus, normally a germ free organism in a sterile environment, is at birth suddenly confronted with a huge and diverse population of micro-organisms which rapidly colonizes the skin and mucosal surfaces. This process is usually achieved without untoward effects and the normal microflora, then established, itself becomes part of the developing defensive system against exogenous infection. The last decade has seen much progress in our knowledge of the ingenious mechanisms by which the fetus and neonate are enabled to resist infection and of methods by which their capacity to do so might be increased. These advances are the subject of this second Beecham Symposium,* held at the Medical Society of London on 19th–21st September 1979.

This book contains the spoken papers, which in most cases have been somewhat amplified by their authors in their written form, because each speaker had been constrained to ten minutes at the lectern. This allowed ample time for the discussions which followed, and formed the main bulk and a most valuable part of the work of the meeting. As in the first colloquium in 1978, the numbers involved were strictly limited, on this occasion to 26, each of whom contributed to the working sessions.

On behalf of the organizing committee, the editors wish to express their thanks to the sessional chairmen, Sir Ashley Miles, Sir Charles Stuart-Harris, Dr Phillip Evans and Dr David Tyrrell; for the pace and liveliness of the meeting if not its content, was largely in their hands. Beecham were once again the organizing force, to whom the participant scientists owe thanks. The editors are particularly glad to acknowledge the valued work of Palantype who, with audio engineers, ensured a rapid transcription service for these discussions.

Sir Charles Stuart-Harris
Professor H. P. Lambert
Professor F. W. O'Grady
Professor J. D. Williams
Professor C. B. S. Wood
The late Mr D. Goodchild

* The first Beecham Symposium on Antibiotic Interactions was edited by J. D. Williams and published by Academic Press, 1979.

ORGANIZING COMMITTEE

Chairman—Sir Charles Stuart-Harris, CBE

Professor H. P. Lambert
Professor F. W. O'Grady
Professor J. D. Williams
Professor C. B. S. Wood
The late Mr D. Goodchild

List of Participants

Matteo Adinolfi, Paediatric Research Unit, The Prince Philip Research Laboratories, Guy's Hospital Medical School, London SE1, UK.

A. C. Allison, International Laboratory for Research on Animal Diseases, P.O. Box 30709, Nairobi, Kenya, Africa.

J. J. Bullen, Laboratory of Bacterial Infectivity, National Institute for Medical Research, Mill Hill, London NW7, UK.

P. J. Cole, Cardiothoracic Institute, Brompton Hospital, London SW3, UK.

Max Cooper, Department of Pediatrics, University of Alabama Medical Center, Birmingham, Alabama, USA.

A. M. Denman, Division of Immunology, Clinical Research Centre, Northwick Park Hospital, Harrow, Middlesex, UK.

Janet M. Dewdney, Beecham Pharmaceuticals, Brockham Park, Betchworth, Surrey, UK.

Philip Evans, 24 Abbey Road, London NW8, UK.

W. Page Faulk, Blond McIndoe Centre for Transplantation Biology, Queen Victoria Hospital, East Grinstead, Sussex, UK.

Anthony Hayward, Department of Pediatrics, University of Colorado, Medical Center, 4200 East Ninth Avenue, Denver, Colorado 80262, USA.

Pekka Kuitinen, Jorvin Hospital, Sairaalen-Kuntainliitto, Jorvin, Finland.

H. P. Lambert, St George's Hospital, Blackshaw Road, Tooting, London SW17, UK.

W. C. Marshall, The Hospital for Sick Children, Great Ormond Street, London WC1, UK.

L. Mellander, Department of Immunology, University of Göteborg, Guldhedsgatan, 10, 413 46 Göteborg, Sweden.

Sir Ashley A. Miles, Department of Medical Microbiology, The London Hospital Medical College, Turner Street, London E1, UK.

F. W. O'Grady, Department of Microbiology, University Hospital, Queen's Medical Centre, Nottingham NG7, UK.

W. G. Reeves, Department of Immunology, University Hospital, Queen's Medical Centre, Nottingham NG7, UK.

Bruno Reiter, National Institute for Research in Dairying, Shenfield, Reading RG2, UK.

J. W. G. Smith, National Institute for Biological Standards and Control, Holly Hill, Hampstead, London NW3, UK.

Sir Charles Stuart-Harris, University of Sheffield Medical School, Beech Hill Road, Sheffield S10, UK.

J. F. Soothill, Institute of Child Health, Guildford Street, London WC1, UK.

H. Stern, Department of Virology, St George's Hospital Medical School, Hyde Park Corner, London SW1, UK.

Adolfo Turano, Instituto di Microbiologia, Spedali Civili, 25199, Brescia, Italy.

D. A. J. Tyrrell, Clinical Research Centre, Division of Communicable Diseases, Watford Road, Harrow, Middlesex HA1, UK.

W. Allan Walker, Pediatric-Gastrointestinal and Nutrition Unit, Massachusetts General Hospital, Boston, Mass 02114, USA.

J. A. Walker-Smith, Department of Child Health, St Bartholomew's Hospital, London EC1A, UK.

J. D. Williams, Department of Medical Microbiology, The London Hospital Medical College, Turner Street, London E1, UK.

C. B. S. Wood, Department of Child Health, Queen Elizabeth's Hospital for Children, Hackney Road, London E2, UK.

Contents

Foreword   v

Preface   vii

List of Participants   ix

Clinical Aspects of Pre and Perinatal Infection   1
W. C. MARSHALL

Ontogeny of Complement, Lysozyme and Lactoferrin in
    Man   19
MATTEO ADINOLFI

Role of the Placenta in Protecting the Fetus from Infection   53
W. PAGE FAULK

Clinical Problems in Postnatal Infection   69
C. B. S. WOOD

The Nature and Role of Mucosal Surface Immunity against
    Infection in the Newborn   83
W. ALLAN WALKER

Development and Maturation of Immunity in the Newborn 107

A. R. HAYWARD

The Role of Milk and Gut Flora in Protection of the Newborn Against Infection 123

J. J. BULLEN

Humoral and Cellular Immunities Transmitted by Breastmilk 139

L. MELLANDER, B. CARLSSON, U. DAHLGREN and L. Å. HANSON

The Contributions of Milk to Resistance to Intestinal Infection in the Newborn 155

BRUNO REITER

Advances in Immunization for Protection of the Fetus and Newborn against Infection 197

J. W. G. SMITH

Damage to the Fetus and Newborn from Prophylactic Procedures

W. C. MARSHALL

Future Prospects for Protection of the Fetus and Newborn 227

A. C. ALLISON

Subject Index 247

Clinical Aspects of Pre and Perinatal Infection

W. C. MARSHALL

The Hospital for Sick Children
Great Ormond Street, London WC1, UK

Infections or febrile illnesses presumed to be due to infection in pregnancy are common but there is little precise information available on their frequency. Prospective clinical studies will underestimate the numbers because of a failure to identify subclinical infections (Sever and White, 1968). Screening of cord blood for immunoglobulin levels depends on infection of the fetus and may not identify perinatal infections or fetal damage consequent on indirect mechanisms such as toxins or fever (Smith et al., 1978). In spite of the frequency of infection the majority seem to be of little significance and the number of agents known to infect and damage the fetus are limited (Table I). Maternal immune status and fetal maturity are known to be important factors in some but not all of these infections, but little is known of the role of the placenta in either preventing or facilitating fetal infection.

With the exception of neonatal chickenpox, when some infants with neonatal herpes or with either congenital rubella or congenital toxoplasmosis require treatment, the clinician relies on serology or identification of the infectious agent to diagnose congenital infections. But for diagnosis to be attempted the

1

TABLE I.
Agents proven or suspected of causing fetal infection and damage.

Proven	Suspected
Rubella virus	Mumps virus
Rubella vaccine virus	Influenza viruses
Cytomegalovirus	Hepatitis A, non A/non B viruses
Varicella-zoster virus	Coxsackie virsues
Epstein-Barr virus	Echoviruses
Vaccinia virus	Measles virus
Variola virus	
Hepatitis B virus	
Poliovirus	
Listeria monocytogenes	
Treponema pallidum	
Mycobacterium tuberculosis	
Toxoplasma gondii	
Plasmodia	
Trypanosomes	
Filaria	

clinical features must arouse the suspicion of congenital or perinatal infection and then the most appropriate specimens must be collected. In this respect the placenta and membranes and amniotic fluid are grossly underutilized.

It is now hoped that congenital rubella is in a transitional state whereby the natural history is being modified by the use of rubella vaccines. The spectrum of clinical disorders associated with congenital rubella is well known and a full description is beyond the scope of this presentation. However attention should be drawn to the longterm effects. It is now accepted that perceptive deafness may develop months or even years after birth, and the most recent report of this phenomenon is contained in the study of Desmond *et al.* (1978). In mid-infancy, skin rashes and pneumonitis may make their appearance and then resolve without any apparent *sequelae*, but the lung disease may cause death (Phelan and Campbell, 1969). A remarkable finding has been the description of progressive rubella panencephalitis, first described by Townsend *et al.* (1975) and by Weil *et al.* (1975). It occurs early in the second decade and is slowly progressive and fatal. The disorder superficially resembles the subacute sclerosing panencephalitis of measles. Serum and CSF rubella antibodies are greatly elevated and rubella IgM antibody is reported to be present in the early stages. Rubella virus has been isolated from the brain by cocultivation techniques, and presumably the virus has gained entry to the nervous system before birth.

As the rubella immunization programmes proceed it is important to re-examine the assumption that congenital rubella is a consequence of primary infection in pregnancy; is the evidence of pre-existing rubella antibody secure? At the present time this assumption would seem to be correct.

There is abundant evidence that cytomegalovirus is the most common infection of the human fetus. Estimates of the number of children damaged as a result of congenital infection have been the major stimulus to develop a cytomegalovirus vaccine (Stern, 1979). Regional differences in the incidence of maternal and fetal infections may exist and warrant further investigations. One group in whom there is a higher risk is the young unmarried woman (MacDonald and Tobin, 1978). CMV resembles rubella with respect to the evidence for continuing or late development of defects. The risk of fetal infection is high, being of the order of 50% (Stern, 1979).

However the subject is a complex one; perinatal infection is not uncommon but the limited data presently available indicate these infections are not a hazard (Reynolds *et al.*, 1973). On the other hand infection of the newborn from blood products can be serious (Benson *et al.*, 1979).

The knowledge that congenital infection may occur in women known to be immune (Stagno *et al.*, 1977; Schopfer *et al.*, 1978) requires a re-evaluation of present estimates on the risk of damage caused by prenatal infections. The present evidence that damage does not occur when fetal infection occurs in an immune woman is encouraging but is limited in both the number of infants who have been identified and duration of observation.

The serious effects of herpesvirus nominis in numerical terms are related to infection occurring at or around the time of delivery. Nahmias and Visintine (1976) have clearly demonstrated the potential for the devastating disease and the extraordinary high mortality rate from infection in the neonate by this virus. The source of the infection has raised the interesting possibility of prevention by avoiding vaginal delivery. It might be hoped that chemotherapy could be effective but the agents which are available at the present time have not had a dramatic impact. It would be interesting to speculate on a role for interferon administered to the mother just before delivery.

TABLE II.
Major features of congenital varicella syndrome (early gestational chickenpox).

Low birth weight for gestational age
Cicatricial skin lesions
Limb atrophy/hypoplasia
Chorioretinitis, optic atrophy
Microphthalmia, cataracts
Cerebral cortical atrophy

TABLE III.

Relationship between onset of perinatal varicella and outcome.

Maternal onset before delivery	Infant onset	Numbers			Fatality rate
		Total	Survived	Fatal	
≥ 5 days	0–4 days	27	27	0	0
≤ 4 days	5–10 days	23	16	7	30·4%

Adapted from De Nicola and Hanshaw (1979).

Chickenpox is infrequent in the pregnant woman but may have widely differing consequences depending on the time of infection. The spectrum ranges from the permanent defects caused by early gestational infection (Table II) to mild or severe chickenpox in the neonate, the neonatal disease being more severe if the maternal rash occurs within four days of delivery (Table III) (De Nicola and Hanshaw, 1979). The other member of the herpesvirus group, Epstein-Barr (EB) virus seems to be remarkable in the almost complete absence of a role in fetal infection (Chang and Seto, 1979).

The risk of hepatitis B infection depends on whether there is overt hepatitis or a carrier state in the pregnant woman. In the former, late gestational infection appears to carry a high risk of transmission to the fetus (Schweitzer *et al.*, 1972). In contrast the risk of pre or perinatal infection in HBsAg carrier mothers is complex and not fully elucidated. The presence of HBeAg is clearly important but anti HBeAg apparently is not necessarily protective. Ethnicity would appear to be another factor. In studies in the UK Derso *et al.* (1978) and Woo *et al.* (1979) have shown higher infection rates in offspring of Chinese mothers. Lee *et al.*, (1978), in Hong Kong, also identified the importance of HBeAg but have drawn attention to the presence of HBsAg in gastric contents of these infants and suggested a universal mechansism of infection by the oral route during delivery. These early childhood hepitits B infections are, with rare exceptions (Kattamis *et al.*, 1974; Dupuy *et al.*, 1975), apparently of little clinical significance but insufficient time has elapsed to determine the effects of longterm carriage of HBsAg (Shiraki *et al.*, 1977). There is a risk to attendants at delivery of HBsAg carrier mother and the care of the carrier infant which has to be recognized.

The role of hepatitis A and the non A/non B hepatitis in pregnancy has yet to be determined. The application of means to identify these agents will probaly confirm the role of hepatitis A in causing premature labour as has been shown with hepatitis B by Hieber *et al.* (1977).

The recent outbreaks of infection with enteroviruses in several nurseries in this country (Nagington *et al.*, 1978) has drawn attention to their potential for damage

TABLE IV.

Incidence of congenital toxoplasmosis per 1000 live births.

Vienna	6·0–7·0
Netherlands	6·5
Gottingen	5·0
Paris	3·0
Mexico City	2·0
Birmingham, Alabama	1·3
New York	1·3
UK	0·05

in the newborn but evidence is lacking for any significant consequence of prenatal infection, other than by poliovirus. On the other hand mumps virus deserves reevaluation, with attention being paid to its possible neurotrophism.

Toxoplasmosis is rare in the UK and there is a striking difference in the incidence of congenital infection in different countries (Table IV). An interesting feature of this infection is that fetal infection following early gestational toxoplasmosis is less frequent than late gestational infection but the incidence of damage is greater (Fig. 1). Periodically the question is raised as to whether congenital infection can occur in subsequent pregnancies. Desmonts is of the opinion that there is no convincing evidence to support this (G. Desmonts, 1978, pers. comm.).

Attention should be drawn to the increasing numbers of malaria in the UK (Table V)—many of these infections are occurring in nonimmune individuals, and thus cases of congenital malaria can be expected to occur from time to time. Since 1950 there have been eight cases of congenital malaria in this country (Bradbury, 1977). The role of malaria in causing fetal growth retardation and low birth weight

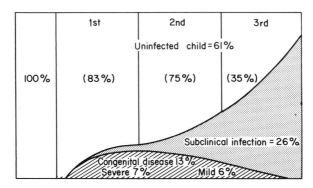

Fig. 1 Frequency of deliveries of infants with clinical congenital toxoplasmosis (hatched area), subclinical infection (stippled area), and with no infection (unshaded area), following acquisition either before or during the three trimesters of pregnancy. (Desmonts and Couvreur, 1978.)

TABLE V.
Notified imported cases of malaria in the UK 1970–1979.*

Year	Number†
1970	101
1971	261
1972	336
1973	541 (1)
1974	662
1975	749 (1)
1976	1220 (3)
1977	1527
1978	1909
1979 (January–June)	711

*From Malaria Reference Laboratory, Ross Institute, London School of Hygiene and Tropical Medicine.
† Figures in brackets denote numbers of cases of congenital malaria.

in areas where malaria occurs in an immune population is well known (Reinhardt, 1978).

The role of drugs must be taken into account when evaluating the possible effects of any infection. A recent example of this concerns tuberculosis in pregnancy. In one area of London 10% of Asian women with tuberculosis had pregnancy coinciding (O. R. McCarthy, 1979, pers. comm.). Rifampicin is now standard chemotherapy in most Western countries and is contraindicated in pregnancy because of a very small number of reports of severe defects of the nervous system. However the incidence of these or other adverse effects of this drug is unknown; studies of women who fail to avoid becoming pregnant when receiving rifampicin should be carried out.

The clinician is heavily dependant on the microbiologist and the immunologist for the diagnosis of the majority of fetal or perinatal infections. The immunological response of the fetus and the newborn to these infections enables the diagnosis to be made in the majority of cases but other materials should also be utilized; from the infant but also from the mother and from the placenta. As termination of the infection in the infant in order to prevent continuing damage would seem to be desirable, rapid diagnosis is necessary for the most effective results of such treatment.

REFERENCES

Benson, J. W. T., Bodden, S. J. and Tobin, J. O'H. (1979). Cytomegalovirus and blood transfusion in neonates. *Archives of Disease in Childhood* **54**, 538–541.

Bradbury, A. J. (1977). Congenital malaria in one non-identical twin. *British Medical Journal* **2,** 613.

Chang, R. S. and Seto, D. Y. S. (1979). Perinatal infection by Epstein-Barr virus. *Lancet* **ii,** 201.

De Nicola, L. K. and Hanshaw, J. D. (1979). Congenital and neonatal varicella. *Journal of Pediatrics* **94,** 175–176.

Derso, A., Boxall, E. H., Tarlow, M. J. and Flewett, T. H. (1978). Transmission of HBsAg from mother to infant in four ethnic groups. *British Medical Journal* **1,** 949–952.

Desmond, M. M., Fisher, E. S., Vorderman, A. L., Schaffer, H. G., Andrew, L. P., Zion, T. E. and Catlin, F. I. (1978). The longitudinal course of congenital rubella encephalitis in non-retarded children. *Journal of Pediatrics* **93,** 584–591.

Desmonts, G. and Couvreur, J. (1975). Toxoplasmosis: Epidemiologic and Serologic Aspects of Perinatal Infection. *In* "Infections of the Fetus and the Newborn Infant" (Eds S. Krugman and A. A. Gershon), p. 118. Progress in Clinical and Biological Research, Vol. 3. Liss, New York.

Dupuy, J. M., Frommel, D. and Alagille, D. (1975). Severe viral hepatitis B in infancy. *Lancet* **i,** 191–194.

Hieber, J. P., Dalton, D., Shorey, J. and Combes, B. (1971). Hepatitis and pregnancy. *Journal of Pediatrics* **91,** 545–549.

Kattamis, C. A., Demetrios, D. and Matsaniotis, N. S. (1974). Australia antigen and neonatal hepatitis syndrome. *Pediatrics* **54,** 157–164,.

Lee, A. K. P., Ip, H. M. H. and Wong, V. C. W. (1978). Mechanisms of maternal-fetal transmission of Hepatitis B virus. *Journal of Infectious Diseases* **128,** 668–671.

MacDonald, H. and Tobin, J. O'H. (1978). Congenital cytomegalovirus infection: a collaborative study on epidemiological, clinical and laboratory findings. *Developmental Medicine and Child Neurology* **20,** 471–482.

Nagington, J., Wreghitt, T. G., Gandy, G., Robston, N. R. C. and Berry, P. J. (1978). Fatal ECHOVIRUS II infections in outbreak in special care baby unit. *Lancet* **ii,** 725–728.

Nahmias, A. J. and Visintine, A. M. (1976). Herpes Simplex *In* "Infectious Diseases of the Fetus and Newborn Infant" (Eds W. B. Saunders, J. S. Remington and J. O. Klein), 156–190.

Phelan, P. and Campbell, P. (1969). Pulmonary complications of rubella embryopathy. *Journal of Pediatrics* **75,** 202–212.

Reinhardt, M. C. (1978). A survey of mothers and their newborns in the Ivory Coast. *Paediatrics Acta Helvetia* **33,** Suppl. 41, 65–84.

Reynolds, D. W., Stagno, S., Hosty, T. S., Tiller, M. and Alford, C. A. (1973). Maternal cytomegalovirus excretion and perinatal infection. *New England Journal of Medicine* **289,** 1–5.

Schopfer, K., Lauber, E. and Krech, H. (1978). Congenital cytomegalovirus infection in newborn infants of mothers infected before pregnancy. *Archives of Disease in Childhood* **53,** 536–539.

Schweitzer, I. L., Wing, A., McPeak, C. and Spears, R. L. (1972). Hepatitis and hepatitis associated antigen in 56 mother-infant pairs. *Journal of the American Medical Association* **220,** 1092–1095.

Sever, J. and White, L. R. (1968). Intrauterine viral infections. *Annual Review of Medicine* **19,** 471–485.

Shiraki, K., Yoshihara, N., Kawana, T., Yasui, H. and Sakurai, M. (1977). Hepatitis B surface antigen and chronic hepatitis in infants born to asymptomatic carrier mothers. *American Journal of Disease in Children* **131,** 644–647.

Smith, D. W., Clarren, S. K. and Harvey, M. A. S. (1978). Hyperthermia as a possible teratogenic agent. *Journal of Pediatrics* **92,** 878–883.

Stango, S., Reynolds, D. W., Huang, E. S., Thanes, S. D., Smith, R. J. and Alford, C. A. (1977). Congenital cytomegalovirus infection. Occurrence in an immune population. *New England Journal of Medicine* **296,** 1254–1258.

Stern, H. (1979). Cytomegalovirus vaccine: justification and problems. *In* "Recent Advances in Clinical Virology" (Ed. A. P. Waterson), Vol. 1, 117–134. Churchill, Livingstone.

Townsend, J. J., Baringer, J. R., Wolinsky, J. S., Malamud, N., Mendick, J. P., Panitch, H. S., Scott, R. A. T., Oshiro, L. S. and Cremer, N. E. (1975). Progressive rubella panencephalitis, late onset after congenital rubella. *New England Journal of Medicine* **292,** 990–993.

Weil, M. L., Itabashi, H. H., Cremer, N. E., Oshiro, L. S., Lennette, E. H. and Carnay, L. (1975) Chronic progressive panencephalitis due to rubella virus simulating subacute sclerosing panencephalitis. *New England Journal of Medicine* **292,** 994–998.

Woo, D., Cummins, M., Davies, P. A., Harvey, D. R., Hurley, R. and Waterson, A. P. (1979). Vertical transmission of hepatitis B surface antigen in carrier mothers in two West Indian hospitals. *Archives of Disease in Childhood* **54,** 670–675.

DISCUSSION

Hayward EB virus infections seem to me to be extremely interesting, and in particular why newborns do not get them. We don't know how early either epithelial cells or B cells in developing fetuses will develop receptors for EB virus.

If the data in mice are true, which indicate that B cells develop C3 receptors relatively late, and Klein's data suggest that the EB virus gets into the B cell by something which is closely associated with the C3 receptor, it is possible that very early B cells in humans, perhaps before 10 weeks of gestation, would not have C3 receptors.

In that context we could ask Max whether he thinks that, in their findings, very early B cells had C3 receptors.

Marshall Does this make this a unique virus as far as the herpesviruses are concerned?

Hayward The others do not get in through C3 receptors, do they?

Wood This leads me to want to ask a rather simpler question: do the viruses which appear to cause quite serious tissue destruction through one means or another have any common properties either immunological or structural or chemical?

Marshall At a very simple level I think if you consider whether they are DNA or RNA viruses, it is found that both DNA and RNA viruses cause widespread damage.

Denman Dr Hayward has drawn our attention to the possibility that until B lymphocytes develop suitable receptors, EB virus might not be able to gain entry into these cells and grow. But is this not really part of a much more general question, namely the extent to which maturation of the reticuloendothelial system in general has to progress before various viruses are able to replicate in the sites of predilection in the adult. I wonder if one can make any broader correlations in terms of those viruses which are pathogenic for the fetus once they enter and replicate in reticuloendothelial cells and the state of maturation of the reticuloendothelial system and the pathogenicity of these viruses? This might apply to virus infection in which tissue damage results from the immune response to the virus and the immunopathological consequences.

Marshall   This would seem not to be true in the case of rubella where even preconception rubella causes infection at the very early implantation stage, and a virus can be isolated from products of conception at the very earliest stage of pregnancy and the virus is presumably replicating in the embryo.

Denman   I suppose you could argue also that viruses grow in tissue culture in relatively immature cells.

Evans   I was going to mention something of the same sort: it does not have to be reticuloendothelial tissue, does it? For example *Bordetella pertussis* will grow in egg when the trachea is differentiated, but not before.

Wood   So when is a fetus nice to grow in, and when does it produce inflammatory response to something growing in it? Is it the inflammatory response which is more destructive than the colonization by the virus?

Allison   There are some examples, for instance lymphocytic choriomeningitis where infection is initiated early in fetal life. It is the immune response to the virus which actually cases the damage.

Wood   To what extent is it an immune response and to what extent is it an inflammatory response which does not necessarily have to have immunological components?

Allison   In the case of lymphocytic choriomeningitis, it appears to be a T cell mediated and immune response, which ends up with an inflammatory component. There are other interesting features as well such as the restriction on the basis of major histocompatibility types, of the destruction of infective cells sensitized T lymphocytes, as well as the nonspecific inflamatory component.

Tyrrell   Some of the work that Andrew Neighbour did indicated that it was not necessary to suggest anything more than that a virus invaded some cells, multiplied them and killed them. His findings in a mouse model were adequately explained, without postulating any immune reponse taking part in the destruction of embryonic cells.

Making a really wide generalization, I think you have to say that a virus susceptible cell is a virus susceptible cell. You can find exceptions to other generalizations. You may have to wait for the respiratory tract to mature for virus infections just as you do for *Bordetella*. On the other hand in experimental infections with enteroviruses, only the young animal, the suckling mouse, for instance, is the classical model of the coxsackie infection. But the trouble is that I think if you look at it at a cellular level, we are still ignorant about what determines whether a virus will enter and infect or not. Dr Marshall was mentioning enteroviruses and if you put nucleic acid in, all sorts of enteroviruses will grow in all sorts of cells. In that case the surface of the cell has to have a site (which we call operationally a "receptor") through which an intact enterovirus can enter. So if we can generalize about that, susceptible cells are those with the right surface structure into which a virus can enter, and within which it can replicate and cause damage. But that may only be a partial explanation for other systems.

Hayward   Do you visualize these viruses as crossing the placenta? Or do you think that they could cross the amniotic sac?

Marshall   I do not know, but I think the words "crossing the placenta" are not very clear. In all intra-uterine infections, there is a placentitis, an infection is set up in the placenta, and then it moves on to the fetus as the next stage. I don't think these agents drift across from the maternal circulation into the fetus, I think placentitis is an integral part of the pathogenesis of these infections.

Tyrrell   But in fact the involvement of the placenta, on the maternal side in general can be sufficient in animal models anyway to explain most of the abnormalities of the fetus. Again, going back to Andrew Neighbour's work, I think it was with the coxsackie system, he found there was no evidence that the virus actually invaded the fetus at all. It was presumably due to nutritional effects mediated through the inflammation and other damage that the fetus was underweight, underdeveloped.

Marshall   What about the role of fever itself in the fetal damage? There has been recent publicity on this aspect, and it was stated that there did not appear to be a higher incidence of congenital malformations in Scandinavian women who took frequent sauna baths. One wonders whether, if you have frequent sauna baths, you adapt yourself to recurrent high environmental temperatures and therefore not likely to have a deleterious effect on pregnant women. Whereas the high fever occurring as a result of an infection there is no adaptation.

Cooper   With regard to receptors for viruses, there is a means of gaining entry into cells, and presumably there are receptors for bacterial and other kinds of infectious agents as well. There probably is not much known about the operation of some of these receptors—or is there? Before finding out whether anyone can answer that, I should like to mention a novel way in which microbes might enter cells which has been put forth by Weissman. One would like to know a great deal more about the antigens of receptors used by bacteria and viruses to gain entry into the fetal cells. One interesting mechanism proposed by Weissman for oncogenic viruses is the use of specific antibodies as receptors. These should be present by the ninth or tenth week of gestation and would allow agents to infect specific clones of immunocompetent cells. How important that might be as a means of disseminating an infectious agent I do not know but it is an interesting phenomenon.

Faulk   I should like to follow up the point just made by Dr Cooper. A very rich source of the so-called antibody receptor which he was talking about, which is generally referred to as an Fc receptor, is the trophoblast; and in fact it is one of the jobs of the trophoblast to transport immunoglobulin, particularly IgG immunoglobulin. If this immunoglobulin is bound to whatever microbiological agent you have in mind, whether it is a virus or not, you will activate Fc into such a configuration that it will fit into trophoblast Fc receptor. I must stress that there is no experimental evidence on this point, to my knowledge, but one would presumably "piggy-back" into the trophoblast the antibody-bound virus complex.

Allison   I have wondered about this point, because some viruses which infect the placenta such as lymphocytic choriomeningitis and herpes virus, have virus antibody complexes which are still infectious. This would be consistent with what has been said. One could set up such a study experimentally, injecting virus intravenously or virus antibody complexes which are still infective. One could then see if there is any increased probability of infecting the placenta.

Turano   I have always been struck, during the period of an epidemic such as the rubella we had a few years ago in Italy, by the fact that there were very few birth defects. Could we take into consideration also the role of interferon in this case?

Marshall   That is an interesting suggestion, particularly in relation to the placenta. As far as rubella virus is concerned, it is associated with viraemia. Many of the respiratory viruses, such as influenza, would not be of this type were viraemia is extremely rare.

Hayward   Do you think that EB viruses could infect the placenta?

Marshall   I think the answers to the EB virus question rest very firmly with technologists, in developing methods of identifying the agent and therefore knowing about its consequences of infection. One can only speculate as to these.

Allison   The nasopharyngeal cells are infected, and in the case of the nasopharyngeal tumours it is possible to recover the complete virus from them, so that the presumption is that EB virus can attach to enter and transform those cells.

Allison   This is recent work done by Epstein's group in Bristol.

Denman   Could we go back to the more general point raised by Dr Marshall that an inflammatory response in the placenta invariably aides the dissemination of virus in the fetus? What do you envisage as being the essential component of this reaction? To what extent is this an immune reaction? Also is there good evidence to support the notion that Fc receptors engendered by infectious complexes or villous or circulating cells are a means of transporting infectious complexes into the fetus, with the subsequent release of virus, with the pathological consequences which follow?

Marshall   Most paediatricians never see the placenta.

Denman   Presumably there must be evidence of some sort. I am asking whether those viruses which induce immunopathological reaction in the placenta are those which are more likely to be disseminated in the fetus and induce pathological *sequelae*, and that the initiating effects are in the placenta.

Faulk Since the word placenta has come up, I should like to say that there is quite a lot of work on this question being done in the USA. In the first instance, one has to consider the route of infection. In the case of an ascending infection, we have to broaden our horizons away fron the placenta to the amnion. In this case, one sees a good many examples where there are inflammatory cells, the so-called chorioamnionitis. Sex chromosome markers on those cells show that they are predominantly maternal. This is somewhere in the neighbourhood of 20% of pregnancies, and one cannot ascribe the infectious agent to it. One sees this in diseases such as pre-eclamptic toxeamia, and in maternal diabetics, where there may be an underlying immunopathological disease but not infectious. On the other hand, in terms of placentitis, this is an inflammation of the placental villus, and in this case the cells that are inflamed in the villus are predominantly fetal in origin. These are almost always ascribable to an infectious aetiology. The highest incidence of nondiagnosed villitis is about 6%. But most people who have spent their career in studying this problem, such as Prof. Harold Fox in Manchester, seem to think that it is somewhere in the neighbourhood of 3%. In other words, when we see placentitis, more often than not the infectious organism can be obtained by culture. If we see chorioamionitis, usually it cannot be obtained.

Adinolfi Is there any risk of infecting the fetus by performing amniocentesis?

Marshall I was not referring to amniocentesis as a method of diagnosis but further examination of amniotic fluid; not only for the identification of an infectious agent but for immunoglobulin levels in the amniotic fluid obtained at the time of delivery. At this stage I was not deliberately proposing that we would use this as a method of diagnosis of intra-uterine infection.

Smith Do you have any idea what proportion of congenital defects can be attributable to infection of the mother?

Marshall Certainly less than 5% of all defects could be attributable to infection in pregnancy.

Could I take up the term congenital defects and perhaps comment on that? I think this has held up much of understanding of intra-uterine infections that they cause any clinical abnormality at birth. I was trying to show that the consequences of these infections may not become manifest for one or two decades after birth. If we are looking for defects of malformations present at the time of birth there will be a great underestimate of the impact of these infections.

Smith I appreciate that they may come out later.

Marshall Many will come later.

Smith One in 37 births at the moment in the UK have some sort of defect apparent at birth, but the proportion due to uterine infection is fairly small.

Chairman Dr Marshall, are you referring to the late effects, for instance, of rubella virus—at birth apparently normal, but deafness occurring within say, six months, a year, two years or so attributable to an infection *in utero*? Is this what you are getting at?

Marshall   Yes.

Walker Smith   Could I ask whether you would advocate screening neonates for infection in the light of this?

Marshall   The initial interest in screening was related to the measurement of immunoglobulins in the cord blood. It is clear that different agents have a different capacity to generate premature synthesis of IgM in the fetus, and perhaps the time of fetal infection is important. For example, in some children with congenital cytomegalovirus infection, IgM cytomegalovirus antibody is not present in the cord blood and may not develop for a week or so later. Alford has shown that there are a number of infections that occur when the levels of IgM are not elevated there are going to be situations where the IgM is going to be raised and it is not due to an infection. Perhaps there has been too much attention paid to the immunoglobulins. I would like to hear some comments about the coexistent premature synthesis of IgA by the fetus as a second marker of a prenatal immunological stimulus.

Cooper   It seems unlikely that IgA would be a good marker until very late in gestation since it has not been shown that one can trigger plasma cells to make and secrete IgA antobodies until well after 30 weeks of gestational age; Although at this time there are plenty of B lymphocytes expressing IgA on their surface, they do not seem to be triggerable by antigen or nitogen.

Tyrrell   Can I get just a point of clarification. You say that you believe a placentitis is part of the means by which the virus gains access to the embryo and it was mentioned elsewhere that placentitis can be found. Is there any evidence that looking for such pathological changes is a way of picking up children who might otherwise be missed with mild infections with gross morphological changes?

Marshall   The *Lancet* very recently has reported fluorescence of placental tissues for cytomegalovirus as a mode of diagnosing congenital cytomegalovirus infection. It was claimed that this would be a short cut to diagnosis where the present method is isolation of virus, which, of course, is time-consuming. But I think it is a field which certainly should be looked at.

Reeves   I would like to extend the discussion concerning IgM levels and other antibody levels into asking the question, what kind of markers should we be looking for in cord blood, or in other fluids, to try to ascertain what the real incidence of intra-uterine infection may be, whether or not there is significant pathology associated with it. About five years ago or more, several authors in the literature were stating categorically that when the cord IgM level was more than 18 or 20 mg % that was indicative of intra-uterine infection. Workers in Canada and a study which we performed in Nottingham did nor confirm this impression and certainly our feeling is that this is a low yield exercise. As Dr Marshall was implying, there are quite a lot of children born who have a cord IgM about that level and who, even with careful follow-up, do not produce any evidence to indicate pathology.

Marshall I would agree entirely that the approach to the identification of the true incidence of infection has not really been attempted at any great extent. It is going to require a multi-disciplinary approach. Most investigators have been interested in one particular aspect. A group studying it on a multidisciplinary basis is more likely to arrive at the true incidence.

Reeves Proceeding to look for specific IgM against toxoplasmosis or cytomegalovirus is a procedure that one does not undertake lightly on vast numbers of cord sera. One needs an entry point, an indication for doing it. It would be nice to know what indices of suspicion should cause one to be looking for specific antibodies against certain organisms.

Wood I wonder whether this is a situation where one could use acute phase reactants, for certainly they have been interesting in relationship to bacterial infections in the newborn. Do they have a role in looking to see whether there is evidence of virus infection?

Adinolfi I think that C9, a later complement, may be a very good candidate as an acute phase protein because it is present in very low concentration in the cord blood. It is the only component of the complement which is present in concentrations around 10–20% of the levels in the adult and behaves as an acute phase protein. Because of infection the levels will increase dramatically. We have seen in children of about 10 or 11 years of age C9 is a very useful marker for infection.

Denman Could we ask Dr Marshall how discriminatory he feels acute phase reactants are in distinguishing between specific infections and tissue damage from any cause.

If, for example, one considers C-reactive protein in a disease like systemic lupus erythematosus it has been shown that blood levels cannot be used to distinguish between secondary bacterial infection, viral infections and exacerbations of the disease process. Thus one wonders whether given the difficulties of interpreting the pathological features in the placenta in such serological assays would be any more discriminating.

Marshall I do not think that we know this. The question of tissue damage by hypoxia or trauma may well be factors that generate these substances and, therefore discrimination could be very low.

Soothill Might I comment on this speculation we are having? Until we know what questions we are answering, we will not be able to select the right test. I am not quite sure what infection is. If the organism gets there but does not get established, is that infection? If it gets there, gets established, but does not cause trouble, is that infection? An example of the latter in fetus infection with rubella who are not damaged. So it is likely that the proportions in their different categories will differ with different organisms. Also hosts will differ. Until the question is expressed precisely, it is not helpful to discuss the tests to investigate it.

Cooper It seems probable than an important response that is seen to exogenous agents is non specific, i.e. having to do with polyclonal responses of immunocompetent cells to mitogens that many of these agents or their products exert, LPS stimulation is a classic example of a good way to trigger clones of antibody producing cells that react with self antigen. This raises several considerations. This would imply that a lot of antibodies or immune cell products that were being made would not be specific for the infection agent. Presumably all kinds of clones would be triggered. Nevertheless the polyclonal immune and inflammatory responses could be important in eliminating an agent. It could be that agents who do not serve as polyclonal mitogens might survive for longer periods of time. It would be curious to know if rubella is a polyclonal mitogen, for example, since it does survive so long, although it obviously seems to be triggering clones that are not reactive with its determinants, antigenic determinants. Thirdly, there is the problem of injuring the fetus with the activation of self-reactive clones or release of biologically active materials that would cause inflammatory disease.

Faulk   May I just say that there are several situations, if we are talking about antigenic bombardment of the fetus, which I think are profitable to bear in mind. In the first place, the mother is transporting IgG into the fetus, and the mother's IgG has genetically determined groups on the heavy chains, known as GM groups, and very rarely indeed—in fact, on a mathematical basis, almost never is the fetus compatible with these antigens on the mother's heavy chains. So from square one in the most normal pregnancy the fetus is being bombarded with antigen. And whether or not these are polyclone stimulated, or what have you, I think has just never been studied. On the other hand, and to agree very much with you John, I think a definition of infection needs very badly to be made. And the reasons I do is that we have recently been looking at the human placenta in malaria. If you want a definition of intra-uterine infection, you can say that 100% of the children born in the Gambia suffer from intra-uterine infection because the placenta is absolutely chock-a-block with plasmodia. So I think that is not a very helpful definition, and that one must go back and think about this one again, so I do entirely agree with you. Also, on the score of scattered sometime clandestine reports, but nevertheless confirmed from many quarters, that anyone who looks for C particles in the human placenta or in the baboon placenta finds them. We have found them; most people have. It is almost a thing you do not report any more. This is a rather common observation. Do you call that infection or do you call that normal part and parcel of pregnancy?

Walker Smith   Could I comment on this question from the clinical aspect? What is infection? If you are going to screen for cytomegalovirus and the baby is well, yet you find the screening is positive, do you in fact tell the mother then and also do you follow the baby for years, or what do you do?

Marshall   I feel reluctant in admitting that the situation with cytomegalovirus is very, very poorly understood, and I think it is because there have not been adequate numbers of pregnancies studied throughout the pregnancy and the consequences when infection has taken place, whether from reactivation or primary infection. We have been talking for years about the possibility of preventing congenital CMV with a vaccine. And it is shameful to admit we know so little about this infection. I think in answer to your question, I think you should tell the mother that the child is infected, but try to explain one can only guess about the consequences.

Chairman Do you want to add to that, Dr Stern?

Stern I would agree that you have to tell the mother that the child is an excreter. We usually tell the mother that the baby is carrying a virus infection, and if the baby is healthy at the time, we say that it will probably come to no harm. But the baby ought to be followed up because there may be some consequences that will develop subsequently. I think we have now, sufficient data available to us on primary infection to know that at least 10% of these babies will be damaged, usually obviously so within six months, and that perhaps a further 10% will show evidence of some sort of damage, within the next few years. With regard to the reactivation of intra-uterine infections of course we do not have enough data. There are probably only about two dozen cases that have been followed up for perhaps a year or so, and none of these have shown signficant damage, but these are very small numbers.

Denman Granted that you have infinite resources, what kind of criteria would you now lay down as constituting evidence of a pathogenic viral infection by virus of a human fetus resulting in disease?

Marshall I think the evidence we have got makes that an unanswerable question.

Wood Could I ask about the interpretation of splenomegaly? In a new born in whom there appears to have been a healthy pregnancy you may find the spleen is enlarged. Is this extramedullary erythropoiesis or is it to be taken as evidence of covert intra-uterine action.

Evans You can feel the spleen in 60% of newborn babies.

Wood Yes, that is what I mean.

Walker Smith I am not sure that this argument with Prof. Soothill raises is productive in the long run. You may define infection with a specific pathogen or define that a particular pathogen can cause an effect, which to show up anyway requires a long follow-up. Surely infection can generally be easily defined as the invasion of the tissues by foreign bodies. Whether that infection goes on and causes an effect may be clinical or sub-clinical for each organism. What you are really concerned with in the long term is the ultimate effect on the fetus and the child.

Walker Smith It is more difficult to define but it is not a harmful effect on an infant as compared with controls, but it can be very difficult to establish because it may require a very long follow-up.

Marshall It is the follow-up period which makes it unanswerable. How long do you have to observe these patients for the late development of defects? I would cite the example of encephalitis and congenital rubella occurring in the second decade of life. These are children known to have congenital rubella by their other types of defects and serological criteria for congenital rubella. When they are about 13 or 14 years of age they develop fatal encephalitic processes in which the rubella virus has been isolated from the brain and in which there are very high titres of rubella antibody both in the serum and the CSF. Now what is going to happen in the third decade of life? And in the fourth decade of life?

Walker Smith   But you can still give a definition of what infection is.

Marshall   I do not think you can define pathogenic infection in the same sense.

Walker Smith   I would like to comment on another aspect of neonatal infection. If you have rota virus in the stools you can have infants in whom there is no clinical manifestation of the disease during the neonatal period and others in whom there is a gastro-enteritis-like illness, whereas later in childhood the identical rotavirus appears to be always associated with clinical illness. We have had the experience in the neonatal unit of finding the rotavirus in identical amounts in the stools of babies in adjacent cots, one baby with a clinical disease, i.e. gastroenteritis and the other baby without, and yet later in childhood this does not seem to be the case.

Chairman   As there is a pause I feel compelled to call on Sir Ashley to give us what he would think would be a helpful comment in relation to Prof. Soothill's poposition.

Sir Ashley   I think you are making unecessary difficulties. If you have something in the tissues which, as somebody said, is a foreign intruder, and in these cases is a replicating foreign intruder, you have a state of infection and you can say it is going to be silent, subclinical, clinical or what you will, but the definition of pathogenicity is whatever you care to say it is. It is what you are interested in and what you may find dangerous and there is no more to it than that. Obviously Dr Marshall is wanting to define what he finds dangerous.

Soothill   I must reply to that. I simply say, decide what you are talking about and then we will talk about tests. We, who might develop tests, will try to do so but cannot until you have told us what we are to test for.

Tyrrell   I think what one wants is as thorough an understanding as possible of what is going on. If you are looking at the interaction between a virus and the host then you have to know both whether the infection is there or not and whether there is a disease present or not. But nobody has mentioned yet that that is not the end of the story, it is often difficult to decide, whether they are, in fact associated with infection which you may have detected; this is a further problem in the design of trials. Somebody mentioned mental defect and deafness and yet there are still other diseases that develop later in life, and in the end I think the answer has to be that in the individual cases you cannot know whether the infection you have detected is actually causing the disease you have detected, you can only draw conclusions on the basis of properly constructed trials which give you the outcome in groups of people with infections and groups of others without. You then have to go back and apply this general sort of knowledge to the individual case. You can then only state probabilities drawn on the basis of these findings of the groups thus studied. In fact, in strict logic if a child from whom you have isolated rubella has a cataract, we cannot in strict logic say that the cataract is a result of the rubella virus. We can only say that it is the most probable cause.

Chairman The ophthalmologists might have some comments on that, otherwise I think I would agree with you. Dr Marshall the last word is with you.

Marshall I think there is an attempt to try and generalize too much. There is such a wide variety of infectious agents and their responses that there is no simple approach to the problem. You have to think in terms of individual infections and the possible effects that they might produce. This makes it exceedingly difficult because the numbers of infections although not massive, are fairly large and beyond the resources of most clinical laboratories who are faced with this problem on a day-to-day basis.

Ontogeny of Complement, Lysozyme and Lactoferrin in Man

Matteo Adinolfi

Paediatric Research Unit,
The Prince Philip Research Laboratories,
Guy's Hospital Medical School, London, UK

INTRODUCTION

Complement, lysozyme, lactoferrin and interferon have been recognized to play an important role in the mechanisms of defence against bacterial and viral infections in association with the cellular and humoral immune response (Miller, 1973). Since the beginning of this century the ontogeny of complement has been the object of several investigations both in human newborns and in experimental animals (Adinolfi, 1972, 1977; Colten, 1976). However, only during the last two decades has clear evidence of the onset and site of synthesis during fetal life of various components of complement (C), lysozyme (LZM), lactoferrin (LF) and interferon been obtained, mainly as a result of the introduction of new methods for the isolation and identification of the plasma proteins forming the C system, the use of short term cultures of fetal tissues in the presence of labelled amino acids and the discovery of the genetic polymorphism of several components of C.

In this paper, the maturation of the C system, of LZM and of LF will be reviewed with particular emphasis on the studies carried out in man.

ONTOGENY OF COMPLEMENT

Nomenclature and Pathways of Activation

In the late nineteenth century it was recognized that the bactericidal activity of fresh serum required the participation of at least two factors: the first, heat-stable, specific for each organism, was identified as an "antibody" and was later shown to belong to the immunoglobulin molecules; the second factor, heat-labile, nonspecific, was designated "complement" (Buchner, 1889; Pfeiffer and Issaeff, 1894; Bordet, 1909).

Soon after its discovery, it became apparent that C consisted of several components which acted in a well-defined order to produce the death and lysis of bacteria (Ferrata, 1907; Mayer, 1961).

At present, more than 20 components have been shown to interact in the complex mechanism of activation of the C system (Müller-Eberhard, 1968, 1972, 1975; Lachmann, 1973, 1979b; Rudy, 1974).

Most of the distinct plasma proteins which form the C system (Table I) are present in blood in an inactive form. The interaction of C system with antigen–antibody complexes (Ag–Ab) or directly with bacterial polysaccharides results in the sequential activation of the various components and the formation of multimolecular structures, some of which adhere on the surface of biological membranes and are responsible for the elimination of foreign materials from the body.

Recent studies have shown that C fulfils various functions, besides acting on the bacterial membrane and causing cell death (Table II). In fact C may also produce activation of specialized cell properties, such as an increased vascular permeability, the release of histamine from mast cells and platelets, the contraction of smooth muscle and the enhancement of phagocytosis.

A unique property of C proteins in their inherent ability to undergo transition from soluble molecules to membrane constituents through the generation of binding regions. In fact, cleavage of a component of C usually results in the formation of a minor fragment, capable, for a short period of time, of binding to an appropriate receptor.

Operationally the activation of the C system has been divided in two pathways (Fig. 1); the first or *classic pathway*, mediated by Ag–Ab complexes, has been grouped into three different units: the recognition, activation and membrane attack systems (Müller-Eberhard, 1968, 1972). The *alternative pathway* activated by IgA or naturally-occuring polysaccharides and lipopolysaccharides has come to

TABLE I.

Some properties of human components of C and their levels in sera from normal adults.*

Protein	Levels in serum† (mg/100 ml)	Electrophoretic mobility	Mol. wt	Major fragments
Classical components				
C1q	18	$\gamma 2$	400 000	
C1r	10	β	180 000	
C1s	11	α	86 000	
C2	2·5	$\beta 1$	117 000	C2a, C2b
C3	130	$\beta 2$	180 000	C3a, C3b, C3c, C3d
C4	43–64	$\beta 1$	206 000	C4a, C4b
C5	8	$\beta 1$	180 000	C5a, C5b
C6	7·5	$\beta 2$	110 000	
C7	5·5	$\beta 2$	95 000	
C8	8	$\gamma 1$	163 000	
C9	23	α	79 000	
Alternative pathway Initiating factor (IF)	2–5	$\gamma 1$		
Properdin (P)	20	$\gamma 2$	150 000	
Factor B (C3 pro- activator, C3PA)	14–22	α	93 000	
Alternative pathway Factor D (C3 proactivator convertase)	0·1–0·5	$\alpha 2$	24 000	
Regulatory proteins C1 inhibitor (C1–INH)	18	$\alpha 2$	105 000	
C3b inactivator (C3b–INA; KAF)	3–5	β	100 000	
Anaphylatoxin inactivator	4	α	300 000	
$\beta 1$H (Factor H)	13·3	β	150 000	

* References quoted in the text.
† Levels from Müller-Eberhard (1975) and Ruddy (1976) and Götze and Müller-Eberhard (1976).

light largely as a result of a suggestion advanced by Pillemer *et al.* (1954) of a nonspecific resistance to infections mediated by properdin, a normal serum protein. Both pathways' activation results in the cleavage of C3 and the formation of C5 convertases which cleave C5 and activate the late components of C.

In addition, the C system includes "regulatory" proteins such as C1 inhibitor (C1–INH), C3b inactivator (C3b–INA), $\beta 1$H and an anaphylotoxin inactivator

TABLE II.

Some of the biological activites of the activated fragments of certain components of C.

C14b	Increases immune adherence and enhances phagocytosis Involved in viral neutralization
C3b	Promotes activation of the alternative pathway; increases immune adherence via receptors on lymphocytes and phagocytic cells; enhances the antibody-dependent cellular cytotoxicity
C5a	Involved in the histamine release, in the increased capillary permeability and the chemotaxis of leukocytes and monocytes
Factor B	Increases phagocytic activity of macrophages

(Table I). These proteins play an important role in the biological control of C activation since the deficiency of any of them is usually associated with severe clinical disorders (Lachmann, 1979b).

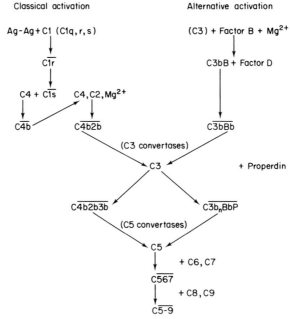

Fig. 1   Classical and alternative pathways of complement. The classical activation starts with the interaction between C1 and Ag–Ab complexes or C reactive protein; it involves the cleavage of C4 and C2. The alternative pathway is regulated by the interaction between the initiating factor (IF), factor B, factor D, properdin (P) and C3. The activation of both pathways results in the cleavage of C3, the formation of C5 convertases and the interaction of the late components of C.

Comprehensive and critical reviews of the C system have been published in recent years (Müller-Eberhard, 1968, 1972, 1975; Lachmann, 1973, 1979b; Ruddy, 1974; Götze and Müller-Eberhard, 1976). In this paper only a brief account of the activation of the classical and alternative pathways will be presented, mainly to remind the reader of the terminology used.

Since a great deal of information on the functional properties of the components of C is derived from studies of its haemolytic activity, the reaction sequence is conventionally expressed starting with the formation of complexes between erythrocytes (E) and antibodies (A), followed by the individual compounds of C that have reacted with EA. For example, $EAC\overline{142}$ designates an intermediate stage of reaction, consisting of antigen, antibody and the first, fourth and second component of C.

The activated forms of the components of C are indicated by adding a bar above the symbol; e.g. $\overline{C1}$ is the enzymatically active form of C1 and $C\overline{567}$ the activated complex of C5, C6 and C7 that takes part in reactive lysis. The fragments are instead described by adding a lower case letter as, for example, for the fragments of C3: C3a, C3b, C3c and C3d.

Subunits of a macromolecular complex are designated adding a lower case letter as, for example, C1q, C1r and C1s.

The *classical* complement activation is initiated by the binding of the first component of C (C1) to an antigen–antibody molecule; activation of C1 may also be induced by C reactive protein (Kaplan and Volanakis, 1974). C1 is present in serum as a cation dependent macromolecular complex of three subunits, C1q, C1r and C1s (Naff *et al.*, 1964; Müller-Eberhard, 1975; Porter and Reid, 1978). C1q is the subunit that possesses the binding site capable of reacting with Ig molecules.

Human IgG and IgM, whose molecular structure has been modified by their interaction with the specific antigens, are capable of binding C1q. The relative binding affinities of C1q for IgG follow this order: IgG3 > IgG1 > IgG2 and IgG4. Although IgG4 was thought to lack reactivity with C, recent studies have revealed a weak but definite interaction between this IgG subclass and C1q.

As a result of C1q binding, C1r acquires the capacity to activate C1s, which in turn will activate C4 and C2; C4 is cleaved into two fragments: the larger, C4b, may become bound to cell membranes or, free in the fluid phase, acts by greatly enhancing the activity of C1s in cleaving its other natural substrate, C2. This leads to the physical uptake of a major fragment of C2 by the cell receptors forming the complex $EAC\overline{42}$ (Müller-Eberhard and Lepow, 1965; Schreiber and Müller-Eberhard, 1974). The $C\overline{42}$ complex, the classical C3 convertase—whether present in the fluid phase or bound to the cellular intermediate—cleaves the third component of C (C3) into two fractions. The major fragment, C3b, either binds to the cell or remains in the fluid phase in an inactive form, C3bi (Müller-Eberhard, 1975; Müller-Eberhard *et al.*, 1966). Nascent C3b modifies the substrate specificity of the activated convertase, rendering it capable of cleaving C5.

C5b, the larger of the two fragments produced by C5 cleavage, interacts with C6 to form $\overline{C56}$ and begins the assembly of the multimolecular C5–C9 complex (Kolb *et al.*, 1972). The reaction of $\overline{C56}$ with C7 leads to the formation of $\overline{C567}$ on the cell membranes; $\overline{C56}$ in fluid phase can also react with C7, forming $\overline{C567}$, which is, for a short period of time, capable of binding directly to the cell surface in absence of antibody or the earlier components of C.

Finally, the $\overline{C567}$ complex interacts with C8 and then with C9, completing the formation of the multimolecular complex C5–C9, capable of damaging the cell membranes (Kolb and Müller-Eberhard, 1974).

Two different approaches have lead, independently, to the discovery of the properdin or *alternative pathway system*. In 1954, Pillemer and his collaborators described properdin as a component of fresh serum which was removed by incubation at 17°C with zymosan, an insoluble extract of yeast cell walls. The absorbed serum was found to lose its capacity to neutralize certain bacteria and viruses and to lyse paroxysmal nocturnal haemoglobinuria (PNH) erythrocytes, while maintaining its C3 haemolytic activity.

Numerous publications appeared in the next five years, dealing with the biological role of the properdin system (for references see Osler and Sandberg, 1973) but all publications on this subject came to almost a standstill around 1960, mainly as a result of the suggestion that most of the activities ascribed to the properdin system could be explained by the presence in normal sera of antibodies against zymosan (Nelson, 1958).

A re-evaluation of the concepts of an alternative pathway and the role of properdin was set up by the observation of C3–C9 activation induced by endotoxins and immune complexes which would bypass the first components of C (Gewurz *et al.*, 1968). A full account of the rediscovery of of the properdin system has been published by Götze and Müller-Eberhard (1976). The terminology and some of the characteristics of the proteins involved in the alternative pathways are shown in Table I.

Uncertainty exists as to the mechanisms of activation of the alternative pathway by fungal and bacterial cell wall polysaccharides or by aggregated IgA. The initial event seems to occur on the surface of the activating particles and, at present, it is assumed that this involves the participation of the intitiating factor (IF) which interacts with Factor B, Factor D and with native C3, in the presence of Mg^{2+}, to generate the first C3 convertase. When Factor B combines with C3b, it becomes susceptible to proteolysis by Factor D, a low molecular weight esterase which resists all protease inhibitors in plasma and is present *in vivo* as a fully active enzyme. The complex $\overline{C3bBb}$ is a powerful C3 splitting enzyme which is attached to the surface of the activating particle and generates a receptor for properdin $(\overline{P})$; upon binding, active $(\overline{P})$ extends the half-life of the alternative C3b-dependent C3 convertase.

There is evidence to suggest that P receptors reside in at least two closely spaced

C3b molecules which, in combination with Bb and $\overline{P}$ fragments, results in the expression of C5 convertase.

Of great importance is the suggestion that in the alternative pathway C3b generated by cleavage of C3 exerts a feedback effect on the activation of this pathway. The control of the alternative pathway activation is finely timed by the rate at which C3b is generated on one hand and the cleavage of C3b operated by C3b–INA (KAF), which occurs only when C3b has undergone substantial modulation following its reaction with β1H; this regulatory protein competes with factor B to bind with C3b (Lachmann, 1979b).

The activation of the C sequence is regulated basically by two factors; the first is that most of the products of the cleavage (e.g. C2a, C4b, C5b etc.) and complexes ($\overline{C567}$) are unstable and decay rapidly (Polley and Müller-Eberhard, 1968; Shin et al., 1971). The second factor is represented by a series of inhibitors and inactivators which may combine with or destroy the activated components of C and thus prevent the progression of the reaction sequence or inhibit the biological function of the activated product. The importance of these regulatory proteins is emphasized by the fact that the absence of any of them may result in an uncontrolled activation of the C system with accompanying disease.

The four regulatory proteins listed in Table I have been well characterized. C1-inhibitor (C1–INH) combines stoichiometrically and inhibits the esterolytic activity of C1 either in fluid phase or bound to a cell (Naff and Ratnoff, 1968). C1–INH is polyspecific since it also inhibits the enzymatic activities of plasmin, kallikrein, lysosomal enzymes and the activated Hageman factor (factor XIIa) Naff and Ratnoff, 1968).

The deficiency of C1–INH is associated with the clinical syndrome of hereditary angioedema (Landerman et al., 1962; Donaldson and Evans, 1963).

Onset and Site of Synthesis of C During Fetal Life

Methods

Several approaches have been used to study the ontogeny of the components of C in man and other mammals (Table III).

First of all, the estimation of the levels of each component of C in sera from fetuses at various stages of gestation and in newborn blood offers preliminary information on the appearance of each component of C during development. Lack of correlation between the levels of a component of C in pairs of maternal and cord samples is suggestive of fetal synthesis, although transfer across the placenta cannot be excluded.

The development of suitable *in vitro* tissue culture techniques to study the synthesis of plasma proteins has made it possible to obtain, simultaneously, information about the onset and site of synthesis of the components of C during fetal life.

TABLE III.
Methods used to study the ontogeny of components of C.

(a)	Estimation of the levels of single components of C in sera from human fetuses at various stages of gestation
(b)	Relationship of the levels of components of C in pairs of maternal and newborn samples
(c)	*In vitro* synthesis of C in the presence of labelled amino acids and detection of newly produced haemolitically active components
(d)	Detection of different genetic variants of components of C in pairs of maternal and cord blood
(e)	Presence of a specific component of C in offspring of C deficient mothers

Basically, the method consists in the incubation at 37°C for a short period of time of fetal tissues in selected media containing labelled amino acids; the culture fluids are then analysed for the presence of the newly sythesized proteins using immunological methods such as the autoradiography of the immunoplates obtained using specific antisera.

Details of the optimal conditions to study the *in vitro* synthesis of various components of C have been described in several papers (see Colten, 1976; Adinolfi, 1977). It is essential that the production of the newly synthesized components of C should be established using more than one method and particular care should be taken to avoid protein–protein interaction during the incubation period.

The discovery of a genetic polymorphism of several proteins forming the C system has also proved to be of great help to study the ontogeny of this group of proteins. The detection of different phenotypic variants of a specific component of C in pairs of maternal and fetal sera, clearly indicates that the protein under study is produced by the fetus under the control of a paternal gene absent in the mother, and that the corresponding maternal molecules do not cross the placenta.

In experimental animals, information about the onset of the fetal synthesis of a component of C has also been obtained by selected breeding of genetically C deficient individuals. In fact, the first evidence of the production of C during fetal life was obtained about 50 years ago in guinea pigs, using a strain with an inherited C deficiency. In 1930, Friedberger and Gurwitz investigated the ontogeny of C in newborn guinea pigs and within the limits of the methods available at that time, they were able to show that both "middle" and "end" pieces of C were present in sera obtained from fetuses at the end of the gestational period. Two years later, Hyde investigated a strain of guinea pigs with the first known inherited serum C defect; this was, in fact, the first record of inheritance of a single non-sex-linked character affecting plasma proteins of a mammal. Animals with the complete defect were homozygotes for a recessive autosomal gene.

By selectively breeding guinea pigs with different genotypes for the C deficiency, Hyde was able to demonstrate that the component of C under study was produced during fetal life. For example, he showed that it was present in guinea pig fetuses obtained from mothers which were homozygotes for the deficiency and had been mated to normal males. These studies also proved that the component of C under investigation was not crossing the placenta barrier from fetuses to the mothers or vice versa.

Occasionally, in humans, C deficient mothers have provided evidence for the fetal synthesis of a specific component of C.

Furthermore, data on the site of the synthesis of components of C may be collected using hybrid cells. This approach has not yet been fully exploited but hybrid cells between human hepatocytes and mouse fibroblasts have suggested that C6 is synthesized in liver cells.

Levels of components of C in fetal and newborn sera

Early work has shown that the mean level of total C in normal newborn sera was about half that detected in maternal samples (Wasserman and Alberts, 1940; Arditi and Nigro, 1957; Fischel and Pearlman, 1961).

In 1961, Fischel and Pearlman made the first attempt to identify the limiting factors responsible for the reduced total C activity of cord sera by measuring the levels of the components of C known at that time (C1, C2, C3 and C4) in pairs of maternal and cord sera, using the classical "R" reagents. Within pairs of maternal and newborn sera, the ratios of the four major components of C were found to correspond to the ratio of total C. Anticomplement activity was not detected in the cord samples tested.

In more recent studies, the levels of single components of C in fetal and cord sera have been estimated using modifications of the radial diffusion technique and haemolytic tests in agar gel.

The first components of C which have been measured in human fetal sera using these methods were C3 and C4; the two plasma proteins have been detected in sera from human fetuses more than 9–10 weeks old (Fig. 2).

The concentrations of C3 and C4 in cord blood have been found to be near 50% of the levels in maternal sera (Fireman *et al.*, 1969; Adinolfi, 1970; Propp and Alper, 1968; Sawyer *et al.*, 1971; Ballow *et al.*, 1974).

The mean levels of C2 in cord blood have also been found to be near half the values in maternal sera (Sawyer *et al.*, 1971; Ballow *et al.*, 1974).

C1q has been detected in all newborn sera tested and in fetuses more than 20 weeks old (Adinolfi, 1970; Mellbye *et al.*, 1971). Using the single radial diffusion technique, the mean cord maternal ratio was found to be near 0·65; at 4 days of age the mean level of C1q was similar to that observed in maternal blood (Ballow *et al.*, 1974).

C5 has been detected in sera from human fetuses more than 5 weeks old and the

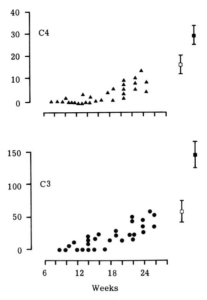

Fig. 2   Individual levels of C4 and C3 (mg/100 ml) in sera from human fetuses (gestational age in weeks). Mean levels of C4 and C3 in newborn (□) and maternal (■) sera (from Adinolfi, 1977).

mean level in cord sera is about half that in maternal blood (Adinolfi, 1970; Ballow *et al.*, 1974). Fireman *et al.* (1969) have also collected data on the levels of C3, C4 and C5 during the first 12 months of life. It was found that levels similar to those observed in samples from adult subjects were reached in infants between 6 and 12 months of age.

Recently, the levels of C6, C7, C8 and C9 have been measured in newborn sera using various techniques (Ballow *et al.*, 1974; Adinolfi and Beck, 1976). The amount of C6 and C8 in the cord sera has been found to be near 50% of the level in maternal blood; C7 is present in concentrations between 60 and 70% of the levels detected in sera from normal individuals (Fig. 3). C9 is the only component of C which is present in low concentrations, approx. 10–25% of the levels in blood from normal individuals (Fig. 3). C7 and C9 have been detected in sera from human fetuses more than 14 and 18 weeks old respectively (Adinolfi and Beck, 1976).

Of the components of C involved in the activation of the alternative pathways, Factor B, Factor D and properdin have been measured in fetal and cord sera. Factor B has been detected in sera from fetuses more than 10 weeks old and in all newborn samples (Fig. 4) (Stossel *et al.*, 1973; Adinolfi and Beck, 1976; Adinolfi and Bradwell, 1980).

In cord sera the levels of Factor B are approx. 70% of the values present in normal sera (Fig. 4). Properdin was shown to be present in cord blood and its mean level is approx. 80% of that in normal sera (Minta *et al.*, 1976).

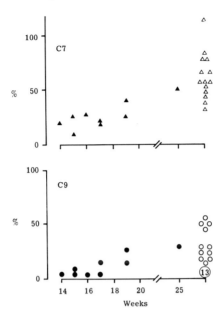

Fig. 3   Levels of C7 and C9 in fetal and cord sera expressed as percentages of the mean levels in sera from normal adults (C7 = 5·5 mg/100 ml; C9 = 23 mg/100 ml). In 13 cord sera the levels of C9 were less than 2 mg/100 ml (from Adinolfi, 1977).

Three of the regulatory proteins of C have been estimated in fetal and cord blood; C1̄–INA has been detected in a fetus 4 weeks old by Gitlin and Biasucci (1969). C3b–INH and β1H have been observed in sera from fetuses more than 14 weeks old and the mean levels in cord blood were found to be approx. 60 and 50% respectively of the mean values present in normal sera (Adinolfi and Bradwell, 1980).

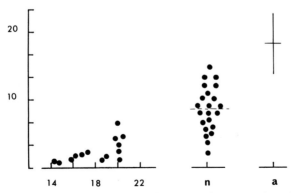

Fig. 4   Levels of factor B (mg/100ml) in sera from normal adult (a), newborn (n) and fetal sera (modified from Adinolfi and Beck, 1975).

TABLE IV.

Levels of components of C in newborns and infants expressed as percentages of mean values in sera from normal adults.

| | Levels expressed as % of adult mean values | | | Levels in adults | | |
	Newborns	1	Infants (age in months) 6	12	units/100 ml	mg/100 ml	Reference
C1q	73	65	65	—	118	—	a
C1q	67		70			18	c
C2	76	102	104	—	141	—	a
C4	58	78	89	100	—	(40)	b
C4	60	73	88	—	—	51	a
C3	54	70	92	96	—	(130)	b
C3	63	69	79	—	—	141	a
C5	56	72	82	98	—	(8)	b
C5	75	67	68	—	—	6·4	a
C6	47	67	95	—	—	21	a
C7	67	—	92	—	—	5·5	c
C9	16	—	80	—	—	23	c
P	53	49	70	--	96	—	a
Factor B	49	72	96	—	—	24	a
β1H	61	71	83	—	98	—	a
β1H	53	—	90	—	—	13	c
C3 INA	60	—	82	—	—	3–5	c
C3 INA	57	68	84	—	104	—	a

(a) Davis *et al.* (1979); (b) Fireman *et al.* (1969): note that the levels of C3, C4 and C5 have been recalculated from normal adult values (expressed in brackets) and that the levels at 1 month were actually collected from babies 1·5 months old; (c) Adinolfi and Bradwell (1980).

Although data on some components of C are still missing or incomplete, it is possible to conclude that all components of C are present in sera from fetuses more than 18–20 weeks old. In infants born at term, most of the components of C are present in concentrations approx. 50 to 70% of the values observed in normal sera, with the exception of C9, whose values are less than 20%. The levels of some components of complement during the first 12 months of life are shown in Table IV.

The levels of C in maternal sera

In many investigations on the ontogeny of C, the levels of the individual components in cord sera have been compared with those present in maternal samples. However, many components of C are present in sera from pregnant women in concentrations higher than those observed in adult individuals. Sawyer *et al.* (1971) observed, for example, that the ratios of maternal:normal standard sera for C3 and C4 were 1·8 and 1·9, while those for C1q and C2 were 0·9 and 1·2.

The data collected from the literature and summarized in Table V show that C5, C9, Factor B and β1H reach mean levels in maternal sera are near 70% of the mean values in normal adults. Certain discrepancies are noticeable; while, for example, our data and those of Kohler (1973) show a modest increase of C3 and C4 in maternal sera, Mak (1978) has observed increases of 48% and 77% respectively. These and other discrepancies are probably due to the different methods used. Mak, for example, has used functional assays for his estimations and his mean values of "adult controls" were 85% and 74% of the levels of C3 and C4 of the "standard", formed by a pool of 20 normal sera; one would expect the controls to be near 100% of the "normal" standard.

The high levels of C9 and factor B in maternal sera are in good agreement with

TABLE V.

Mean levels of some components of C in newborn sera.

Components of C (% of standard or mg/100 ml)		Control (c)	Mother (m)	Newborn (n)	Ratios c/n	m/n	Reference
C1q		18·5	16·4	12·4	1·3	1·3	a
C4			29·3	15·8		1·8	b
C4		25·6	28·1	16·1	1·6	1·7	c
C4		48·1	53·3	29·9	1·6	1·8	a
C3			178·3	88·8		2·0	d
C3	(mg/100ml)		139·3	75·7		1·8	b
C3		130	143·4	54·4	2·4	2·6	c
C3		150	152	86	1·7	1·7	a
C5			11·9	5·8		2·05	b
C5		7·6	10·3	6·2	1·2	1·6	a
C7 (%)		98·2		67·3	1·4		e
C9 (%)		93·9	176·6	16·5	5·7	10·7	e
Properdin		19·3	23·1	15·6	1·2	1·5	f
Factor B (mg/100ml)		15·4	27·1	11·4	1·3	2·4	e
Factor B		33		17	1·9		g
β1H (%)		96·3	170	53	1·8	3·2	h
C3–INA (%)		105	14	60	1·7	2·3	h

(a) Kohler (1973); (b) Fireman *et al.* (1969); (c) Adinolfi (1970); (d) Propp and Alper (1968); (e) Adinolfi and Beck (1976); (f) Minta *et al.* (1976); (g) Stossel *et al.* (1973); (h) Adinolfi and Bradwell (1980).

the role of acute phase proteins attributed to these two components of C (Adinolfi and Lehner, 1976) and the increased levels of C reactive protein detected in maternal blood.

The significance of the increased levels of β1H and C3b–INA in maternal sera is not clear, since modest increases of β1H and C3b–INA have been shown to lead to a severe damping of the alternative pathway (Lachmann and Halbwachs, 1975; Nydegger et al., 1978).

Site of synthesis: in vitro *cultures*

Direct evidence that specific components of C are produced during fetal life has been obtained by incubating fetal tissues in media containing labelled amino acids. The culture fluids were then analysed for the presence of specific newly synthesized components of C, either using haemolytic tests or by the autoradiography of the immunoelectrophoretic plates (Table V) (Thorbecke et al., 1965; Adinolfi et al., 1968; Gitlin and Biasucci, 1969; Kohler, 1973; Colten, 1973, 1976; Rosen, 1974; Hochwald et al., 1961; Stecher et al., 1967; Stecher and Thorbecke, 1967).

In many studies, the newly synthesized components of C have been tested for either their biological or their physiological properties. In general, there has been little controversy on the site of synthesis of the various components of C. The only exception is C1; early studies by Colten et al. (1966, 1968) suggested that in guinea

TABLE VI.

Site of synthesis of human components of C during fetal life.

Component	Main tissue	Age (weeks)*	Reference†
C1	Intestinal epithelium; macrophages	19	Colten et al. (1968) Morris et al. (1979)
C1q	Spleen (?)	14	Kohler (1973)
C2	Liver; macrophages	8	Colten (1972)
C4	Liver; macrophages	8	Adinolfi et al. (1968) Gitlin and Biasucci (1969) Colten (1972)
C3	Liver cells	8	Adinolfi (1972)
C5	Liver	9	Colten (1973)
	Spleen, liver	8–14	Kohler (1973)
C6	Unknown	—	
C7	Liver (?)	14	Adinolfi (1977)
C8	Unknown	—	
C9	Liver	—	Adinolfi (1977)
C1–INH	Liver	4	Gitlin and Biasucci (1969)

* Early detection using *in vitro* cultures.
† For further references see Adinolfi (1972) and Rosen (1974).

pigs and in man macromolecular C1 was synthesized primarily, if not exclusively, in the small and large intestines. At about the same time, Thorbecke and collaborators (Stecher and Thorbecke, 1967; Stecher *et al.*, 1967) reported the *in vitro* production of C1q by human and monkey liver, spleen, bone marrow and lung, as well as in macrophages isolated from the peritoneal cavity and lung. None of their results suggested synthesis of C1 by lymphocytes; however, Day and coworkers (Day *et al.*, 1970) later suggested that C1q was synthesized mainly by tissues rich in lymphoid cells. This was supported by the claim that the synthesis of C1q and IgG were linked: this suggestion was based on the observation that bone marrow transplantation for severe combined immunodeficiency often results in an apparent reconstitution of the C1q serum levels (Ballow *et al.*, 1973). Two observations seem to rule out this hypothesis: first of all, metabolic studies have shown an accelerated catabolism of C1q in patients with immunoglobulin deficiency (Köhler and Müller-Eberhard, 1969); secondly, it has been shown that administration of exogenous Ig in these patients coincides with an increase of the serum levels of C1q (Atkinson *et al.*, 1978).

Interest in the epithelial cells as a site of C1 synthesis was renewed by the elegant experiments by Bing *et al.* (1975) showing production of macromolecular C1 and C1s in longterm cultures of normal human colon, adenocarcinoma of the colon and the transitional epithelial cells of the bladder and urethra.

The controversy concerning the site of synthesis of C1 has been at least in part solved by recent studies by Morris *et al.* (1978), who have demonstrated that epithelial and mesenchymal cells synthesize all three subcomponents of C1. Quantitatively, however, columnar and transitional epithelial cells secrete from 400 to 3700 × more haemolytically active C1 than monocytes and fibroblasts. Only columnar epithelial cells synthesize C1 subcomponents with subunits structures similar to their serum counterparts.

In human fetuses, it seems that the majority of C1 macromolecules are indeed produced in the columnar cells of the small intestine and colon (Colten *et al.*, 1968; Morris, 1978). Production of C1 has also been detected in culture fluids of a human embryo intestine cell line (MA177). However, synthesis of C1 in other sites cannot be excluded, since, for example, Köhler (1973) detected newly produced C1q in culture fluids of human fetal spleen.

Several investigations suggest that in adults the macrophage is the site of synthesis of C2 (for references see Colten, 1976). These cells are also responsible for the synthesis of C2 in human fetuses (Colten, 1976). In fact *in vitro* synthesis of C2 by human fetal liver has been shown to be attributable to large mononuclear cells, probably macrophages.

Newly synthesized C3 and C4 have been detected in the liver culture fluids from fetuses more than 8 weeks old by the autoradiography technique. In addition, haemolytically, *de novo* synthesized C3 has been recovered from the supernatants of fetal liver cultures (Adinolfi *et al.*, 1968; Gitlin and Biasucci, 1969). Human peritoneal cells and alveolar cells from fetuses more than 14 weeks old have been shown to produce C3 and C4, *in vitro*. These findings are in agreement with the evidence that these components of C are produced by liver, lung and peritoneal cells from adult monkeys, rats, rabbits and guinea pigs (Hochwald *et al.*, 1961; Stecher and Thorbecke, 1967; Stecher *et al.*, 1967; Littleton *et al.*, 1970; Rosen, 1974). In man and experimental animals, macrophages collected from adult tissues seem to be capable of synthesizing *in vitro* C4 as well as C2 (Colten, 1976). When human fetal liver macrophages were separated from other hepatic cells on a discontinuous albumin gradient, C4 was found to be produced in a fraction rich in macrophages (Colten, 1976).

In vitro synthesis of C5 has been observed in the culture fluids of liver tissues obtained from fetuses more than 8 weeks old (Köhler, 1973; Colten, 1973, 1976). However, biosynthesis of C5 has also been observed in some culture fluids from fetal spleen, colon, lung, thymus, placenta, peritoneal cells and bone marrow.

The evidence that spleen cells produce C5 is substantiated by studies in C5 deficient mice (Phillips *et al.*, 1969). In fact, transplantation of bone marrow and spleen cells from normal co-isogenic or allogenic donors to C5 deficient mice were found to result in the transient appearance of haemolytic complement in the recipient's sera.

There are no data as yet on the site of production of C6 and C8 during fetal life, although at least on one occasion newly synthesized C6 was detected in the culture fluid of liver from a 20-week-old fetus (unpublished observation). However, final conclusions about the site of synthesis of C6 and C8 during fetal life must await additional studies.

Preliminary studies also suggest that C7 and C9 are produced by fetal liver (Adinolfi, 1977). So far the types of cells reponsible for C7 and C9 synthesis during fetal life have not been identified. A few years ago, a longterm rat hepatoma cell strain was shown to produce C9 (Rommel *et al.*, 1970); the same cell line was found to synthesize albumin, C3 and C1 inhibitor but not C1 and C4 (Strunk *et al.*, 1975). Recently, Breslow and collaborators (see Colten, 1976) have observed synthesis of C9 in primary rat liver cells; after separation by centrifugation, substantial haemolitically active C9 was detected in cultures of enriched parenchymal cells.

The fetal synthesis of C1–INH was first investigated by Gitlin and Biasucci (1969) using *in vitro* culture and the autoradiography technique. Newly synthesized C1–INH was detected in the culture fluids of liver tissues from a 4-week-old human fetus. Early production of C1–INH in fetal liver, as assessed by the functional inhibition of EAC1, has been confirmed by Colten (1976). The rate of synthesis of C1–INH in 11-week-old fetuses appeared to be similar to that observed in normal adult subjects.

Genetic polymorphism of components of C in maternal and cord samples

Another approach to investigating the origin of components of C in newborn blood stems from the existence of a genetic polymorphism of some of these proteins (Alper and Rosen, 1971). The genetic variants of C3 are controlled by two common allelic genes and their products are termed F (for fast electrophoretic mobility) and S (for slow). The S allele has a frequency near 0·7; the three common phenotypes are FF, FS and SS. In 1968, Propp and Alper (1968) noticed that out of 25 pairs of maternal and newborn sera, eight pairs showed discordant phenotypes. Discordant genetic variants of human C4 have also been oberved in pairs of maternal and cord samples (Bach *et al.*, 1971). Alper *et al.* (1975) have detected a genetic polymorphism of human C6, controlled by two common alleles, $C6^A$ and $C6^B$. When pairs of maternal and córd samples were tested, in several cases, the phenotype of the newborn was found to be different from that of the corresponding mother, thus suggesting fetal C synthesis of this component of C and lack of its transfer across the placenta.

Maternal deficiency of a component of C may also be useful in demonstrating fetal synthesis. In humans, Ruddy *et al.* (1970) have confirmed the synthesis of C2 during fetal life by the detection of this component of C in the cord blood of a baby born to a C2 deficient mother.

Ontogeny of C in Other Species

As mentioned, the first evidence of fetal synthesis of C was obtained in guinea pigs with an inherited deficiency of one component. Recent studies have shown that in many other mammals, such as the monkey, lamb, goat, rabbit and mouse, various components of C are produced before birth (Adinolfi, 1972; Rosen, 1974). For example, total C activity has been detected after 125 days of gestation in fetal lamb (Rice and Silverstein, 1964) and after 114 days in goat fetuses (Adinolfi, 1972). Colten *et al.* (1968) have detected C1 in sheep embryos 39 days old; two days after delivery, the levels of total C were found to reach adult values.

It is of interest that neither thymectomy of the fetal lamb nor antigenic stimulation leading to synthesis of specific antibodies have been found to be associated with variation of the production of C.

Total C activity has also been detected in fetal calf at the end of the first trimester of gestation and in fetal piglets after 40 days of fetal life (Day *et al.*, 1969). Synthesis of C8 was observed in culture fluid from fetal kidney and lymph nodes (Geiger *et al.*, 1972).

Studies of genetically deficient C5 mice have also demonstrated that these components of C are produced during fetal life (Day *et al.*, 1969). When homozygote C5 deficient females were mated with either heterozygotes or homozygote normal males, C5 was detected in fetuses more than 11 days old. Using appropriate matings between normal and C5 deficient mice, maternal–fetal transfer of this protein could be excluded.

Phillips *et al.* (1969), making use of mice deficient in C5, have shown that transplantation of bone marrow from normal to deficient adult mice resulted in a transient appearance of haemolytic C in sera of the recipient animals. Spleen cells from the transplanted mice were also found to produce C5 *in vitro*.

Information on the synthesis of C6 in rabbit fetuses has also been obtained using appropriate matings of C6 deficient rabbits.

Ontogeny versus Phylogeny of C

Studies of the phylogeny of C have shown that a well-developed C system—subsequentially similar to that seen in mammals—is already present in the earliest vertebrates, such as sharks, investigated in any detail (Gigli and Austen, 1971; Rosen, 1974). Although cyclostoma sera contain a lytic factor against human red cells, its relation to any recognizable component of C is still uncertain. Equally doubtful is the association between the lytic factors present in invertabrates and their couterparts in the C system in high vertebrates.

The analysis of the maturation of the C system in mammals throws little light on the evolution of C, particularly on the question as to whether the components of the alternative pathways are evolutionary older than those of the classical pathway.

In a recent paper, Lachmann (1979a) has suggested a two-component, C3 and Factor B, "archeo-complement" system. Cleavage of C3 can be brought about by several enzymes, with the formation of two biologically active fragments, C3a and C3b. C3a play an important role as anaphylatoxin, while the nascent C3b has a briefly activated site which can bind firmly to a variety of specific receptors on the cell surface. The interaction of C3b with the specific receptor of cell membranes promotes phagocytosis and/or exocytosis, and for some cells, notably macrophages, it is a mechanism for their activation (Schorlemmer and Allison, 1976; Schorlemmer *et al.*, 1977).

As suggested by Lachmann (1979a), it seems plausible to assume that C3 on its own could serve as a mediator of nonspecific immunity in a simple system where phagocytic cells are present. In conjunction with Factor B, C3b provides a positive feedback amplification of the inflammatory reactions and/or cell activation. Controls of C3 activation are provided by β1H and C3b–INA, which represent the next step in the degree of complexity of the evolution of the C system.

Unfortunately, at present, insight into the sequence of the evolution of C cannot be derived from the analysis of the ontogeny of the single components. It appears, however, that some of the regulatory proteins, notably C1–INH, are produced at an early stage of fetal life in man. Of course the function of these proteins may not be exclusively linked to the control of C activation and their evolution may be independent.

It is also of interest that the synthesis of C9 is markedly reduced during fetal life; this supports the claim that on the terminal components of C is an acute phase protein and its synthesis is stimulated by environmental factors.

The question of the evolution of C may only be solved in the years to come, once the physicochemical structures of the various components are fully known and can be compared.

ONTOGENY OF LYSOZYME AND LACTOFERRIN

Lysozyme

In 1922 Alexander Fleming discovered that various tissues and secretions, as well as hen egg white, could lyse common Gram positive saprophytes. He termed the lytic factor lysozyme (LZM), that is, an enzyme capable of lysing bacteria. By measuring the extent of the lysis of heat killed *Micrococcus lysodeikticus* in agar, Fleming showed that LZM was present in tissue homogenates of cartilage and stomach, and in tears, saliva, sputum, nasal secretions, pathological urine, serum and leukocytes, but not in normal urine, cerebrospinal fluid or sweat (Fleming, 1922). Later studies not only confirmed these early observations but also disclosed the extensive distribution of LZM in nature: in vertebrates, invertebrates, plants bacteria and viruses (Imoto *et al.*, 1972; Jollès *et al.*, 1974).

Because it occurs so widely, LZM is considered to be a constituent of primitive unspecific dcfence mechanisms, associated with the monocyte–macrophage system, phylogenetically older than the more specific lymphocyte–plasma cell–immunoglobulin system (Osserman, 1976). It is of great interest that LZM and secretory IgA show a similar distribution in various body fluids. Both IgA and LZM are present in abundance in such external secretions as tears, saliva, tracheobronchial secretions and gastric juice, and in only small amounts in such internal secretions as serum, pleural fluid and cerebrospinal fluid (Lorenz *et al.*, 1957; Brandtzaeg and Mann, 1964; Adinolfi *et al.*, 1966; Tomasi and Bienenstock, 1968; Schumacher, 1974).

The amount of the enzyme in serum is correlated with the total leukocyte count (Barnes, 1940; Flanagan and Lionetti, 1955; Jollès, 1960; Briggs *et al.*, 1966; Senn *et al.*, 1970). Using partially purified preparations of peripheral blood cells and exudate cells, Senn *et al.* (1970) demonstrated that normal human granulocytes contain approximately 7 μg of lysozyme per 10^6 cells (values expressed using egg white lysozyme as a standard). These results were in good agreement with those of Noble and Fudenberg (1967) who detected 6·2 μg of lysozyme per 10^6 "nonlymphocytic" blood leukocytes.

In 1970 Glynn and collaborators measured the levels of lysozyme in sera from 66 normal fullterm newborns and their mothers and found that the mean concentrations of the enzyme, measured by the lysis of *Micrococcus lysodeikticus* were 9·65 μg ml^{-1} in maternal sera and 12·59 μg ml^{-1} newborn samples. The difference of the two means was statistically significant ($P < 0.001$). When the individual concentrations of lysozyme in pairs of maternal and newborn sera were compared, no correlation between the values was observed; in 14 cases the concentration of lysozyme in cord serum was at least twice that observed in the corresponding maternal serum.

The level of lysozyme was also measured in 14 human fetuses between 9 and 18 weeks old and values similar to those observed in normal adults were detected in fetuses more than 14 weeks old.

In another group of 42 human fetuses from 9 to 24 weeks of age, the presence of lysozyme in the sera was studied by double diffusion in agarose gel, using specific antisera raised in rabbits. Lysozyme was detected in three out of nine fetuses between 9 and 12 weeks old and in eight out of 14 fetuses between 13 and 16 weeks old. The enzyme was detected in six out of seven fetuses from 21 to 24 weeks (Adinolfi, 1972).

The level of lysozyme during perinatal life was studied in two groups of infants. In the first group of 12 pairs of mothers and newborns, the concentrations of lysozyme were measured in serum collected from the mother at the time of delivery, from cord blood and in samples obtained from the newborns 2 and 7 days after delivery. None of the infants in this group was breast fed. The mean level of lysozyme in cord sera was higher than that in maternal samples (Table VII); the highest mean concentration was detected in 2-day-old newborns; in the 7-day-old infants the mean level was similar to that detected in cord sera (Adinolfi, 1972).

The lack of correlation between the amount of lysozyme in pairs of maternal and newborn sera and the constant levels in sera collected during perinatal life both suggested synthesis of the enzyme during fetal life. Evidence for the fetal synthesis of the enzyme was obtained by showing intracellular activity of lysozyme in leukocytes from human newborns (Adinolfi, 1972).

Using the immunoperoxidase method, major changes in the distribution of LZM have been shown to occur during fetal life in man (Klockars et al., 1977). In the youngest fetus studied, 10 weeks old, LZM was observed in renal tubules (Fig. 5). The cytoplasmic LZM staining of the proximal tubules was both fine granular and diffuse. In older fetuses, the intensity of the staining and the number of LMZ-

TABLE VII.

Mean lysoyzme concentrations and white cell, neutrophil and monocyte counts in 12 pairs of maternal and cord sera.

Samples	Lysozyme* (μg ml^{-1})	White cells (mm^3)	Neutrophils (mm^3)	Monocytes (mm^3)
Maternal	8·97	9780	7400	380
Cord	10·30	10520	7010	720

* Lysozyme was estimated by the lysoplate technique.

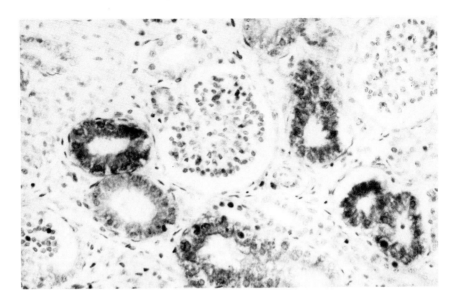

Fig. 5   Human LZM staining of renal tubules of a human fetus 20 weeks of age × 490. LZM in the kidney is derived from serum via the glomerular filtrate (from Klockars *et al.*, 1977).

positive proximal tubules were found to increase and to be correlated with the maturation of the nephrons in the corticomedullary area. Glomeruli, distal tubules and collecting ducts were LZM-negative. The fetal lung showed no LZM-positive cells until 12 weeks of gestation. After 12 weeks, LZM-positive granulocytes and mononuclear cells were observed in the loose connective tissue. The cuboidal epithelium of the trachea and bronchial tree were LZM-negative. At 20 weeks LZM was seen in serous tracheal glands.

In the gastrointestinal tract, LZM was first observed in the gastric glands in fetuses at 14 weeks. In the small intestine, LZM appeared in granulocytes and mononuclear cells of the lamina propria at 14 weeks and in Paneth cells at 20 weeks (Fig. 6). At this time of fetal development LZM was also seen in serous glands of the tongue.

At 16 weeks, clusters of mononuclear cells, strongly LZM-positive, were seen in the region of large veins of the liver. Liver parenchymal cells, blood vessels and biliary capillaries were free of LZM. Large mononuclear cells, scattered in the spleen sinusoids and strongly stained for LZM were present in fetuses more than 16 weeks old. In the thymus, granulocytes and some large LZM-positive mononuclear cells were observed first in fetuses 20 weeks old. The lymphoid cells were LMZ negative in all fetuses investigated. The time sequence of the appearance of LZM in various organs during fetal life is summarized in Fig. 7.

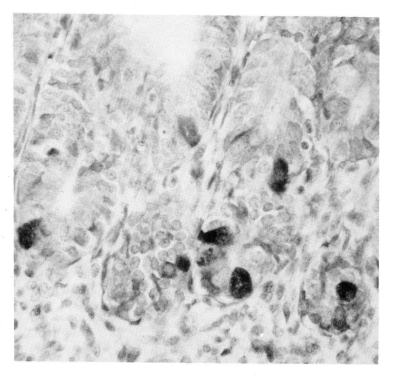

Fig. 6   Human LZM staining of the small intestinal Paneth cells from a fetus 20 weeks old × 490 (from
Klockars *et al.*, 1977).

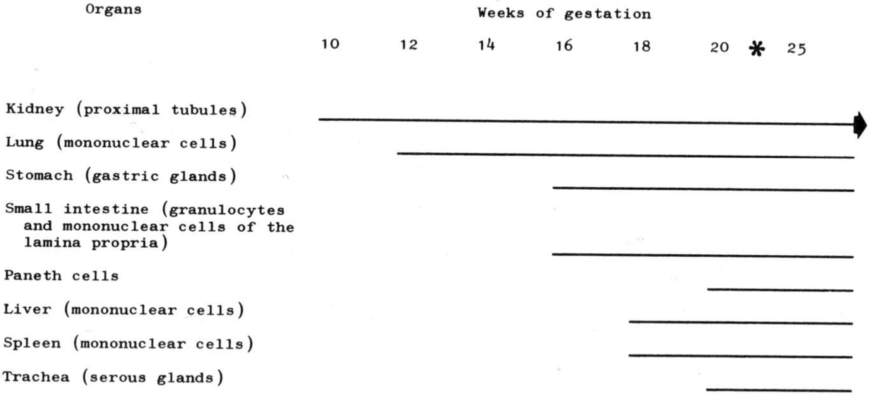

Organs			Weeks of gestation					
	10	12	14	16	18	20 ✱	25	
Kidney (proximal tubules)								
Lung (mononuclear cells)								
Stomach (gastric glands)								
Small intestine (granulocytes and mononuclear cells of the lamina propria)								
Paneth cells								
Liver (mononuclear cells)								
Spleen (mononuclear cells)								
Trachea (serous glands)								

Fig. 7   Onset of detection of LZM in human fetal tissues by the immunoperoxidase technique.

Lactoferrin

Lactoferrin is a protein present in colostrum and milk from many species (Masson and Heremanns, 1971); its function is that of inhibiting the growth of certain micro-organisms by chelating iron (Kirkpatrick *et al.*, 1971; Bullen *et al.*, 1972). Human lactoferrin has a molecular weight near 75 000 and it appears to consist of a single polypeptide chain since no change in the molecular weight is observed when the reduced and alkylated protein is investigated in 6M urea.

Recent studies suggest that lactoferrin present in the specific granules of mature granulocytes may play an important role in the physiological regulation of granulopoiesis (Broxmeyer *et al.*, 1978).

In collaboration with Dr Y. Konttinen and Dr S. Reitamo we have started a systematic investigation on the site of synthesis of lactoferrin during fetal life using an immunoperoxidase method. Preliminary results suggest that lactoferrin is already present in fetuses 12 weeks old in liver, spleen, thymus and lung. The distribution of lactoferrin is similar to that of LZM; however of great interest is the observation that in young fetuses lactoferrin is present in pancreas.

CONCLUSIONS

The results of the studies of the development of the C system in man and other mammals show that all components of C are produced at an early stage of fetal life and that they are present in sera from normal newborns. Their synthesis occurs in different organs and cell types, independently of antigenic stimulation.

The levels in cord sera of the components of the classical and alternative pathways are high enough to provide the human newborn with a fully active C system. In association with the maturation of the humoral and cellular immune responses and the sythesis of LZM and lactoferrin, the human newborn is therefore endowed with a full range of mechanisms of defence against bacterial and viral infections.

To what extent partial deficiencies of single components of C may affect the biological defences of the infant is not yet known; as in older children, it could be expected that certain deficiencies may be tolerated, while others may have more important pathological consequences.

Further studies should also help to elucidate the role that certain components of C, such as C9 and factor B, may play in the diagnosis and prognosis of interauterine or perinatal infections.

ACKNOWLEDGEMENTS

I would like to thank Miss Carolyn Beech for her help in the preparation of the manuscript and Miss Nicola Dobson for her skillful technical assistance.

The original work mentioned in this paper was supported by Birthright.

REFERENCES

Adinolfi, M. (1970). Levels of two components of complement (C'4 and C'3) in human fetal and newborn sera. *Developmental Medicine and Child Neurology* **12**, 306–308.

Adinolfi, M. (1972). Ontogeny of components of complement and lysozyme. *In* "Ontogeny of Acquired Immunity" 65–81. Ciba Foundation Symposium. Associated Scientific Publishers, Amsterdam.

Adinolfi, M. (1977). Human complement. Onset and site of synthesis during fetal life. *American Journal of Diseases of Children* **131**, 1015–1023.

Adinolfi, M. and Beck, S, (1976) Human complement—C7 and C9—in fetal and newborn sera. *Archives of Disease in Childhood* **50**, 562–564.

Adinolfi, M. and Bradwell, A. R. (1980). Synthesis of two components of human complement, β1H and C3bINA during fetal life. *Acta Paediatrica Scandinavica*, in press.

Adinolfi, M. and Lehner, T. (1976). Acute phase proteins and C9 in patients with Bechet's syndrome and aphthous ulcers. *Clinical and Experimental Immunology* **25**, 36–39.

Adinolfi, M., Glynn, A. A., Lindsay, M. and Milne, C. M. (1966). Serological properties of γA antibodies to *Escherichia coli* present in human colostrum. *Immunology* **10**, 517–526.

Adinolfi, M., Gardner, B. and Wood, C. B. S. (1968). Ontogenesis of two components of human complement. β1E and β1C–1A globulins. *Nature, London* **219**, 189–191.

Alper, C. A. and Rosen, F. A. (1971). Genetic aspects of the complement system. *Advances in Immunology* **14**, 252–290.

Alper, C. A., Hobart, M. J. and Lachmann, P. J. (1975). Polymorphism of the 6th component of complement. *In* "Isoelectric focussing" (Eds. J. P. Arbuthnott and J. A. Beeley), 306–312. Butterworth, London.

Arditi, E. and Nigro, N. (1957). Ricerche sul comportamento serico nell' immaturo. *Minerva Pediatrica* **9**, 921–928.

Atkinson, J. P., Fisher, R. I., Reinhardt, R. and Frank, M. M. (1978). Reduced concentrations of the first component of complement in hypogamma globulinaemia: Correction by infusion of γ-globulin. *Clinical Immunology and Immunopathology* **9**, 350–355.

Bach, S., Ruddy, S. and Maclaren, A. J. (1971). Electrophoretic polymorphism of the fourth component of human complement in paired maternal and fetal plasma. *Immunology* **21**, 869–878.

Ballow, M., Good, R. A., Biggar, W. D., Park, B. H., Jount, W. J. and Good, R. A. (1973). Reconstitution of C1q following bone marrow transplantation in patients with severe combined immunodeficiency. *Clinical Immunology and Immunopathology* **2**, 28–35.

Ballow, M., Fang Faye, Good, R. A. and Day, N. K. (1974). Developmental aspects of complement components in the newborn. *Clinical and Experimental Immunology* **18**, 259–266.

Barnes, J. M. (1940). The enzymes of lymphocytes and polymorphonuclear leucocytes. *British Journal of Experimental Pathology* **21**, 264–275.

Bing, D. H., Spurlock, S. E. and Bern, M. M. (1975). Synthesis of the first component of complement by primary cultures of human tumors of the colon and urogenital tract and comparable normal tissue. *Clinical Immunology and Immunopathology* **4**, 341–351.

Bordet, J. (1909). Recherches sur la destruction extracellulaire des bacteries. Annales de l'Institut Pasteur, June 1895. "Studies in Immunity" (Ed. J. Bordet), p. 81. Collected and translated by F. P. Gray. Chapman and Hall, London.

Brandtzaeg, P. and Mann, W. V., Jr (1964). A comparative study of the lysozyme activity of human gingival pocket fluid, serum and saliva. *Acta Odontologica Scandinavica* **22**, 441–455.

Briggs, R. S., Perillie, P. E. and Finch, S. C. (1966). Lysozyme in bone marrow and peripheral blood cells. *Journal of Histochemistry and Cytochemistry* **14**, 167–170.

Broxmeyer, H. E., Smithyman, A., Eger, R. R., Meyers, P. A. and De Sousa, M. (1978). Identification of lactoferrin as the granulocyte-derived inhibitor of colony-stimulating activity production. *Journal of Experimental Medicine* **148**, 1052–1067.

Buchner, H. (1899). Uber die bakterientodtende Wirkunk des zellenfrien Blutserums. *Zentralblatt für Bacteriologie, Parasitenkunde, Infektionskranheiten und Hygiene* **6**, 561–565.

Bullen, J. J., Rogers, H. J. and Leight, L. (1972). Iron-binding proteins in milk and resistance to *Escherichia coli* infection in infants. *British Medical Journal* **1**, 69–75.

Colten, H. R. (1973). Biosynthesis of the fifth component of complement (C5) by human fetal tissues. *Clinical Immunology and Immunopathology* **1**, 346–352.

Colten, H. R. (1976). Biosynthesis of complement. *Advances in Immunology* **22**, 67–118.

Colten, H. R., Borsos, T. and Rapp, H. J., (1966). *In vitro* synthesis of the first component of complement by guinea pig small intestine. *Proceedings of the National Academy of Science, U.S.A.* **56**, 1158–1163.

Colten, H. R., Silverstein, A. M., Borsos, T. and Rapp, H. J. (1968). Synthesis of the first component of human complement *in vitro. Journal of Experimental Medicine* **128**, 595–604.

Davis, C. A., Vallota, E. H. and Forristal, J. (1979). Serum complement levels in infancy: age related changes. *Pediatric Research* **13**, 1043–1046.

Day, N. K., Pickering, R. J., Gewurz, H. and Good, R. A. (1969). Ontogenetic development of the complement system. *Immunology* **16**, 319–326.

Day, N. K., Gewurz, H., Pickering, R. J. and Good, R. A. (1970). Ontogenetic development of C1q synthesis in the piglet. *Journal of Immunology* **104**, 1316–1319.

Donaldson, V. H. and Evans, R. R. (1963). A biochemical abnormality in hereditary angioneurotic edema: absence of serum inhibitor of C′1 esterase. *American Journal of Medicine* **35**, 37–44.

Ferrata, A. (1907). Die Unwirksamkeit der komplexen Hâmolysine in salzfreien Losaungen und ihre Ursache. *Berliner klinische Wochenschrift* **44**, 366.

Fireman, P., Zuchowski, D. A. and Taylor, P. M. (1969). Development of human complement system. *Journal of Immunology* **103**, 25–31.

Fischel, C. W. and Pearlman, D. S. (1961). Complement components of paired mother-cord sera. *Proceedings of the Society for Experimental Biology and Medicine* **107**, 695–699.

Flanagan, P. and Lionetti, F. (1955). Lysozyme distribution in blood. *Blood* **10**, 497–501.

Fleming, A. (1922). On a remarkable bacteriolytic element found in tissues and secretions. *Proceedings of the Royal Society* **93**, 306–317.

Friedberger, E. and Gewurz, J. (1930). Weitere Beiträge zum immunologischen Verhalten des Normalserums. III. Die Entstehung des Komplements. *Zeitschrift für Immunitätsforschung und experimentelle Therapie* **68**, 351–363.

Geiger, H., Day, N. K. B. and Good, R. A. (1972). The ontogenetic development of the later complement components in fetal piglets. *Journal of Immunology* **108**, 1098–1104.

Gewurz, H., Shin, H. S. and Mergenhagen, S. E. (1968). Interactions of the complement system with endotoxic lipopolysaccharide: consumption of each of the six terminal complement components. *Journal of Experimental Medicine* **128**, 1049–1057.

Gigli, I. and Austen, K. F. (1971). Phylogeny and function of the complement system. *Annual Review of Microbiology* **25**, 309–332.

Gitlin, D. and Biasucci, A. (1969). Development of γG, γA, γM, β1C, β1A, C1 esterase inhibitor, ceruloplasmin, transferrin, hemopexin, haptoglobin, fibrinogen, plasminogen, α_1-antitrypsin, orosomucoid, β-lipoprotein, α_2-macroglobulin and prealbumin in the human conceptus. *Journal of Clinical Investigation* **48**, 1433–1446.

Glynn, A. A., Martin, W. and Adinolfi, M. (1970). Levels of lysozyme in human foetuses and newborns. *Nature, London* **225**, 77–78.

Götze, O. and Müller-Eberhard, H. J. (1976). Alternative pathway of complement activation. *Advances in Immunology* **24**, 1–35.

Hochwald, G. M., Thorbecke, G. J. and Asofsky, R. (1961), Sites of formation of immune globulins and of a component of C'3. I. A new technique for the demonstration of the sythesis of individual serum proteins by tissues *in vitro*. *Journal of Experimental Medicine* **114**, 459–470.

Hyde, R. R. (1932). The complement deficient guinea pig: a study of an inheritable factor in immunity. *American Journal of Hygiene* **15**, 824–836.

Imoto, T., Johnson, L. N., North, A. C. T., Phillips, D. C. and Rupley, J. A. (1972). Vertebrate lysozymes. *In* "The Enzymes" (Ed. P. D. Boyer), pp. 665–868. 3rd edn. Academic Press, New York.

Jollès, P. (1960). Lysozyme. *In* "The Enzymes" (Eds. P. D. Boyer, H. Lardy and K. Myrback), pp. 431–445. Academic Press, New York.

Jollès, P., Bernier, I., Berthou, J., Charlemagne, D., Faure, A., Hermann, J., Jollès, J., Perin, J.-P. and Saint-Blancard, J. (1974). From lysozymes to chitinases: structural, kinetic and crystallographic studies. *In* "Lysozyme" (Eds. E. F. Osserman, R. E. Canfield and S. Beychok), pp. 31–54. Academic Press, New York.

Kaplan, M. H. and Volanakis, J. E. (1974). Interaction of C-reactive protein complexes with the complement system. I. Consumption of human complement associated with the reaction of C-reactive protein with pneumococcal C-polysaccharide and with the choline phosphatides, lecithin and sphinogmyelin. *Journal of Immunology* **112**, 2135–2147.

Kirkpatrick, C. H., Green, I., Rick, R. R. and Schode, H. L. (1971). Inhibition of growth of *Candida albicans* by iron-unsaturated lactoferrin: relationship to host defecnce mechanisms in chronic microcutaneous candidiasis. *Journal of Infectious Diseases* **124**, 539–544.

Klockars, M., Reitamo, S. and Adinolfi, M. (1977). Ontogeny of human lysozyme. Distribution in fetal tissues. *Biology of the Neonate* **32**, 243–249.

Köhler, P. E. (1973). Maturation of the human complement system. I. Onset time and sites of fetal C1q, C4, C3 and C5 synthesis. *Journal of Clinical Investigation* **52**, 671–677.

Köhler, P. F. and Müller-Eberhard, H. J. (1969). Complement-immunoglobulin relation: Deficiency of C'1q associated with impaired immunoglobulin G synthesis. *Science* **163**, 474–475.

Kolb, W. P. and Müller-Eberhard, H. J. (1974). Mode of action of human C9: adsorption of multiple C9 molecules to cell-bound C8. *Journal of Immunology* **113**, 479–488.

Kolb, W. P., Haxby, J. A., Arroyave, C. M. and Müller-Eberhard, H. J. (1972). Molecular analysis of the membrane attack mechanism of complement. *Journal of Experimental Medicine* **135**, 549–566.

Lachmann, P. J. (1973). Complement. *In* "Defence and Recognition" (Ed. R. R. Porter), 361–397. Butterworth, London.

Lachmann, P. J. (1979a). An evolutionary view of the complement system. *Behring Institute Mitteilungen* **63**, 25–37.

Lachmann, P. J. (1979b). Complement. *In* "The Antigens" (Ed. M. Sela), Vol. 5. Academic Press, New York.

Lachmann, P. J. and Halbwachs, L. (1975). The influence of C3b inactivator (KAF) concentration on the ability of serum to support complement activation. *Clinical and Experimental Immunology* **21**, 109–114.

Landerman, N. S., Webster, M. E., Becker, E. L. and Ratcliffe, H. E. (1962). Hereditary angioneurotic edema. II. Deficiency of inhibitor of serum globulin permeability factor and/or plasma kallilrein. *Journal of Allergy* **33**, 330–341.

Littleton, C., Kessler, D. and Burkholder, P. M. (1970). Cellular basis for synthesis of the fourth component of guinea pig complement as determined by haemolytic plaque technique. *Immunology* **18**, 693–704.

Lorenz, T. H., Korst, D. R., Simpson, J. F. and Musser, M. J. (1957). A quantitative method of lysozyme determination. I. An investigation of bronchial lysozyme. *Journal of Laboratory and Clinical Medicine* **49**, 145.

Mak, L. W. (1978). The complement profile in relation to the "reactor" state: a study in the immediate post-partum period. *Clinical and Experimental Immunology* **31**, 419–425.

Masson, P. L. and Heremans, J. F. (1971). Lactoferrin in milk from different species. *Comparative Biochemisty and Physiology* **39**, 119–129.

Mayer, M. M. (1961). Complement and complement fixation. *In* "Kabat and Mayer's Experimental Immunochemistry" (Ed. E. A. Kabat), 133–240. 2nd edn. Thomas, Springfield.

Mellbye, O. J., Natvig, J. B. and Krarstein, B. (1971). Presence of IgG subclasses and C1q in human cord sera. *In* "Protides of Biological Fluids" (Ed. H. Peeters), Vol. 18, 127–131. Pergamon Press, Oxford.

Miller, M. E. (1973). Natural defence mechanisms: development and characterisation of innate immunity. *In* "Immunologic Disorders in Infants and Children" (Eds. E. R. Stiehm and V. A. Fulginiti), 127–141. W. B. Saunders.

Minta, J. O., Jezyk, P. D. and Lepow, I. H. (1976). Distribution and levels of properdin in human body fluids. *Clinical Immunology and Immunopathology* **5**, 84–89.

Morris, K. M., Colten, H. R. and Bing, D. H. (1978). The first component of complement. *Journal of Experimental Medicine* **148**, 1007–1019.

Müller-Eberhard, H. J. (1968). Chemistry and reaction mechanisms of complement. *Advances in Immunology* **8**, 1–80.

Müller-Eberhard, H. J. (1972). The molecular basis of the biological activities of complement. *Harvey Lectures* **66**, 75–104.

Müller-Eberhard, H. J. (1975). The complement system. *In* "The Plasma Proteins" (Ed. F. W. Putnam), Vol. 1, 394–432. 2nd edn. Academic Press, London and New York.

Müller-Eberhard, H. J. and Lepow, I. H. (1965). C' esterase effect on activity and physiochemical properties of the fourth component of complement. *Journal of Experimental Medicine* **121**, 819–833.

Müller-Eberhard, H. J. and Dalmasso, A. P. and Calcott, M. A. (1966). The reaction mechanism of β1c-globulin in immune hemolysis. *Journal of Experimental Medicine* **123**, 33–54.

Naff, G. B. and Ratnoff, O. D. (1968). The enzymatic nature of C'1. Conversion of C's to C'1 esterase and digestion of amino acid esters by C'1. *Journal of Experimental Medicine* **128**, 571–593.

Naff, G. B., Pensky, J. and Lepow, I. H. (1964). The macromolecular nature of the first component of human complement. *Journal of Experimental Medicine* **119**, 593–613.

Nelson, R. A. (1958). An alternative mechanism for the properdin system. *Journal of Experimental Medicine* **108**, 515–535.

Noble, R. F. and Fudenberg, H. D. (1967). Leucocyte lysozyme activity in myelocytic leukemia. *Blood* **30**, 465–473.

Nydegger, U. E., Fearon, D. T. and Austen, K. F. (1978). The modulation of the alternative pathway of complement in C2-deficient human serum by changes in concentration of the component and control proteins. *Journal of Immunology* **120**, 1303–1308.

Osler, A. G. and Sandberg, A. L. (1973). Alternative complement pathways. *Progress in Allergy* **17**, 51–92.

Osserman, E. F. (1976). Postulated relationships between lysozyme and immunoglobulins as mediators of macrophage and plasma cell functions. *Advances in Pathobiology* **4**, 98–165.

Pfeiffer, R. and Issaeff, R. (1894). Ueber die specifische Bedentung der Choleraimmunität. *Zeitschrift für Hygiene und Infektionskrankheiten* **17**, 355–400.

Phillips, M. E., Rother, V. A., Rother K. O. and Thorbecke, G. J. (1969). Studies on the serum proteins of chimeras. III. Detection of donor-type C'5 in allogenic and congenic post-irradiation chimeras. *Immunology* **17**, 315–321.

Pillemer, L., Blum, L. and Lepow, I. H. (1954). The properdin system and immunity: I. Demonstration and isolation of a new serum protein, properdin and its role in immune phenomena. *Science* **120**, 279–285.

Polley, M. J. and Müller-Eberhard, H. J. (1968). The second component of the human complement: its isolation, fragmentation by C′1 esterase and incorporation into C′3 convertase. *Journal of Experimental Medicine* **128**, 533–551.

Porter, R. R. and Reid, K. B. M. (1978). The biochemistry of complement. *Nature, London* **275**, 699–704.

Propp, R. P. and Alper, C. A. (1968). C′3 synthesis in the human fetus and lack of transplacental passage. *Science* **162**, 672–673.

Rice, C. E. and Silverstein, A. M. (1964). Haemolytic complement activity of sera of foetal and newborn lambs. *Canadian Journal of Comparative Medicine* **28**, 34–41.

Rommel, F. A., Goldlust, M. B., Bancroft, F. S., Mayer, M. M. and Tashjian, A. H. (1970). Synthesis of the ninth component of complement by clonal strain of rat hepatoma cells. *Journal of Immunology* **105**, 396–403.

Rosen, F. S. (1974). Complement: ontogeny and phylogeny. *Transplantation Proceedings* **6**, 47–50.

Ruddy, S. (1974). Chemistry and biological activity of the complement system. *Transplantation Proceedings* **6**, 1–7.

Ruddy, S., Klemperer, M. R., Rosen, F. S., Austen, K. F. and Kumate, J. (1970). Hereditary deficiency of the second component of complement (C2) in man: correlation of C2 haemolytic activity with immunochemical measurements of C2 protein, *Immunology* **18**, 943–954.

Sawyer, M. K., Forman, M. J., Kuplic, L. and Stiehm, E. R. (1971). Developmental aspects of the human complement system. *Biology of the Neonate* **19**, 148–162.

Schorlemmer, H. U. and Allison, A. C. (1976). Effects of activated complement components on enzyme secretion by macrophages. *Immunology* **31**, 781–788.

Schorlemmer, H. U., Bitter-Suermann, D. and Allison, A. C. (1977). Complement activation by the alternative pathway and macrophage enzyme secretion in the pathogenesis of chronic inflammation. *Immunology* **32**, 929–940.

Schreiber, R. D. and Müller-Eberhard, H. J. (1974). Fourth component of human complement: description of a three polypeptide chain structure. *Journal of Experimental Medicine* **140**, 1324–1335.

Schumacher, G. F. B. (1974). Lysozyme in human genital secretions. *In* "Lysozyme" (Eds. E. F. Osserman, R. E. Canfield and S. Beychok), 427–447. Academic Press, New York.

Senn, H. J., Chu, B., O'Malley, J. and Holland, J. F. (1970). Experimental and clinical studies on muramidase (lysozyme). I. Muramidase activity of normal human blood cells and inflammatory exudates. *Acta Haematologica, Basel* **44**, 65–77.

Shin, H. S., Pickering, J. and Mayer, M. M. (1971). The fifth component of the guinea pig complement system. II. Mechanism of SAC̄12435b formation and C5 consumption by EAC̄1423. *Journal of Immunology* **106**, 473–479.

Stecher, V. J., Morse, J. H. and Thorbecke, G. J. (1967). Sites of production of the primate serum proteins associated with the complement system. *Proceedings of the Society for Experimental Biology and Medicine* **124**, 433–438.

Stecher, V. J. and Thorbecke, G. J. (1967). Sites of synthesis of serum proteins. I. Serum proteins produced by macrophages *in vitro*. *Journal of Immunology* **99**, 643–652.

Stossel, T. P., Alper, C. A. and Rosen, F. S. (1973). Opsonic activity in the newborn: role of properdin. *Pediatrics* **52**, 134–137.

Strunk, R. C., Tashjian, A. H. and Colten, H. R. (1975). Complement biosynthesis *in vitro* by rat hepatoma cell strains. *Journal of Immunology* **114**, 331–335.

Thorbecke, G. J., Hochwald, G. M., Van Furth, R., Müller-Eberhard, H. J. and Jacobsen, E. B. (1965). Problems in determining the sites of synthesis of complement reactions. *In* "Ciba Foundation Symposium on Complement" (Eds. G. E. W. Wolstenholme and J. Knight), 99–114. Churchill, London.

Tomasi, T. B. and Bienenstock, J. (1968). Secretory immunoglobulins *Advances in Immunology* **9**, 1–96.

Wasserman, P. and Alberts, E. (1940). Complement titre of blood of the newborn. *Proceedings of the Society for Experimental Biology and Medicine* **45**, 563–564.

DISCUSSION

Hayward Does anyone know what happens to complement levels in germ-free animals or babies such as those with severe combined immunodeficiency who have been kept germ free?

Adinolfi I do not know of any study where all components of complement have been estimated in germ-free babies. I think it will be quite interesting to see whether the levels of factor B and C9 are high or near normal values. I do not know if Prof. Soothill has any data.

Soothill I think we estimated C3 on the only child we have done this to, a healthy child and I think the C3 was of normal for age (a few days old). I have not heard of complement abnormalities in other infants treated in this way.

Reeves You have mentioned that some complement components behave as acute phase proteins. Can the fetus display an acute phase? Are some of the levels that you may be measuring higher than they might be because of this?

Adinolfi C9 and factor B behave very much as acute phase proteins. It is interesting that they are produced in the liver, which is the site of synthesis of most acute phase protein. I know of only one experimental study which has been done to see whether the levels of components of complement are affected following antigenic stimulation during fetal life in the lamb. Silverstein (1972) has shown that the components of a complement he tested, C3 and C4, were not affected by the antigenic stimulation. The synthesis of these components of complement seems not affected by environmental factors. It would be interesting to see if the levels of C9 or factor B increase as a result of intra-uterine infection.

Reeves Perhaps I could press you further. What is the ontogeny of the development of the ability to mount an acute phase reaction? When do you first become able to display that phenomenon? Does it happen before birth?

Adinolfi Synthesis of acute phase proteins such as α, 1-antitrypsin starts at an early stage of fetal life infections.

Faulk I was interested in the slide of the sites of synthesis there was a blank beside C6. Why do you think there has been some trouble?

Adinolfi The reason is that nobody as yet investigated the site C6 synthesis during fetal life in man. With an antiserum which we were given by Dr Müller Eberhard we were unable to detect C6 in any of the fetal tissues tested *in vitro*.

Basically it is a technical problem since different media should be used to study the *in vitro* synthesis of each component. A medium which is good for the synthesis of C3 or C4 is not good for the study of the synthesis of C9.

Faulk   Atlantic Antibodies in Maine make a very good anti C6 which we have confirmed as being monospecific. We have used this antibody to study the sites of C6 localization in human placentae and our finding to date indicate that this component identified as granules within endothelial cells of fetal stem vessels, almost as though it is being either synthesized or stored in these cells. Fetal stem vessel endothelium cells are however rather peculiar in as much as they also react the antisera to clotting factor VIII and they also have Fc receptors. This is why I asked the question because I was fascinated that the site of synthesis seems not to be known and I wondered if you might like to study placental endothelial cells to see if they are synthesizing C6.

Adinolfi   This is intriguing. Synthesis of C6 has been investigated using hybrid cells, human hepatoma and mouse fibroblast. These cells produced C6. It seems that the liver is one site of synthesis, but it would be interesting to see if the placenta produces it.

Faulk   No, it does not, as far as we can determine. In adults the Cambridge group studied C6 synthesis in a liver transplant patient and their results indicated that C6 was produced by the donor liver.

Adinolfi   Yes, you are right, they tested one patient with a liver transplant and were able to show that the C6 of the donor appeared in the recipient.

Faulk   I am amused by the idea that fetal stem vessel endothelial cells might enter the fetal liver, where they would be accepted as isogenic cells and initiate C6 synthesis.

Reeves   How much do you think the times at which you can first detect a complement component during fetal development are a reflection of the sensitivity of the techniques you have for each of the individual components? There is a very marked difference in the concentration ranges of individual complement components.

Adinolfi   This is a very interesting point, because I was trying to correlate the sequence of the synthesis of the various components of complement during the ontogeny with the phylogeny of complement. The problem is that it is easier to detect C3 than C9 because of the rate of synthesis is greater than that of many other components of complement. However, I still think that the observed difference between C3 and C9 is real, C9 being synthesized later than C3, while C1–INH is synthesized earlier in gestation.

Cooper   What do the low levels mean? From time to time people have made a great deal about the fact that a newborn has less complement than the mother does. You point out that that could be spurious in part because the mother's complement levels are higher than normal. Just looking at the whole thing, the data you show, it would appear that with the possible exception of C9, the fetus can make all the components right from the time he can first make antibodies. I am curious to know if any of those lower levels are actually limiting amount for the things that the fetus might want to do with regard with phagocytosis, chemotaxis and so forth, in order to get rid of an organism.

Adinolfi If in infants there is a correlation between the low levels of one components of complement and infection is not yet clear.

Wood I think there is some data now about eight years old by Stein showing a correlation between opsonic index of plasma of low birth rate infants in relationship to gestation and to the C3 level, and relating this also to immunoglobulin IgG level.

Cooper Is that clinically important?

Wood I would guess it might be. Deficiencies of some components of complement may be well tolerated, for example, a deficiency of C2 may be well tolerated since the infant can use the components of complement of the alternative pathway. Macrophages and components of the alternative pathway should be quite effective in the mechanisms of defence against several infections in the absence of C4 or C2.

Reeves At least two methods are in current use for measuring opsonizing capacities. As I understand, it is more commonly found to be deficient in younger individuals and may or may not be of pathological import. It seems to tie in with the alternative pathway of complement activation and there are two key factors either or both of which may be deficient. Have we any information about the ontogeny of opsonization capacity?

Soothill Miller has shown that in cord and early blood opsonization functions are lower than in adults, I think he showed that preterm infants were lower but I do not think he looked at fetal material. I support Dr Cooper's remark that we do not know whether any of these measurements of minor differences have a functional signficance. The differences observed in individuals with sustained defects which are more important than others. The deficiency of C2 is quite common. It is not associated with frequent infection because of the bypass of the alternative pathway. But deficiency of a regulatory protein is more important. Deficiencies of C1–IHN or KAF are associated with severe disease. Variations of levels of B^1H and KAF produced alternations of the whole complement system, due to the consumption of many components. If there is a bypass mechanism, the individual can cope quite well. It has been shown that antibodies can react with C1 bypass C2 and C4 and continue the reaction with C3 etc.: this is a bypass C4–C2.

Soothill For the sake of completeness it is important to stress that C2 deficiency is associated with lupus and all sorts of nasty things other than straightforward infection. Even intermediate values of C2 are associated with arthritis—as Scher has shown and we have shown that it is associated with atopy. We should therefore not limit our discussion to infection.

Adinolfi But how often do C2 deficient patients have lupus or severe disease?

Cooper Have complement deficiencies been observed in neonatal or in congenital infections?

Adinolfi The entire range of complement estimation in normal infants or presumed infected infants has not been yet carried out. Many of the components have not been investigated.

Walker-Smith I should like to mention a practical point. There are a number of immunoglobulins to use for preventing infections such as hepatitis B and hepatitis A, and to translate the results obtained in older children into newborn babies perhaps ought to be done with caution. There is need for specific evidence that these antiglobulins are effective against disease in neonates. Lower opsonic capacity and complement levels could influence their effect appreciably, I imagine.

Hayward There is at least one case in which cord serum haemolytic complement titres were compared with unrelated adults rather than the maternal sera, where the mean was over 75% I think. As was rightly commented earlier, there is little evidence that haemolytic complement titres are really very significantly low. Whether C9 is the limit is unclear. As has been hinted all along, there is not a lot of evidence to suggest that the haemolytic complement is low in newborns. In a large number a babies the titre is the same in cord sera as it is in unrelated adults.

Adinolfi As I have said, most of the components of complement, are present in cord blood in concentration near 50 or 70% of mean levels in adults. The limiting factor for the total complement values in cord blood may be C9.

Denman How many data are there relating fetal complement levels specific infections such as toxoplasmosis?

Adinolfi There are no data at all.

Bruno Reiter Ungulates are born with a full amount of complement and no antibodies. Does it mean that the placenta which is impermeable to immunoglobulins—in the calf, pig and so on—provides a barrier against infection? Is it therefore a good method of studying the mode of infection in general? As far as I am aware, there are no more fetal infections and very little antibodies produced in any of the ungulates at birth.

Faulk There have been over the years several reports, largely in the paediatric literature but not entirely, showing that cord blood has an anticomplementary effect. It is not too well known why cord blood is anticomplementary but it is a fairly well established observation that most human mothers who become pregnant will make antibodies to incompatible allotype inherited by the fetus from the father. The mother usually makes IgG antibody. It would be expected that maternal IgG antifetal allotype would meet its antigen upon entrance into the placenta or cord blood, and the the resulting immune complexes would fix complement thus appearing to be anticomplementary. In the ungulates where there is no transmission of maternal IgG to the fetus, one would not expect to find immune complexes in the cord blood. Because of that, one might reasonably speculate that cows etc. would have reasonably normal cord blood complement levels and absence of antiallotype antibodies and immune complexes. But that is only a guess.

Chairman Are there any more questions?

Kuitunen As everyone knows, human milk contains lysozyme, lactoferrin and other components, which have an anti-infective effect. When baby food factories are developing formulae for those infants who cannot get breast milk, should they also add some of these in their formulae? If so, do you believe that such things as lysozyme and lactoferrin in the case of other species would have as good effect as in the case of human milk?

Adinolfi I think that this is a subject we are going to discuss at length tomorrow. There is no doubt that colostrum and milk contains several factors which interact, such as IgA, lysozyme, lactoferrin etc., and also contain components of complement of the classical and alternative pathways. I think that these factors interact and play a very important role in the mechanism of defence of the newborn. Whether it is enough to add only one of these components to artificial milk I doubt. I do not think that it would be useful because if one adds only egg white, lysozyme or IgA, complement will still be absent. Other factors will also be missing, particularly T cells which are present in large numbers in colostrum and milk.

Wood Would Matteo say something about the development of lactoferrin in polymorphs?

Adinolfi Once again, I think that we may hear more about the functions of lactoferrin tomorrow. We found it mainly in fetal granulopoietic cells, not in the monocytes. This is in agreement with the observation that there is a dichotomy between the site of synthesis of lactoferrin and lysozyme. Lysozyme is produced in macrophages and monocytic cells. We have found lactoferrin in several tissues, in fetuses more than 10 or 12 weeks old and observed very good correlation between the site of synthesis of the lysozyme and lactoferrin with one exception, lactoferrin granulopoietic cells were detected in the fetal pancreas.

Reiter I understand that lysozyme has been added to baby feed with little success. However, it is little known that, in fact, egg white lysozyme has a much lower rate of activity in lysis and a much smaller spectrum of antibacterial activity than lysozyme isolated from milk. That has been known in the dairy literature for many years, but it has now been confirmed in a recent paper "Infection and Immunity" that the lysozyme is really what was called once betalysin, and also that the spectrum from the blood lysozyme is much wider and, therefore, a replacement with egg white lysozyme is hardly likely to produce any results. But the whole role of intestinal lysozyme needs much more investigation. Biochemically all the lysozymes have the same effect on the bacterial cell walls, but since the spectrum and the rate of lysis and so on is quite different. So it is useless to use egg white.

REFERENCES

Selsted, M. E. and Martinez, R. J. (1978). *Infection and Immunity* **20,** 782.
Silverstein, A. M. (1972). *In* "Ontogeny of Acquired Immunity" 17–25 Ciba Foundation
  Symposium. Associated Scientific Publishers, Amsterdam.
Wakil, J. R., Chandon, R. C., Parry, R. M. and Shahani, K. M. (1969). *Journal of Dairy Science*
  52, 1192.

Role of Placenta in Fetal Protection from Infection

W. PAGE FAULK

Blond McIndoe Centre for Transplantation Biology,
Queen Victoria Hospital,
East Grinstead, Sussex, UK

INTRODUCTION

The two major routes of placental infection are via the maternal birth canal and via the maternal circulatory system. In the former one finds inflammatory cells of maternal origin primarily infiltrated into the amniotic membranes, and the latter is characterized by the appearance of fetal inflammatory cells within the mesenchymal stroma of chorionic villi, although many exceptions to these general conditions can be found. Fox (1978) has reviewed the various microbiological agents which can infect the placenta and extraplacental membranes, but it is clear that many instances of chorioamnionitis probably have a noninfective etiology, although this is uncommonly the case with placental villitis. This paper will not deal with either the microbiology or pathology of placental infections, but instead shall focus on the role of the placenta in protecting the fetus from infection.

Not a great deal is known about placental mechanisms which are responsible for fetal protection. Certainly, placentae do not contain lymphoid aggregates and any immune cells or antibodies which find their way into extra-embryonic tissues must be of either maternal or fetal origin. In contrast, several discrete processes are available to combat infections; for instance, cultured placental tissues infected with rubella virus produce much greater amounts of interferon than do cultures of other fetal tissues (Banatvala *et al.*, 1973). In recent years, several nonspecific factors of resistance have been discovered in human placentae, and some of these will be discussed in the following paragraphs. These will be considered according to the anatomical flux of mother to fetus; namely, the intervillous spaces, the trophoblast, cells within the mesenchymal stroma, and the fetal stem vessels.

The Intervillous Spaces

Blood cells within the intervillous spaces (IVS) are maternal, and the *in vitro* identification of these is a precarious undertaking, for IVS are open spaces, most cells thus wash free during fixation. Nevertheless since the Hunter Brothers described IVS in the eighteenth century, a good deal of experience has accumulated to suggest that the amount and type of blood cells within IVS do not differ significantly from those in the mother's peripheral circulation, although investigations of this point are rare. A striking and perhaps informative exception to these observations can however be seen in maternal malaria, where the IVS are filled with many macrophages (Garnham, 1938). Interestingly, this aggregation of maternal monocytes and macrophages within the placental bed is not reflected in the mother's peripheral blood, although there is considerable damage to the chorionic villi represented principally by masses of perivillous fibrin and greatly thickened trophoblastic basement membranes. These findings appear as immuno-pathology represented by positive immunohistological reactions with antisera to immunoglobulins and complement (Galbraith *et al.*, 1978). Inasmuch as malaria parasites rarely reach the fetus and heavy malarial infestation of the placenta is often associated with an unduly small baby (Jelliffe, 1967), it is possible that perinatal mortality and morbidity are due to compromised placental function secondary to immunopathology (Galbraith *et al.*, 1979). Thus qualitative and quantitative changes in the population of maternal cells in the IVS may protect the fetus from infection but ultimately result in metabolic harassment and impeded fetal development.

The Trophoblast

There are several properties of the trophoblast which may be important in the fetus, but their role in host defences is drawn by analogy from other cells and have not been tested in trophoblast *per se*. Two such examples are phagocytosis (Johnson and Faulk, 1978) and phagolysosome formation, both of which decrease with trophoblastic age (Fox, 1979). These are well known, and until they are more extensively studied it is not particularly informative to deal further with them. Contemporary research into trophoblast biology has revealed new and exciting aspects of the trophoblast, and it does seem appropriate to detail these in this overview. Two examples will be discussed, these being the role of antigens of the major histocompatibility complex (MHC) and the presence of transferrin receptors.

Antigens of the major histocompatibility complex

Zinkernagel and Doherty (1977a) have put forward the idea that a population of thymus dependent (T) lymphocytes carry out an immunosurveillance function which is best represented by their cytotoxicity for virus infected target cells, and the degree or competence of their surveillance function is dependent upon some degree of transplantation antigen compatibility between the cytotoxic cell and the target. The idea is that a virus infected cell undergoes a measurable degree of self alteration, and that this antigenic drift is detected through the specific surveillance mechanism of a particular subpopulation of T cells (Zinkernagel and Doherty, 1977b). Thus if the plasma membrane of the trophoblast shares certain transplantation antigens with the mother, particularly if these cells become infected with a virus, as is possible through the haematogenous route, then it is likely that cytotoxic maternal immunosurveillance T cells with information for the virus will recognize an antigenic modulation of transplantation antigens on the trophoblast and a cytotoxic reaction will occur, thereby causing death of the trophoblast and subsequent rejection or loss of the fetus. However, this mechanism seems to be notwithstanding for trophoblast, because these cells do not manifest transplantation antigens (Faulk and Temple, 1976). Indeed, extensive studies with human trophoblast membranes have failed to show any antigens of the major histocompatibility complex (Faulk *et al.*, 1977), thereby denying the mechanism of Zinkernagel and Doherty (1977a) for virus infected trophoblast in human pregnancy. This elegant adaptive process may also be important in the maintenance of immunobiological equilibrium in the normal materno-fetal relationship.

Transferrin receptors

Another recently observed mechanism which might be important in placental protection of the fetus is one which has apparently been successfully employed by certain parasites for many years. This has to do with the production of a membrane receptor by the parasite which specifically binds an antigen of the host and thereby allows the parasite to escape immunosurveillance, because the host's immune cells recognize the parasite as self antigens. This "wolf-in-sheep's-clothing" trick is used for instance by schistosomes because this parasite coats itself with host blood group antigens (Smithers *et al.*, 1969). A similar process seems to be operating in the host-parasite relationship of human pregnancy, because Faulk and Galbraith (1979) have shown that the trophoblast (the "parasite") produces a receptor which specifically binds transferrin from the mother (the "host"), and this opens several possibilities for placental protection of the fetus from infection. This could operate by limiting the amount of free iron in the intervillous spaces and thereby inhibit either growth or toxin production by iron-requiring micro-organisms (Editorial, 1974), or, it could function by limiting the amount of maternal transferrin within the intervillous spaces, thus arresting the transformation of maternal lymphocytes at the G1 phase of their cell cycle (Tormey *et al.*, 1972; Tormey and Mueller, 1972). The more classical function of this receptor is its role in iron transport.

Cells bearing Fc Receptors

Receptors for a particular region (Fc) of the immunoglobulin G (IgG) molecule are found on the plasma membranes of certain specialized cells. Several years ago it was thought that these receptors were unique to macrophages and a population of bone marrow derived lymphocytes (B cells) as well as certain cells, such as the trophoblast, which are involved in immunoglobulin transport. It is now known that several different types of nonlymphoid cells manifest Fc receptors although the functions of these are not especially clear. One property of the receptor is its ability to bind antigen–antibody complexes, and it is in this regard that they may be important in infections during pregnancy. One consequence of most infectious diseases is the generation of immune complexes, and certain molecular configurations of these complexes cause a type of immunopathology and tissue damage. Interestingly, the placenta has three different levels of Fc receptors, and these will be considered separately.

Fc receptors of the trophoblast

Brambell (1966) proposed, as a result of his extensive studies of antibody transport from mother to fetus, that the trophoblast manifests receptors for maternal IgG, and that bound IgG was thus transported across the plasma membrane into phagosomes, being sterically protected from lysosomal damage throughout transport to the mesenchymal stroma of the chorionic villus. This idea has proven on balance to be correct, although more recent studies by Wild (1975), a student of Brambell, have broadened the concept to include transport by coated vesicles. Whether these receptors transport immune complexes *in vivo* is not clear, but *in vitro* studies employing enzyme–anti-enzyme complexes or antibody coated erythrocytes have shown that these complexes are bound by trophoblast Fc receptors, suggesting that immune complexes as well as monomeric immunoglobulin may be transported from the intervillous spaces into the connective tissue stroma of chorionic villi. The immunopathological consequences of this are not presently known.

Fc receptors of Hofbauer cells

In 1903 Hofbauer reported a unique cell in the mesenchymal stroma of human chorionic villi, and today this is thought to be a type of tissue macrophage (Boyd and Hamilton, 1970). The cells are more frequently found in early or preterm placentae and are common in term placentae that have sustained an infection. Studies employing the use of sex chromatin markers have revealed that these cells are of fetal origin. Like fibroblasts and other stromal cells, placental macrophages have HLA antigens. Several different investigators have found that Hofbauer cells bind both labelled IgG aggregates and immune complexes, indicating the presence of Fc receptors (Moskalewski *et al.*, 1975; Johnson and Matre, 1979), and it has been suggested that these receptors may serve to protect the fetus from soluble immune complexes produced following placental transfer of maternal IgG antibody to antigens within chorionic villi (Johnson *et al.*, 1977).

Fc receptors on fetal stem vessel endothelium

Most endothelial cells do not manifest Fc receptors, but Johnson *et al.*, (1976) have shown that the endothelium of fetal vessels within placental villi have the ability to bind immune complexes, labelled IgG aggregates and antibody sensitized erythrocytes (Johnson and Matre, 1979). These data strongly suggest that fetal stem vessel endothelium is endowed with Fc receptors, again possibly serving to protect the fetus from immune complexes that were either transported into or formed within chorionic villi. It is interesting that the endothelial plasma membrane is the last placental structure through which an antibody or complex must pass before entering the fetal circulation, and at this strategic location is found the third and final array of immune complex receptors. Alternatively, endothelial Fc receptors are well situated to bind complexes formed within the fetal stem vessels by either maternal or fetal antibody, but their precise role in the protection of the fetus from infection remains to be established.

The Placental Sink and Immunopathology

From the above discussions it is likely that certain micro-organisms might make their way into placentae, and in so doing will encounter either specific resistance from the maternal or fetal immune systems or nonspecific resistance from the placenta. Nonetheless, those organisms which reach the placental stroma will encounter an impressive array of Fc receptors, and antibody sensitized organisms will be bound by trophoblast, Hofbauer cells or fetal stem vessel endothelium.

Such complexes offer a substrate on which complement fixation can occur, and this has the possibility of setting into motion the vicious cycle of immunopathological damage within the placenta. Indeed, it is known that a good deal of immuno-pathology can be identified in both term and preterm placentae (Faulk and Johnson, 1977, 1980; Johnson and Faulk, 1978) and accentuation of this has the possibility of causing enough placental damage to compromise nutrient transfer and fetal growth. Thus, unsatisfactory or suboptimal development of the fetus following clinical or subclinical infections could be due to immunopathology within the placenta rather than to direct damage caused by the micro-organism. At least, this possibility seems to merit consideration, particularly in light of the above several recent observations that the placenta exerts primarily a nonimmunological role in protecting the fetus from infection, and that immunological responses to infection by either mother or fetus are likely to result in immune reactions occurring within the placental bed.

ACKNOWLEDGEMENTS

Work represented in this paper was supported in part by the East Grinstead Research Trust and the Medical Research Council.

REFERENCES

Banatvala, J. E., Potter, J. E. and Webster, M. J. (1973). Foetal interferon responses induced by rubella virus. *In* "Intrauterine Infections", 77–79. Associated Scientific Publishers, Amsterdam.

Boyd, J. D. and Hamilton, W. S. (1970). "The Human Placenta", 232–239. Heffer, Cambridge.

Brambell, F. W. R. (1966). The transmission of immunity from mother to young and the catabolism of immunoglobulins. *Lancet* ii, 1087–1093

Editorial (1974) Iron and resistance to infection. *Lancet* ii, 325–326.

Fox, H. (1978). "Pathology of the Placenta", 286–325. Saunders, London.

Faulk, W. P. and Galbraith, G. M. P. (1979). Transferrin and transferrin receptors in the host parasite relationship of human pregnancy. *Proceedings of the Royal Society (B)* 204, 83–97.

Faulk, W. P. and Johnson, P. M. (1977). Immunological studies of human placentae: Identification and distribution of proteins in mature chorionic villi. *Clinical and Experimental Immunology* 27, 365–375.

Faulk, W. P. and Johnson, P. M. (1980). Immunological studies of human placentae: basis and practical implications. *Recent Advances in Clinical Immunology* 2, 1–31.

Faulk, W. P. and Temple, A. (1976). Distribution of B2-microglobulin and HLA in chorionic villi of human placentae. *Nature* 262, 799–802.

Faulk, W. P., Sanderson, A. and Temple, A. (1977). Distribution of MHC antigens in human placentae. *Transplantation Proceedings* 9, 1379–1384.

Fox, H. (1979). Placenta as a model for organ ageing. *In* "Placenta—A Neglected Experimental Animal", 351–378. Pergamon Press, Oxford.

Galbraith, R. M., Faulk, W. P., Galbraith, G. M. P. and Bray, R. S. (1978). Placental immune complexes in malaria. *Protides of the Biological Fluids* **26**, 229–232.

Galbraith, R. M., Hsi, B., Galbraith, G. M. P., Bray, R. S., Fox, H. and Faulk W. P. (1979). The human materno-fetal relationship in malaria: II. Histological, ultrastructural and immunopathological studies of the placenta. *Transactions of the Royal Society of Tropical Medicine and Hygiene* **74**, 61–72.

Garnham, P. C. C. (1938). The placenta in malaria with special reference to reticulo-endothelial immunity. *Transactions of the Royal Society of Tropical Medicine and Hygiene* **32**, 13–34.

Jelliffe, E. F. P. (1967). Placental malaria and foetal growth failure. *In* "Nutrition and Infection", 18–35. Churchill, London.

Johnson, P. M. and Faulk, W. P. (1978). Immunological studies of human placentae: Identification and distribution of proteins in immature chorionic villi. *Immunology* **34**, 1027–1035.

Johnson, P. M. and Matre, R. (1979). Membrane receptors for IgG in the human placenta. *In* "Protein Transmission through Living Membranes", 45–54. Elsevier/North-Holland Biomedical Press, Amsterdam.

Johnson, P. M., Faulk, W. P. and Wang, A. C. (1976). Immunological studies of human placentae: Subclass and fragment specificity of binding of aggregated IgG by placental endothelial cells. *Immunology* **31**, 659–664.

Johnson, P. M., Natvig, J. B., Ystehede, U. A. and Faulk, W. P. (1977). Immunological studies of human placentae: The distribution and character of immunoglobulins in chorionic villi. *Clinical and Experimental Immunology* **30**, 145–153.

Moskalewski, S., Ptak, W. and Czarnik, Z. (1975). Demonstration of cells with IgG receptor in human placenta. *Biologica Neonatorum* **26**, 268–73.

Smithers, S. R., Terry, R. J. and Hockley, D. J. (1969). Host antigens in schistosomiasis. *Proceedings of the Royal Society (B)* **171**, 483–494.

Tormey, D. C. and Mueller, G. C. (1972). Biological effects of transferrin on human lymphocytes *in vitro*. *Experimental Cell Research* **74**, 220–226.

Tormey, D. C., Imrie, R. C. and Mueller, G. C. (1972). Identification of transferrin as a lymphocyte growth promoter in human serum. *Experimental Cell Research* **74**, 163–169.

Wild, A. E. (1975). Role of the cell surface in selection during transport of proteins from mother to foetus and newly born. *Philosophical Transactions of the Royal Society (B)* **271**, 395–407.

Zinkernagel, R. M. & Doherty, P. C. (1977a). Major transplantation antigens, viruses, and specificity of surveillance T cells. *Contemporary Topics in Immunobiology* **7**, 179–220.

Zinkernagel, R. M. and Doherty, P. C. (1977b). The concept that surveillance of self is mediated via the same set of genes that determines recognition of allogenic cells. *Cold Spring Harbor Symposium on Quantitative Biology* **41**, 505–510.

DISCUSSION

Adinolfi　You said in the beginning you were talking exclusively about human material. Is that right?

Faulk　Yes.

Adinolfi　Do you have any evidence that in the placenta of other species there is a receptor for transferrin?

Faulk The baboon and the macaque both have transferrin receptors. The transferrin receptor is cross-substitutable, that is, you can use baboon transferrin in a macaque or in a human. Interestingly, the rabbit, the guinea pig, the rat and the mouse do not have transferrin receptors but the structure and function of those placentae are so different that I am not very surprised that they do not.

Adinolfi Am I right to assume that transferrin and transferrin receptors have nothing to do with the trophoblastic specific antigen you have described in the past year.

Faulk The trophoblast glycoprotein which inhibits mixed lymphocyte culture reactions, has a rather similar distribution, but it is certainly not transferrin, and we do not think it is transferrin receptor either.

Soothill Can I ask a question about the three different Fc receptors? The ones on the fetal vessels have the characteristics of reacting with an aggregated IgG, which is similar to the one of lymphoid cells etc. Am I right in assuming that the ones responsible for the IgG transfer react with monomer IgG, and if so, have you any more information about the nature of this very interesting specificity.

Faulk Monomeric IgG binds the Brambell receptor but not the endothelial receptor, as you said. Aggregates and immune complexes bind the endothelial receptor but not the Brambell receptor, and antibody sensitized erythrocytes will bind both.

Bullen This observation you have made about the transferrin and the placenta looks very interesting indeed, but I did want to ask one thing. You postulated that you might get very low iron concentrations on the outside of the fetal membrane. Would it be possible to measure the saturation of the transferrin in the arterial and venous flow on the maternal side in the placenta, because you would not normally expect that there would be any difference in the saturation of the transferrin? What this reminds me of is the situation in the gut where we think that the IgA and the lactoferrin act as very powerful protective mechanisms on the gut membrane. The material you describe is definitely transferrin not lactoferrin.

Faulk The trophoblast receptor binds transferrin, not lactoferrin.

Bullen But you do not know anything about the saturation of the plasma transferrin on the maternal side of the placenta?

Faulk No.

Bullen There would be plenty of IgG about on both sides of the membrane, so this might be a very effective mechanism. If you have got high concentrations of transferrin on the membrane, would you in fact expect to get any alteration in the saturation in the immediate vicinity? *A priori*, one would not, but obviously it is worth finding out.

Faulk I do not know the answer to that, but I might tell you that we have looked at a lot of human tumour cells with the idea that these cells are confronted with a similar type of host–parasite relationship to that of the trophoblast, and we find that most human tumour and transformed cells maintained *in vitro* have the transferrin receptor. In addition, primary cultures of human fibroblasts do not have transferrin receptors, but after about 10 subcultures *in vitro* they begin to bind transferrin, and after about 20 subcultures they seem to be as efficient as the trophoblast in their ability to bind transferrin.

Bullen Very interesting.

Turano Could this model of pathogenicity also be applied to *Toxoplasma*? And another question which I would raise is this. Does the transferrin receptor apply to *Leptospira* infection and what happens to *Brucella* which we know very much affects the fetus in human and in bovine? What do you think about viruses at the level of the trophoblast?

Faulk I do not really have any ideas about transferrin and iron control in viruses. Perhaps Dr Bullen does.

Bullen No.

Turano Maybe you have experience about *Toxoplasma*?

Faulk Not enough to actually talk about, no.

Allison The interesting thing about *Toxoplasma* is that as in malaria, there are large numbers of parasites in the placenta and very few, if any, in the fetus. It looks as though the placenta must be a privileged site for the multiplication of these parasites. I do not know whether the type of change which you were discussing in malaria, deposition of fibrin and so on, occurs in a *Toxoplasma* infected placenta. Does anybody know?

Faulk We could answer that if we had the tissues.

Allison This is a common phenomenon in Africa. I understand that Prof. Turano sees such infection also in Italy.

Faulk Do you think that organisms which require iron for their metabolism would tend to focus in the placental bed?

Allison It is an interesting possibility, but I certainly do not know of any evidence. Incidentally, in relation to the origin of binding transferrin, you do have genetic markers in transferrins, if you were able to dissociate them under relatively mild conditions you could establish the maternal origin.

Faulk You are correct, it is maternal.

Adinolfi When did you start to detect the receptor in the fetal placenta?

Faulk We have studied abortion tissues which we are fairly sure is trophoblast from 3·5 to 4 weeks gestation, and these have transferrin receptors. It is the syncytiotrophoblast which manifest transferrin receptor; cytotrophoblast either does not have receptors, or it does not have very many transferrin receptors. We have looked at this another way by means of looking at the chorion side of the amniotic membranes. In this location one finds almost pure population of cytotrophoblast and no transferrin receptors. Thus, the development of receptor occurs with maturation from cytotrophoblast to syncytiotrophoblast. This is similar but opposite to the situation in maturing red cells, where the reticulocyte manifest transferrin receptor but the mature erythrocyte does not. Interestingly, red cells also lose HLA antigen at about the same time.

Soothill   Might I ask that we record and describe ages of fetuses in a standard way. Are we speaking of age derived from length, are we relating to the date of last menstrual period or date of calculated ovulation?—different groups use different nomenclature.

Faulk   The last menstrual period.

Cooper   About transferrin receptors on lymphocytes, I believe de Souze has postulated that they might be involved in governing the migration of lymphocytes via concentrations of iron. Is that not so?

Faulk   My understanding of transferrin receptors on lymphocytes is that lymphoblastoid cell lines bind transferrin. In addition, peripheral blood lymphocytes may show transient receptor activity following culture with phytohaemagglutinin. These data change somewhat if one uses radio-immuno assay to determine receptor activity, as this technique is more sensitive than membrane fluorescence, and with this greater sensitivity one obtains data that indicate that several different cells seem to specifically bind transferrin, but not very much. Finally, the work done in Dr Amos's laboratory indicate that T and B cells have different densities of transferrin receptors.

Cooper   Taking this information, could you speculate about how transferrin receptors on the trophoblast might either keep lymphocytes away or influence their behaviour once they are there?

Faulk   One way this could operate in the immunobiology of pregnancy is by coating the materno-fetal interface with maternal protein. In this way, maternal lymphocytes would be impeded in their ability to recognize and respond to fetal antigens on the trophoblast. This type of masking effect is employed in conditions of host–parasite relationship in for instance schistosomiasis, where the schistosome produces a receptor for human blood group antigens. A second way that the trophoblast receptor could tend to protect the placenta from maternal lymphocytes is by limiting the amount of free transferrin in the intervillous spaces. This could be important because transferrin is required for lymphocyte proliferation in response to lectin stimulation, and could presumably also impede maternal recognition of allogeneic antigens on the trophblast. Finally, there could be physical properties and charge relationships that might be altered but I do not think that there are very solid data on these possibilities.

Allison   Will the cells stripped of transferrins stimulate lymphocyte proliferation *in vitro*?

Faulk   We find they do not. For example, we work with the Be Wo trophoblast cell line which is maintained in a human serum free medium supplemented with fetal calf serum. Fetal calf serum does not react with antiserum to human transferrin. Cells from these cultures do not stimulate in MLC reactions, but there is no good evidence that the human trophoblast manifest either Ia or HLA-D antigens, in fact, there is fairly good evidence that they do not.

Reiter There is so much new to me that perhaps I did not understand it. Are those receptors for transferrin tangible? Can you isolate them?

Faulk Yes.

Reiter Because lactoferrin and transferrin are both very basic proteins, they will attach to the (bare) surface of bacteria and there is no need for other receptors.*

Faulk The transferrin receptor has been extensively studied for many years on rabbit reticulocytes, and to my knowledge there is no information to support the concept that receptor activity is dependent upon basic proteins. In addition, we now have a crude preparation of transferrin receptor isolated from trophoblast, and there are other groups who are trying to isolate transferrin receptors with a certain degree of success.

Allison The species specificity of the binding suggests again that not only charge is involved.

Faulk I think so, yes.

Allison But they have roughly the same charge.

Faulk Yes, electrophoretically measured.

Allison In relation to the general point of whether transferrin could be protective it is a kinetic problem because you must have so much maternal blood bathing the system that there must be an excess of free transferrin. But one thing must be very intriguing is the role of this in iron transport. Again, this is a kinetic problem because presumably there is transfer of iron from the transferrin to the placental cells. Iron then passes through to the fetus, and this would be an interesting equilibrium situation to study, using labels.

Faulk We would be quite interested in studying that. At the moment it is thought that the iron–transferrin complex binds to its receptor and is endocytosed. Following which, in tandem with carbonate ions, the ferric atoms are released and bound by trophoblastic ferritin, which is isotypically specific for placentae. That is how it is possible to transport iron uphill, as it were. Interestingly, one also finds isotypes of placental ferritin in certain tumours, as you probably know.

Allison Presumably, then, this would imply that the level of free ferric iron in the placenta would be very low and this could be protective in the way that Dr Bullen and others have shown.

Wood I wonder if you could comment on the condition of the placenta when it gets to the stage of degeneration, that is in late or even post-term pregnancies. Are these mechanisms still to be observed there?

Faulk One sees transferrin receptor in trophoblast that had been maintained in

*Steel (1975). *Immunology* **29**, 31.

culture for years. Usually we study Caesarian tissue simply because it has less artefacts, so we are rarely able to study pregnancies beyond 40 weeks.

Cooper Could you straighten me out on what all those Fc receptors are actually doing? Specifically, do they transport from the intervillus spaces, either complexes of IgG or antigen–antibody complexes, across into the fetal circulation?

Faulk I do not think there would be a very good chance of that, because once they got into the villus they would have to get past two other types of Fc receptors. The evidence that complexes are transported is rather bad: there is no evidence against it, but the evidence in favour of it is not very strong. Maternal antifetal allotype for IgG (Gm) is for example transported as monomer into the mesenchymal stroma via the Brambell receptor, and fetal Gm antigens are to be found in this stroma by virtue of leakage of fetal IgG from the fetal stem vessels. This has been shown by using double marker reactions for paternal (fetal) Gm groups and maternal Gm groups. So what is happening all the time in the connective tissue of the villus is the formation of allotype–anti-allotype complexes. Some of these complexes can also be shown to have fixed complement and are thereby presumably coprecipitated in the tissue, although I know of no careful study of this point. In addition, those complexes which are not coprecipitated by complement would in all likelihood be bound by the Fc receptors manifest by endothelial cells of the fetal stem vessels. This can also be shown by using appropriate markers. These observations have introduced a new idea which I initially found to be quite puzzling, because I was always taught that the fetus makes very little IgG. Indeed, the mass of cord blood IgG is maternal and not fetal in origin, but if we look in the placenta we find impressive amounts of IgG bearing fetal (paternal) IgG allotype markers. We interpret these observations in terms of the placenta serving as a type of physiological sink for immune complexes. Whether they are transported into or form within the sink, they seem to on balance never leave the sink. This puts forward several interesting points for discussion, one of which is the possible protective or buffering role of placental Fc receptors in impeding the entrance of immune complexes into the fetal circulation. Another is the point you and your colleagues have raised regarding the possible activation of suppressor cells by such complexes.

Cooper One can think of the placental set of Fc receptors as a way of preventing complexes from reaching the baby, but are there really good data available to show that IgG complexes stick in the placenta and go no further? It is not only a matter of transfer of infectious agents, but the suppressor population of T cells seem to be rich in Fc receptors, and they serve as one of the triggers for activating their suppressor activity.

Faulk There is no doubt that the cord blood is a gold mine for suppressor T cells. Whether it has anything to do with placental immune complexes, and your idea of what activates suppressor T cells, I do not know.

Walker I should like to extend the point to which Dr Cooper has been alluding. Do we know for a fact that the Fc receptors for aggregate IgG block the transport of immune complexes or do they facilitate the transport of immune complexes across the endothelium? With regard to the Fc receptors for monomeric IgG mentioned earlier, presumably this receptor is a facilitated transport mechanism for uptake of immune globulins from maternal to fetal circulation.

Faulk We have not been able to isolate receptor from fetal endothelial cells although we have not focused intensively on the biochemical aspects of this. However, when one reviews the studies of others with trophoblast Fc receptors one. usually finds that intact and nonfractionated membranes were used. By the same logic, if one uses fetal endothelial cells harvested from the umbilical cord, one can show that those cells will bind complexes. Immune complexes or aggregate bound to endothelial cells are also mobile, capping at 37°C and not capping at 5°C. Finally you are absolutely right to point out that Hofbauer cells might contain complexes which they have apparently phagocytosed and are not necessarily on their cell membranes. To see these, one would have to fix the cell in order to remove the plasma membrane, but the results I have shown today were obtained from unfixed tissues and are a fair representation of what one might expect to find on the surface of the cell.

Walker Is there any evidence that hormones affect the maturation of these receptors, as Waldman and others have shown with respect to the monomeric Fc receptors on the intestine of the suckling rat? In other words, can you differentiate between the receptors by the effects of hormones on their maturation?

Faulk With the suckling rat gut it has been reasonably well shown that one can block transport by giving an injection of cortisol. When one gives cortisol to these animals both gut transport and alkaline phosphatase activity are affected. It is a reasonably recent invention that this affects the Fc receptors.

Walker Do you shut off the effect of alkaline phosphatase or do you stimulate the effect? I thought it had been shown that there is an increased maturation of the alkaline phosphatase levels on the surface of the intestinal cell, which was an indication of maturation of the cell membrane.

Faulk You are correct. Let us agree, for purposes of discussion, that something happens to the alkaline phosphatase. Is this an effect on Fc receptor, or is this an effect on some other transport system in which the Fc receptor is involved? I do not know.

Walker I raise this issue because there are many parallels between the transport of immune globulins across the intestine of the rodents that have modified transplacental passage of immunoglobulins and the transplacental passage of immunoglobulin in man. I am curious to know whether or not there was a persistence of receptors on endothelial cells for aggregated and monomenic IgG as compared to receptor on endothelial cell in other vascular compartments.

Faulk We have not observed Fc receptors on other fetal endothelium.

Denman Are there any studies on the placentas of fetuses born to mothers with immune complex disease comparing the composition of complexes in the placenta with those in the maternal sera. This would enable the transport role of cells with Fc receptors to be analysed. Furthermore, is there any evidence that such bound complexes interfere with the normal transfer of maternal immunoglobulin.

Faulk One normally finds a certain amount of immunopathology in the mature chorionic villus. We view this as a physiological concomitant of normal pregnancy. This point is well supported by reports of C3d and C9 on the trophoblastic basement membranes of normal term placentae. In maternal SLE, one finds very much more. In addition, one normally finds C4 in the intervillous fibrin areas, but in the SLE mother there is more C4 than in normals. One also sometimes finds C1q in the walls of fetal stem vessels, but again in the placentae from SLE mothers one finds more of this complement component, suggesting that the physiological process of complement activation is amplified in maternal SLE. It does seem that there are more complexes in the SLE placenta, and it is well known that the pregnancy outcome in those mothers is much worse than in normal controls. They sustain a very high incidence of miscarriage and perinatal pathology. It is thus our impression that maternal SLE represents an example of maternal-fetal immunopathology. You wanted to also know if transferrin or the transferrin receptor was involved in the placental immunopathology of SLE mothers, and I must say that I do not know. Those kind of tissues are really very rarely obtained.

Cooper How do organisms get from the mother to the fetus across the placenta?

Faulk I do not really know. There is a review of this in "Pathology of the Placenta", published by Saunders, where the author, Prof. H. Fox, goes through most known infections in an effort to make sense of this. It is perhaps fair to say that if an organism is present in the placental bed, unless it is a special example like malaria, it will probably get over into the fetal circulation. The mechanism for this isn't clear.

Cooper In terms of the mechanism that you have discussed with us today, do infectious agents go across the placenta by themselves, complexed to antibodies, ride over in a cell, or do you have any notion of how organisms do breach this barrier?

Faulk There is not one intelligent study which really casts light on the question.

Miles Are there lymphocytes in the placental villi?

Faulk This was argued for hundreds of years. It seems to be fairly well settled now that there are not.

Miles How often during a pregnancy would you postulate that damage could happen so that you would not have rupture of this perfect intermediary trophoblast?

Faulk I think it must happen in all pregnancies.

Sir Ashley But that might be one of the ways your infections could get across, with an actual breach.

Faulk That is the usual answer, but I am not able to determine how much of this is fact versus opinion.

Stern How do fetal red cells cross the placenta to enter the maternal circulation.

Faulk The usual answer is placental tears, but there is no good evidence to support that, unless you go in and tear it yourself.

Stern But fetal red cells do get across.

Faulk Absolutely, most fetal cells do get across as demonstrated by observations that mother make antibodies to them. This does not however tell us how it happens.

Chairman On that note of mystery perhaps we ought to wind up this session.

Clinical Problems in Postnatal Infection

C. B. S. WOOD

Medical College of St Bartholomew
and the London Hospital and
Queen Elizabeth Hospital for Children, London, UK

My purpose is to outline the nature, prevalence and problems associated with postnatal infections. It is not possible to separate antenatal and postnatal infections totally one from another, but infections due to bacterial invasion seem more likely to be acquired during or after birth, and may be transmitted from the mother, as well as nosocomially. The incidence from a number of series is about 1·5 per 10^3 live births (Jeffery et al., 1977). Bacterial infections may be intensely destructive, but are potentially treatable and hence there is a pressing need for urgent and accurate diagnosis. Because clinical decisions have to be taken before laboratory results are available an empirical approach to likelihood is needed, assisted by inference from epidemiological findings and insight into developmental immunology.

Among the newborn, 6% are of low birth weight either because of short gestation or because of impaired intra-uterine growth. These and others who are delivered in circumstances of obstetric abnormality and are admitted to neonatal special and intensive care units seem to be particularly vulnerable to bacterial infection. Low birth weight infants are also among those least well endowed with maternal IgG immunoglobulin but their immunological apparatus appears otherwise to be responsive if inexperienced, with the possible exception of leukocyte chemotaxis (Miller, 1971), which may be tardy in development.

Staphylococcal infections and cross-infection are fortunately less of a problem than hitherto. Environmental factors such as the personalization of the babies' nursing materials, and the provision of 5 m² for each cot in nurseries, and rooming in with the mother wherever possible, have contributed to the major fall in staphylococcal infection. Skin colonization still occurs rapidly however. Vaginal staphylococcal carriage is limited to about 5% and hence it must be concluded that colonization results from transfer of the organism from the hands of attendants and the ward environment. (Gillespie et al., 1958; Wolinsky et al., 1960).

The risk of clinical infection is related to the rate of previous colonization and was much reduced when hexachlorophane was used for bathing. This was associated with a slight increase in Gram negative infections. Anxiety about cerebral dystrophy due to hexachlorophane has reduced its use in most units to a dusting powder (0·3%) applied to the cord. This is however useful, and staphylococcal infections have not really re-emerged.

Currently, chlorhexidine, which is not absorbed and therefore presents less of a threat of toxicity and has perhaps a slightly wider antibacterial spectrum, is being considered as an alternative antibacterial agent for skin cleansing and care (Cowen et al., 1979).

The pattern of infection with staphylococcal organisms has been reported as follows:

Conjunctivitis	60%
Superficial skin	20%
Umbilicus	10%
Deep infection	4%

The rate of colonization can be very strikingly reduced by nursing preterm infants in open dry incubators (compensation for fluid loss by evaporation is achieved by increasing the fluid intake) rather than in traditional enclosed humid incubators. (Chang et al., 1979).

It is now 15 years since group B streptococcal infections were first recorded to be important in the newborn (Eickhoff et al., 1964). Hitherto the organism was thought rarely to be the cause of human disease and was ordinarily associated with bovine mastitis. An increasing number of neonatal cases has now established the infection as equal in importance to that due to Escherichia coli (Kjems et al., 1978). The majority of infants infected are born to mothers who carry the organism vaginally and only a minority seem to acquire it by cross infection in the nurseries (Pass et al., 1978). The acute early form of infection is associated with apnea, or tachypnoea similar to the respiratory distress syndrome, and collapse, in the first day of life. (Cowen et al., 1977; Ablow et al., 1978). This form of illness is virtually untreatable because of the rapidity with which the organism is invasive. It may be due to any of the three main serological types, but type three is more associated with a slightly latent pattern of disease appearing at or after the end of the first week of life and often involving meningitis.

It is most useful to know that in the care of such infants that Gram positive cocci can be obtained from gastric aspirate. The peripheral blood granulocyte count is often deceptively low (Menke *et al.*, 1979) and this is important because the early form of illness may mimic the respiratory distress syndrome although the inflation pressure required to achieve artificial ventilation is lower. Surprisingly, diagnosis is not particularly assisted by determination of "C-reactive" protein (acute phase proteins) (Phillips, 1979) but the rapid synthesis of the protein seems to be more indicative of the capacity to survive than of the presence of infection.

Hill *et al.* (1978) showed that there were problems with humoral and cellular immunity and their relationships to this infection and Baker and Kasper (1979) had shown that of infants born to carrier mothers who remained well, 76% had antibodies to group B streptococci but among those who were ill, antibody was absent. A method of predicting high risk of infants has been propounded by Berquist *et al.* (1979) who found that by developing a score relating to antenatal and perinatal events, such as prolonged rupture of membranes etc., it was possible to predict 55% of the septicaemic group and so an epidemiological approach may prove to be helpful.

Coliform infections are second only to group B streptococcal disease as a major threat to the newborn. Epidemic gastroenteritis due to specific serological types of *E. coli* is recognized as is the importance of those carrying the K1 antigen in neonatal bacterial meningitis. This capsular antigen appears to be linked with virulent infection. Infection by *Pseudomonas* spp. has long been recognized as a natural enemy of the newborn. Infection rates have varied from between 3% to 28% and other organisms occasionally found in this context to be associated with disease include *Citrobacter alcanigene*.

Neonatal infection by *Listeria monocytogenes* is at times a transplacental infection but also has a late and probably acquired form which is different from the intra-uterine granulomatous illness and is yet always severely damaging.

Listeria monocytogenes thus appears to cause two kinds of illness in the perinatal period. About half of recognized cases are ill within 2 day of birth, with a septicaemic condition in which there may be respiratory difficulty, circulatory failure, fits and purpura. Many of the infants with this early, acute form of *Listeria* infection are premature or of low birth weight. Often the *liquor amnii* has been found to be infected, and organisms found in the genital tract of the mother, in whom antibodies may also be found.

A smaller group has been recognized in which a meningoencephalitis appears after about one week after a normal term delivery. Mononuclear cells predominate in the CSF, but the mother is healthy and the amnionic fluid not infected. An intermediate group also exists in both in timing and mixed pathology, and yet others result in stillbirth or abortion, and appear to the examples of the early form.

Listeria monocytogenes is probably responsible for 1 in 1000 perinatal mortalities, and the factors which determine individual vulnerability are unknown. Among survivors, handicap is prominent.

Recent interest has been generated by the problems of chlamydial infection. Forty-four per cent of infants with this infection acquire it as part of a maternal–child pair, presumably in the birth canal, and both eyes and the lungs may be involved. Micropannus is found in the eye but this infection is not as destructive as the other infection described above. (Frommell *et al.*, (1979).

Infection rates for gonococci vary from centre to centre. Neonatal gonococcal ophthalmia no longer contributes much to the relatively large proportion (20%) of blindness arising in the newborn period. Some are resistant to penicillin and produce a β lactamase, although the organism is rarely invasive other than in the eye. The infection is still increasing in adult population and hence more neonatal infections are to be expected.

Wide variations in pathological consequences are found in the spectrum of virus diseases in the newborn. Thus, rotavirus (Murphy *et al.*, 1977) has been found in a number of apparently well newborn, although this virus is clearly associated with gastroenteritis later. In this very early epoch the RSV group is probably more associated with catarrhal than bronchiolitic infections. Serious problems have arisen with enteroviruses and Echo 11 type has been associated with a catastrophically destructive illness in the newborn not unlike that due to the group B staphylococcus (Naglinton *et al.*, 1978).

Central current problems concern the pathogenesis and epidemiology and hence prevention of group B streptrococcal and other bacterial infections, and their early diagnosis and treatment, and in parallel is the need to find quick methods of diagnosing bacterial infections in newborn, before irretrievable damage is done.

REFERENCES

Ablow, R. C., Driscoll, S. D., Effman E. L., Gross, I., Jolles, C. J. G., Uauy, R. and Warshaw, J. B. (1976). A comparison of early onset of Group B streptococcal infection and the respiratory distress syndrome. *New England Journal of Medicine* **294**, 65–70.

Baker, C. J. and Kasper, D. L. (1979). Immunological investigation of infants with septicaemia and meningitis due to Group B streptococci. *Journal of Infectious Diseases* **130**, Suppl. 898–904.

Berquist, G., Eriksson, M. and Zetterstrom, K. (1979). Neonatal septicaemia and perinatal risk factors. *Acta Paediatrica Scandinavica* **68**, 337–339.

Chang, C. R., Glass, L., Evans, H. E. and Pierog, S. H. (1979). Bacterial colonisation of infants raised in incubators under radiant heat. *Archives of Disease in Childhood* **52**, 507–509.

Cowen, J., Ellis, S. H. and McAinish, J. (1979). Absorption of chlorhexidine from intact skin of newborn infant. *Archives of Disease in Childhood* **54**, 379–383.

Eickhoff, T. C., Klein, J. D. and Daly, A. K. E. (1964). Neonatal sepsis and other infections due to Group B beta haemolytic streptococci. *New England Journal of Medicine* **271**, 1221–1228.

Frommell, G. T., Rottenburg, R., Wang, S. P. and McIntosh, K. (1979). Chlamydial infection of mothers and their infants. *Journal of Pediatrics* **95**, 28–32.

Gillespie, W. A., Simpson, K. and Tozer, R. C. (1958). Staphylococcal infections in a maternity hospital: epidemiology and control. *Lancet* **ii**, 1075–1080.

Hill, H. R., Shigeoka, A. O., Hemming, V. G. and Allred, C. D. (1978). Cellular and humoral aspects of host defence mechanisms against Group B streptococci. *In* "Pathogenic Streptococci" (Ed. M. I. Parker), pp. 157–159. Reed Books, Chertsey, England.

Jeffrey, H., Mitchison, R., Wigglesworth, J. S. and Davies, P. A. (1977). Early neonatal bacteraemia. *Archives of Disease in Childhood* **52**, 83–86.

Kjems, S. E., Perch, B. and Henrichsen, J. (1978). Incidence of serious neonatal infection due to Group B streptococci in Denmark. *In* "Pathogenic Streptococci" (Ed. M. I. Parker), pp. 173–174. Reed Books, Chertsey, England.

Menke, J. A., Giacoia, G. P. and Jockin, H. (1979). Group B beta haemolytic streptococcal sepsis and the indiopathic respiratory distress syndrome: A comparison. *Journal of Pediatrics* **94**, 467–474.

Miller, M. E. (1971). Chemotactic function in the human neonate: humoral and cellular aspects. *Pediatric Research* **5**, 487–492.

Murphy, A. M., Albrey, M. B. and Crewe, E. B. (1977). Rotavirus infections of neonates. *Lancet* **ii**, 1149–1150.

Naginton, J., Wreghlitt, T. G., Gandy, G., Roberton, N. R. C. and Berry, P. J. (1978). Fatal Echovirus 11 infections in outbreak in special care baby unit. *Lancet* **ii**, 725–728.

Pass, M. A., Gray, B. M., Khare, S. and Dillon, H. C. (1978). Epidemiological studies of Group B streptococcal infection in the neonate. *In* "Pathogenic Streptococci" (Ed. M. I. Parker), pp. 175–177, Reed Books, Chertsey, England.

Phillips, A. G. S. (1979). Protective effect of acute phase reactants in neonatal sepsis. *Acta Paediatrica Scandinavica* **68**, 481–483.

Wolinsky, E. W., Lipsitz, P. J., Mortimer, E. A. and Rammelkamp, C. H. (1960). Acquisition of staphylococci by newborns. *Lancet* **ii**, 620–622.

DISCUSSION

Dewdney Would you comment on the use of antibodies in these pyogenic infections? I think that antibiotics can only be fully effective if polymorph function is intact. The slide showed that in many of the very young children polymorphs are obviously not functioning very efficiently. What is general experience about the use of antibiotics to control, for example, staphylococcal and streptococcal infection?

Wood One's experience has been that high dosage of appropriate antibiotics is reasonably effective for staphylococcal infection and for group A streptococcal infection. One can think of clinical instances where we know that polymorph function has been abnormal on a genetic basis, where careful high dose cloxacillin has worked in dealing with abscess formation. Coliform infections of the central nervous system are still a problem, in that antibiotic treatment is often not adequate. As for the group B *Streptococcus*, I have to admit that I have had very few patients who have done well even with high dosage of penicillin G combined with gentamicin. Nevertheless, our approach is to try to treat very early and to use high doses. This means treating long before we have confirmation of the nature of the infection, on the basis of the likelihood to which I have referred.

Bullen   Are the children that go down with streptococcal infection breast fed or bottle fed? You mentioned the importance of maternal IgG. Have you measured this and is it possible to boost it in any way? Is it absolutely crucial, do you know?

Wood   There is such a heavy predominance of babies born by operative or abnormal deliveries among those with the group B streptococci that it is only a minority who are breast fed. This group of infected infants are almost all in special care units. If they receive breast milk it will probably be breast milk that has been stored. In any case, the acute illness in the first 24 hours is before lactation has really become established. The giving of breast milk does not seem to weight heavily in the occurrence or otherwise of the early septacaemic form.

With regard to IgG, there has been debate in clinical paediatrics about whether infants should be given immunoglobulin by injection if they are of very low birth weight.

In general the concensus has been against this because it was felt that these infants were immunologically competent, and that if we protected them, environmentally, it was perhaps better than loading them with immunoglobulin not knowing what would be the consequences to subsequent endogenous IgG synthesis and whether sensitization could occur.

Hayward   A trial of Kempe and others showed that there was little evidence of protection, although there was some suggestion some years later that children who were treated prophylactically had IgG levels somewhat lower than those who were not treated.

Faulk   Are you sure that maternal antibody to group B streptococcus is protective for the newborn? Has anyone looked into the possibility of a vaccine against group B streptococcus which could be given during pregnancy to the mother to allow protective antibody to be transported across the placenta to the fetus?

Wood   I do not know whether an effective vaccine can easily be produced. There has been some interest in bacteriological screening of pregnant women, who are numerous, and this presents a logistic problem for laboratories. Giving the mothers chemotherapy when they are found to be positive does not apparently always eradicate the group B streptococcus from the vagina or eradicate it for a long period of time. That does not really answer your question; it comments on another aspect of it.

Allison   I am just going to comment on that fact that nowadays it is possible to get very specific antibodies, for example by the monoclonal technique, and I was wondering whether groups such as those we have been discussing might not be suitable for this purpose. Presumably an antibody administered to the newborn might be helpful?

Wood Yes.

Marshall Is there not some evidence that antibody is of value once infection has taken place? I am citing the report of exchange transfusion for the treatment of children with early onset of disease. The children who survived were those children who received exchanged blood which contained antibody to the type of group B streptococcus with which they were infected, deaths in this group of children were those children in whom the donor blood did not contain the antibody to their infecting organism (Shegeoka *et al.*, 1978).

Wood Yes that is right.

Smith I think the prospects for vaccination are fairly optimistic in this field. The type 3 organism is, I believe, responsible in the USA for over 50% of the cases. In the UK, I think the figure is about 42%. If you were to add type 1A and 1B polysaccharide to a type III vaccine about 85% would be covered by those three antigens. The protective antigen in each case appears to be the polysaccharide capsule, and very effective polysaccharide vaccine have been made, particularly in the last few years. It should be possible to screen mothers' blood for the presence or absence of antibodies to these organisms and to vaccinate those with low levels, because, Baker's evidence suggests very strongly that mothers with low levels of antibodies are the ones who tend to have infected babies. It is also possible to show in mice with type 1 and type 2 organisms that the capsular antibody is protective against group B infection. I know there is a lot of interest in such a vaccine in the USA, but I do not think anybody has yet got to the stage of clinical trial. It could well have an important role to play if used specifically in defined patients, which is an attractive way of using a vaccine.

Tyrrell I should like to make a few points about the chlamydia and viruses. First, the chlamydia are actually bacteria, second I wondered what your experience had been of therapy, partly because in adults tetracyclines are such good drugs and you obviously would not want to use them, and partly because it seemed to me that the immune response of the host is a very important element in controlling these agents and that it might be that it was a deficiency there which lay behind the fact that the patient had become ill. Can I just tack on one other thing concerned with enteroviruses.

People have been talking about immunoglobulins as a way of controlling some of these infections. One of the problems with enteroviruses is that the epidemic echovirus is usually one which has not been around for some years, therefore people have not raised antibodies against it, and therefore antibody is not found in the usual pooled immunoglobulin which is supplied by blood transfusion services for this sort of purpose. I think there might, therefore, be difficulties, particularly as you would not necessarily know ahead of time which enterovirus is going to be your problem, shall we say, in 1980, in having immunoglobulins available which would be really useful.

Williams Immunological defence mechanisms are valuable in preventing infection, but in neonatal units with normal children, we have the problem of preventing the acquisition of pathogens by the child. Some thought might be given to this aspect. Professor Wood showed the usual way of classifying organisms which are causing infection: Gram positive, Gram negative, viruses etc. There is another way of classifying these organisms, and that is from their origin: one group which has been derived from the mother, the group B streptococci, the rotaviruses (probably), herpesvirus, chlamydia, *E. coli*; the other group is derived from the environment, the *Pseudomonas, Klebsiella–Enterobacter*, the staphylococci, *Staphylococcus aureus*, for example. The two groups present quite different problems of prevention of infection. How much of the group B streptococcal infection is due to the move away from one form of vaginal disinfectant to another? Chlohexidine kills anaerobic organisms rather poorly compared to iodine compounds. To mention one environmental problem, in some units where they stopped using hexachlorophane the incidence of staphylococcal sepsis rose to levels which had occurred a few years previously, in units where they continued using hexachlorophane staphylococcal infection has remained at a low level.

*Hill** I would point out for your information that we are sponsoring two studies now specifically aimed at the development and testing of a group 3 group B polysaccharide, essentially an extension of Carol Baker's work. Carol has, in fact, put this into a few adults in phase 1 studies. We are also doing another study at Temple University in Philadelphia. Also we are looking at the possibility of the dangerous effects of giving polysaccharides, because in the USA we do not usually recommend the use of any vaccines in pregnant females. We are looking at the use of several polysaccharide vaccines in pregnant models in a study at Tulane University.

Smith Could I comment on the use of specific immunoglobulins? It seems because of the point Dr Tyrrell mentioned that a specific infection may only occur rather rarely and the corresponding antibody may not be in normal immunoglobulin pools, one might tackle this by the use of monoclonal antibodies. It would, I suppose, be theoretically possible now to produce human monoclonal antibodies in tissue culture and have them available against a range of pathogens. I would like to ask if this is a practical possibility now and would it work in real life? Are not monoclonal antibodies so specific that they may not be very good, for example, for virus neutralization or for perhaps sensitizing to phagocytosis.

Allison In answer to the first question, some antiviral monoclonal antibodies neutralize very efficiently, so I do not think that would necessarily be a problem. I do not know of any work which has been done with monoclonal antibacterial antibodies in relation to opsonization, if this has been done, I should be interested to know what the answer is.

Smith I can inform you of one virus which is not neutralized; I cannot

* Dr J. C. Hill, National Institute of Allergy and Infectious Diseases, National Institutes of Health, Bethesda, Maryland 20205, USA.

remember its name but I can look it up. I think you cannot necessarily assume it will always work.

Marshall   Could I ask Dr Tyrrell to comment on another approach to the control of neonatal enteroviral infections? That is the use of a monovalent polio vaccine virus to block the infection. In doing this presumably one assumes that the child's polio virus infection or immune function is quite adequate to cope with.

Tyrrell   I would not be too happy about this, as it seems that a virus interference is the mechanism which actually implements the protection you are talking about. One virus gets into an animal or a cell and multiplies, therefore another one cannot. It can be quite efficient in laboratory set-ups, but it depends very much on timing. Interference is transitory and in certain cases the second virus is only kept out of tissues into which the first virus has gained access. If you use a very attenuated virus, as you would have to do, like an attenuated type 2 polio virus, it would probaly stay in the gut and not protect other tissues. I think it is a possible procedure as you say but I would only use it when one was really worried that one had nothing else to offer. I do not regard it as a desirable final way of handling the situation.

Hayward   It seems to me that one of the problems we have is one of numbers. The frequency of group B strepococcus is, even in fairly severely affected nurseries only 2 to 3 per 10^3, and planning to immunize the mother in advance may be difficult because very often the affected children are the ones born prematurely: commonly without prenatal care. Or at least that is true in Denver. So I do not see that it will be easy to identify them, particularly towards the end of pregnancy when your immunization is likely to be most effective.

Obviously what we need is a system for very rapid diagnosis and, as you point out, looking for C reactive protein has its limitations. Another possibility which I believe the National Institute of Health is funding research on is looking for group B antigens in the urine affected children, but above all one has the problem that the actual frequency of children who are likely to benefit is extremely low. Do you really want to treat a thousand children for the possibility of dramatically changing the outlook in two or three? So intervention, if it is to take place, should be prompt and directed to those who are likely to be affected.

Wood   May I comment on that? It is very much the crux of the problem. A quick latex slide agglutination method detecting bacterial antigen in plasma which produces a sensitive and immediate result, has been published but is limited to type 3, at the moment. That may be of some interest because it is probably quicker than any other diagnostic method. The fact that symptomatic group B infection is not terribly common makes a large scale approach to the national population difficult, plus the additional fact that perhaps 15% of young women looking after babies in the nursery will probably also carry the organism vaginally. One cannot be certain that there is not cross infection taking place through this route.

Going back to Dr Tyrrell's question, we have used local tetracycline applied to the eye safely, and have sometimes used chloramphenicol and erythromycin for more generalized infections, but the generalized infections with chlamydia have not, so far as I am aware, been anything like as catastrophic as the other bacterial infections.

Turano I would like to come back to what Prof. Williams said, because I have the impression that according to how we treat the vagina and the baby we have different incidence of isolation of group B streptococcus. This is the case in Brescia where hexachlorophene has been banned. In 500 pregnant women the percentage of group B streptococci was only 7%. My coworker, M. Colombata and I followed up the 500 newborns from the mother and also this group was 7% positive, and we had not problems of septicaemia, which we could not have missed. We noticed an increase in the number of *E. coli* and also in the other groups of streptococci. There was quite a large increase in group D, faecium, faecalis, sometimes bovis, and as I said very low group B. Concerning the feeding, this is mostly breast feeding.

Dewdney I was going to come back to the polymorph question, if I might, and ask one question and make one comment. The question is whether you feel there is any role for granulocyte infusion in these very young children. The comment was that I think we are very used to looking at the effect of antibiotic on the bacterium we want to kill, but I wonder whether we pay enough attention to the possibility that the antibiotic might affect the function of the polymorph. I am referring to studies both in the clinic and in animals, and the gist of these seems to be that some antibiotics—and the Japanese, for example, have published on α carboxy penicillins—may indeed stimulate polymorph function, whereas other antibiotics, for example the tetracyclines, have inhibitory effects, for instance on chemotaxis, and on the bactericidal effect of serum. I am wondering if we pay enough attention to the choice of antibiotic with respect to polymorph function, particularly where this is likely to be immature or deficient in some way.

Wood I think you are reminding us of the work published by Miller in 1971, which was referred to yesterday, where it seemed that the normal newborn had abnormal chemotactic functions in polymorphs in relationship to staphylococcal and coliform toxins and antibody–antigen complexes. I must admit I think this has been a neglected field, and one has assumed that because the oxidative metabolism of the polymorph in the newborn is apparently normal, other aspects of its function were also all right. In addition to an antibody problem in group B streptococci but there may be a chemotactic problem as well. Certainly I think it is possible problems occur with other bacteria, particularly pyocyanea.

With regard to antibiotics, I do not think I am qualified to talk about the effect that they may have on polymorph function. I had thought that the ampicillin and penicillin group were probably harmless in this respect.

Adinolfi I would like to go back to the question of the neutralizing effect of virus antibodies and the interesting suggestion of using monoclonal antibodies. Suffin *et al.* (1979) have recently published a paper in which they suggest a model in ferrets which is useful for the study of protection of human infants against the respiratory syncytialvirus. They have shown that the infant ferret is protected from the virus challenge if the mother is immunized; but the passive transfer of the maternal serum containing the neutralizing antibodies does not occur. What is effected is a nonantibody product which is present in the milk, in fact it is through lactation that the infant ferret is protected. So it seems that the neutralizing antibody is not effective against respiratory syncytialvirus that there is something else in the milk, a sort of lipoprotein, which has this neutralizing and protective effect.

Soothill I would like to suggest that we are running into a serious risk of interfering with the highly complicated process of establishing a flora. The medical profession has already blundered badly in permitting artificial feeding of babies and introducing supplementary feeds. If we are talking about the treatment of an ill child, that is fine. But some of this discussion is apparently to talk about the management of children in general, and we just do not know enough physiology to interfere much. We already interfere by having babies born in hospital. Prof. Wood told us that there was a relationship between these infections and abnormalities of the babies and suggested this may be a feeding effect. They also stay in hospital a long time. Has anyone done a breakdown on the prevalence of infections in normal babies according to length of stay.

How often do these organisms come from the mother, and how often do they come from other patients or staff of the hospital? The host factors are also important, not only because of prematurity or gross abnormality. Polymorphs may well be important. The only immunodeficient children, who die of infection in the first days of life are those with reticular dysgenesis; infants with severe combined immunodeficiency are well for three months. Infants with a syndrome Hayward, Wood and I recently described in whom there was failure of umbilical cord separation and defective neutrophil mobility, they have catastrophic infections in the early days of life strongly pointing to the importance of the neutrophils at this time.

We must also consider whether modification of the intestinal flora may lead to late immunopathological effects. Our demonstration that exclusive artificial feeding does protect the child with minor immunodeficiency from later atopic disease that interference at this stage might have later immunopathological effects, to suggest that all the complicated manipulations you are discussing should be applied first to the clearly abnormal and their application to healthy infants should be very cautious with appropriate small-scale controlled trials.

Wood May I comment on that? I think Prof. Soothill is absolutely right to draw a distinction between the abnormal newborn, the child who has to be in a special care unit, and the newborn in whom one hopes that medical interference is minimal and who is not separated from his mother but is, if possible, separated from other patients. The hospital stay should also be as short as possible. In the special care unit the newborn is colonized by staphylococci at a rate of something like 20% and then 40% as each 24 hours goes by; this can be modified by altering the environment in that the dry open incubator is much less likely to encourage colonization. The closed damp incubator has these very high infection rates. The trouble about the open incubator is that the child tends to dry up as well, and that requires a much larger fluid intake.

Having said this I do not think there is any escape from the fact that some infants are going to require special care and that their bacteriological hazards have to be taken on with their other problems relating to hypoxia and respiratory distress. Among normal healthy term infants, serious bacterial infections are now rare, but risks of infection are greater in low birth weight babies who have been subject to operative deliveries or complications of pregnancy and delivery. They may have experienced a lot of interference in delivery and procedures subsequently where a greater risk of infection occurs.

Reeves I would like to return to the interesting question that has been raised about possible interactions between antibiotics and antibacterial agents and the host reponse in contradistinction to primary effects on the invading micro-organisms. In Nottingham in conjunction with Francis O'Grady, we have performed some preliminary studies on the antibiotic nocardicin, using a radiometric assay for opsonization capacity. We have found that a concentration which is not too far away from what one might expect to obtain *in vivo*, there is consistent enhancement of the opsonization capacity of normal human serum. Serum for some patients in an acute phase of bacterial illness is pneumonia and before they have received an antibacterial agent, has an opsonization capacity well below the normal range. In that situation we have observed an even greater enhancement in the presence of an antibiotic such as nocardicin.

Denman Could you clarify, Prof. Wood, what you mean by the term "granulocyte deficiency" with respect to those patients who are at risk? In other words, can you distinguish two situations. The first would be one where granulocyte deficiency is proportional to the degree of immaturity in these infants who are at risk of developing infections which would be simply related to the possibility that they would encounter bacteria to which they are particularly at risk. The second situation involves infants with a more specific defect involving granulocytes over and above what might be expected from that degree of immaturity. With respect to these points, I have some specific questions. The first is: have the siblings of babies who have succumbed to the kind of infections you have been describing been examined for evidence of granulocyte deficiency? The second related question concerning children who recover from overwhelming sepsis in the first few days of life is what is their subsequent natural history? Finally, if belief that mothers who carry group B streptococci and have a relative deficiency of antibody, to the agent does this reflect specific lacuna deficiency—to use Wood's immunodeficiency in respect to this agent, or is there evidence of more immunodeficiency to those mothers?

Wood Commenting of the first, as you know, there are families in which there are deficiencies of granulocyte number, mobility and killing capacity. It is easier to define those in the neonatal period who have deficiencies of number. They are fairly rare, and they are sometimes associated with deficiencies of chemotactic and spontaneous mobility as well. Such infants seem to be vulnerable to both Gram negative and Gram positive infections, although I have wondered whether the Gram negative infection have an additive effect in depressing polymorph function. I do not think that the abnormal chemotactic function demonstrated by Miller 1971 has been further studied in the otherwise normal newborn. Perhaps Prof. Soothill can comment on this.

Hayward I just wanted to make two general comments, one about the effect of antibodies on neutrophils. We need to bear in mind that we mostly treat these children with either cephaloridine or aminoglycosides and rarely I think with tetracycline. I cannot think of any who are given nocardicin. There is a report of a neutrophil mobility defect caused by aminoglycosides, but curiously the pattern of infection that the newborn has is not that which is associated with defects in neutrophil mobility. We are dealing mostly with catastrophic septicaemias, not with spreading surface infections. One other point to comment on what Dr Denman said about the results of infection, I think one of the intriguing observations from Carol Baker's work was that the children who had early group B infection tended not to make antibodies. Only ten infants who were studied, and all failed to make antibody to the polysaccharide, whereas, there are other studies from Gold *et al.* (1978) suggesting that antibodies can be made to other polysaccharides.

REFERENCES

Baker, C. J. and Kasper, D. L. (1976). Correlation of maternal antibody deficiency with susceptibility to neonatal Group B streptococcal infection. *New England Journal of Medicine* **294,** 753–756.

Gold, R., Lepow, M. L., Goldschneider, T., Draper, T. F. and Gotschlich, E. C. (1978). Antibody responses in human infants to three doses of group A Neisseria meningitidis polysaccharide vaccine administered at 2, 4 and 6 months of age. *Journal of Infectious Diseases* **138,** 731–735.

Shegeoka, A. O., Hall, R. J. and Hill, H. R. (1978). Blood transfusion in group B streptococcal sepsis. *Lancet* **i,** 636–638.

Suffin, S. C., Prince, G. A., Muck, K. B. and Porter, D. D. (1979). Immunoprophylaxis of respiratory syncytial virus infection in the infant ferret. *Journal of Immunology* **123,** 10–14.

The Nature and Role of Mucosal Surface Immunity Against Infection in the Newborn

W. ALLAN WALKER

Pediatric Gastrointestinal and Nutrition Unit,
Massachusetts General Hospital,
Harvard Medical School, Boston, Massachusetts, USA.

INTRODUCTION

An important adaptation of the gastrointestinal tract to the extra-uterine environment is its development of a mucosal barrier against the penetration of harmful bacteria and bacterial toxins (enterotoxin and endotoxin) present with the intestinal lumen. At birth, the newborn infant must be prepared to deal with bacterial colonization of the gut and with formation of toxic byproducts of bacteria and viruses (enterotoxins and endotoxins). These potentially noxious substances if allowed to penetrate the mucosal epithelial barrier under pathologic conditions can cause inflammatory reactions which may result in gastrointestinal and systemic infectious or toxic disease states (Walker and Isselbacher, 1975).

83

To combat the potential danger of invasion across the mucosal barrier, the infant must develop an elaborate system of defense mechanisms within the lumen and on the luminal mucosal surface which act to control and maintain the epithelium as an impermeable barrier to uptake of micro-organisms. These defences included a unique local immunologic system adapted to function in the complicated milieu of the intestine as well as other nonimmunologic processes such as a gastric acid barrier, intestinal surface secretions, peristaltic movement and natural antibacterial substances (lysozyme, bile salts) which also help to provide maximum protection for the intestinal surface (Walker, 1976).

Unfortunately, during the immediate postpartum period, particularly for premature and small-for-dates infants, this elaborate local defense system is incompletely developed. As a result of the delay in the maturation of the mucosal barrier, newborn infants are particularly vulnerable to enhanced bacterial adherence to the mucosal surface and to penetration by these harmful intraluminal organisms. The consequences of altered defense are susceptibility to infection, potential for inflammatory reactions and for formation of pathologic immune complexes. With these reactions come the potential for developing life-threatening diseases such as necrotizing enterocolitis, sepsis and hepatitis. Fortunately "nature" has provided a means for passively protecting the "vulnerable" newborn against the dangers of a deficient intestinal defense system, e.g., human milk. It is now increasingly apparent that human milk contains not only antibodies and viable leukocytes but many other substances which can interfere with bacterial colonization and prevent microbial penetration.

BACTERIAL PENETRATION IN THE SMALL INTESTINE

Several clinical studies suggest that micro-organisms and other intestinal antigens can cross the mucosal barrier under normal physiologic conditions in man (Walker, 1975). Since the pinocytotic process of antigen absorption most likely represents a residual and premature absorptive mechanism in the alimentary canal (Clark, 1959), the capacity to absorb large molecules may be more extensive in the immature small intestine than in mature and more highly developed intestine. In fact, this observation is supported by evidence suggesting that premature and newborn infants can absorb greater quantities of ingested food antigens than older infants or adults (Anderson *et al.*, 1925). Rothberg (1969), for example, has measured bovine serum albumin (BSA) in the serum of premature infants fed quantities of this protein normally present in the daily milk requirement. In contrast, circulating BSA could not be detected in serum samples from older children fed equivalent quantities of protein. He and others (Katz *et al.*, 1968); Korenblat *et al.*, 1968), have also reported a larger percentage of infants with serum samples containing antibodies to food antigens suggesting that food proteins are absorbed intact into the circulation of infants in sufficient quantities to evoke a systemic immune response. In like manner, enteropathogenic micro-organisms may adhere to the newborn intestinal surface in larger numbers than the mucosa of mature animals (Hirschberger *et al.*, 1977). Since bacterial adherence is associated with bacterial penetration, newborn infants are therefore more vulnerable to bacterial infections and mucosal surfaces than older individuals.

The implication of these studies is that the neonatal intestine may absorb larger antigenic quantities of ingested protein and proliferating micro-organisms than the more mature adult intestine. To support this hypothesis, Lev and Orlic (1973) in recent morphological studies with fetal monkeys, and Moxey and Trier (1975) with human fetuses, have shown excessive uptake of large molecules by intestinal epithelial cells. They also described morphologic features of epithelial cells suggesting structural immaturity. This same immaturity of gastrointestinal function and structure may persist beyond fetal life into the newborn period, at a time when the small intestine is exposed to increased quantities of both bacterial and food antigens. In addition to increased antigen uptake, it is also possible that a greater quantity of protein ingested by intestinal epithelial cells escapes intracellular proteolysis as a result of immature lysosomal function, and therefore more protein becomes available for subsequent transport out of the cell and into the circulation.

Although infants may absorb greater quantities of antigens, evidence also exists to suggest a limited but nonetheless measurable absorption of macromolecular antigens from the small intestine of older children and adults. Korenblat *et al.* (1968) showed that an appreciable percentage (15–30%) of normal adults developed milk precipitins after a physiologic load of milk proteins. In earlier studies, Wilson and Walzer (1935) reported uptake and transport of undigested protein (egg albumin) using immunologic methods to measure circulating food proteins; they also demonstrated precipitins to food proteins in serum of adults fed physiologic quantities of the same proteins.

FACTORS CONTRIBUTING TO PATHOLOGIC ABSORPTION OF ANTIGENS (MICRO-ORGANISMS) AND DEVELOPMENT OF HOST DEFENCES

Although macromolecular antigens can traverse the intestinal mucosa of man in small, nutritionally insignificant quantities, the vast majority of humans show no ill effects as a result of this apparently natural phenomenon. However, when increased quantities of antigenic or toxic substances gain access to the body because of an alteration in the intraluminal digestive process, or because of a defect in the mucosal barrier, micro-organism penetration may be increased to

TABLE I.

Factors contributing to pathologic absorption of intestinal antigens.

Selective immunoglobulin A deficiency
Alteration in mucosal barrier
  increased adherence of antigens
  inflammation
  ulceration
Lysosomal dysfunction
Abnormal intraluminal digestion
  achlorhydria
  pancreatic insufficiency

pathologic proportions which may in turn contribute to the pathogenesis of either local intestinal or systemic clinical infection. It would now appear that certain factors may in fact predispose to abnormal or pathologic transport of macromolecules (Table I).

The factors listed above are meant to be representative and not comprehensive. Many of the factors to be discussed are altered during the neonatal period when gastrointestinal defense mechanisms are incomplete and when the developing enterocyte may retain an enhanced capacity to engulf large molecules. The increased intestinal permeability to antigens noted during this period may therefore be potentially dangerous to the neonate.

Immunologic Defenses

The mature gastrointestinal tract is replete with lymphoid tissue capable of mounting an immunologic response to protect against the penetration of antigens across the epithelial barrier. Lymphocytes and plasma cells are present in abundance either as aggregates in Peyer's patches in the ileum and appendix or as a diffuse population of cells in the lamina propria of the small and large intestine. During the past decade, several classical studies have established the local immunologic system as a unique, protective process present at all epithelial surfaces in direct contact with the external environment (bronchial tree, genitourinary tract, and the intestine) (Tomasi *et al.*, 1965). Research studies have demonstrated that the local immunologic response is governed by an antigen stimulus at the epithelial surface. Furthermore, the plasma cell population responsible for antibodies in external secretions is in large part located in close proximity to the epithelial surface. In addition, the antibodies produced by local plasma cells are delivered to the epithelial surface by a unique transport system. These antibodies have properties adapted for optimum function in the complicated milieu of intestinal secretions containing proteolytic enzymes and other digestive substances. These observations suggest the immunologic defenses of the gastrointestinal tract are uniquely suited for protecting the host against the penetration of micro-organisms and antigenic materials at that site (Walker and Isselbacher, 1977).

Secretory Immunoglobulin A (SIgA)

Although all classes of immunoglobulins are represented in intestinal secretions, the predominant secretory immunoglobulin is IgA, which exists in a dimeric form. In the absence of IgA, (e.g. selective IgA deficiency), there is a compensatory increase in the luminal secretion of another polymer immunoglobulin, namely, IgM. These observations suggest that polymeric immunoglobulins are the preferred form of secretory antibody. The delivery process of polymeric antibodies into intestinal secretions involve transport through the intestinal epithelium by a specific intracellular glycoprotein–carrier system (secretory component, SC) localized to secretory columnar cells in the crypt region of the intestinal villus. Strong evidence suggests that dimeric IgA and polymeric IgM are completely assembled within local plasma cells and the joining chain (J chain) participates in the formation of polymeric immunoglobulins. After release from the plasma cells in the crypt region of intestinal villi and diffusion across the basement membrane, these antibodies linked to SC, either during contact with this protein on the basal–lateral surface of the epithelial cells or during passage through the epithelial cell. Following combination with SC, the completed secretory immunoglobulin is released from the epithelial cell by reverse pinocytosis. Linkage of SC to the IgA dimer protects it against breakdown by lysosomal enzymes on the intestinal surface. The co-operation between plasma cells producing the IgA dimer and epithelial cells producing SC represents an unusual cellular interaction to provide most mammals with antibody molecules that can co-exist with the proteolytic enzymes of intestinal secretions (Lamm, 1976). Figure 1 depicts this process in a conceptual manner.

Although a number of mechanisms of action have been suggested for secretory antibodies, including opsonization and complement fixation, there is now substantial evidence that a major function of intestinal antibodies is the process of immune exclusion at the mucosal surface (Walker and Isselbacher, 1977). Several specific properties of secretory antibodies enhance their effectiveness within the gastrointestinal tract. After transport from the lamina propria onto the intestinal surface, secretory antibodies are retained within the mucous coat on the surface of epithelial cells by interaction with cystine residues contained in mucins present within the glycocalyx (Beinenstock, 1975). This stationary location of antibodies in juxtaposition to the intestinal epithelial cell allows for more effective interaction with intestinal antigens coming in contact with the mucosal barrier. This property of secretory antibodies has lead to the term "antiseptic paint" to describe the

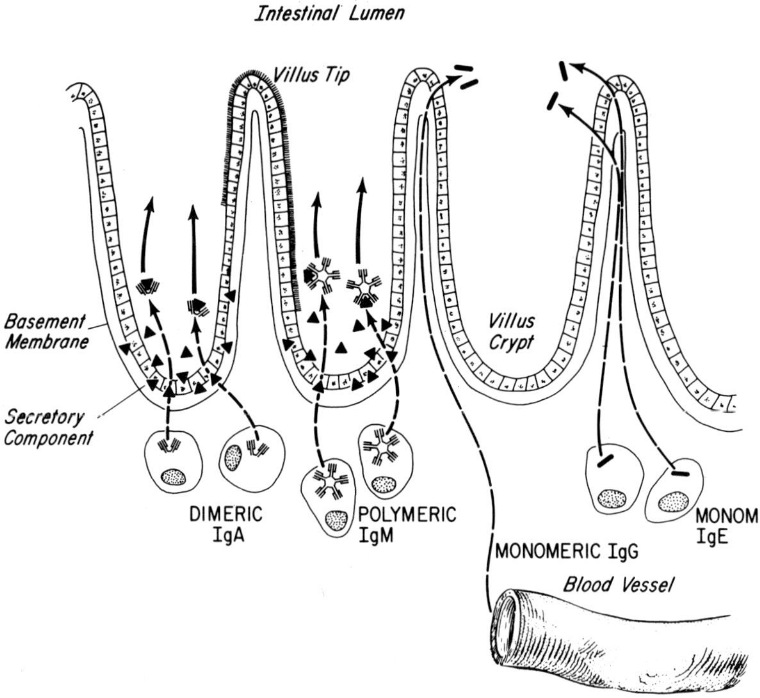

Fig. 1 Transport mechanisms for intestinal antibodies. Polymeric immunoglobulins (IgA and IgM) are assembled and secreted in polymeric form by local plasma cells adjacent to crypt secretory cells. After diffusion across the basement membrane, these molecules interact with a receptor, secretory component, on the surface of or within intestinal cells, and are transported as complete secretory antibodies by a specific carrier process through the cell onto the intestinal surface. Monomeric immunoglobulins are synthesized locally (IgE) or transported to the lamina propria via the circulation (IgG and IgD) and diffuse across the villus epithelial cells by a nonspecific mechanism common to other plasma proteins entering the intestinal lumen. From Walker, W. A. and Isselbacher, K. J. (1979). *New England Journal of Medicine* **297**, 767.

mucous barrier of gastrointestinal tract (Walker and Isselbacher, 1977). Recent investigations have provided direct evidence for the immune exclusion function of intestinal antibodies. Williams and Gibbons (1972) examined the adherence properties or oral pathogens, such as *Streptococcal viridans*, to epithelial cells before and after exposure to these organisms to specific SIgA antibodies. They observed a significant decrease in adhesion of these bacteria after exposure to secretory antibodies. They concluded that SIgA–antibodies block specific binding sites on the bacterial adherence to epithelial surfaces. A decrease in adherence results in decreased colonization as well as enhanced clearance of the bacteria by surface secretions. The presence or absence of intestinal antibodies capable of interfering with specific bacterial adherence may also be important in determining the nature of indigenous bacterial flora of the gut.

Intestinal antibodies can also protect against the effects of toxic bacterial by-products, e.g. enterotoxins. Secretory antitoxins complexing with cholera toxin can prevent toxin binding to receptors on intestinal microvillus membranes and thereby interfere with the activation of adenylate cyclase, a necessary step in the active secretion associated with toxigenic diarrhoea (Wu and Walker, 1976). In like manner, intestinal antibodies interfere with the uptake of nonviable antigens introduced directly into the gastrointestinal tract (Walker *et al.*, 1972).

Cell-Mediated Immunity (CMI)

Although considerably less attention has been focused on the nature of CMI, this aspect of intestinal immunity may also be independent from a comparable systemic CMI response. Research in this area has been largely experimental and, therefore, extrapolation into clinical areas remains highly speculative. Nevertheless, the data suggest that epithelial surfaces develop an independent CMI response, and the nature of the immune response depends on the mode of immunization (oral v. parenteral). Although investigations in this area have largely involved the lung, recent studies reported by Müller-Schoop and Good (1975) suggest that lymphocytes committed to CMI are present in Peyers's patches of the ileum and are capable of responding to antigens present within the intestinal lumen.

Role of Secretory Immunity in Local Defences

Monomeric immunoglobulins (IgG, IgD, IgE) also present in intestinal secretions, appear to function in a secondary capacity as secretory antibodies since their concentrations in secretions reach protective levels only with intestinal inflammation (Walker and Isselbacher, 1977). In contrast to polymeric intestinal antibodies monomeric immunoglobulins are transported into secretions by a nonspecific process shared with other proteins entering the intestinal lumen from the systemic circulation (Fig. 1). IgG and IgD antibodies, synthesized by peripheral lymphoid tissues, as well as local lymphoid cells enter by transudation or by direct diffusion across the epithelial surface. However, IgE antibodies are produced locally by IgE-producing plasma cells present along epithelial surfaces. Regardless of the site of synthesis, all monomeric immunoglobulins are transported across epithelial surfaces at the villus tip. These antibodies do not interact with SC and therefore are not protected from intracellular and intraluminal degradation as are polymeric immunoglobulins. As a result of nonspecific transport and degradation, minimal monomeric immunoglobulins can be detected in secretions. When the gastrointestinal tract becomes inflamed, increased quantities of monomeric immunoglobulins, particularly IgG, are noted in secretions. This increase in secondary secretory antibodies probably results from chemotactic factors released by inflammatory cells which enhance exudation of immunoglobulins from the intravascular space. The process has been referred to as the "secondary line of defense" of intestinal epithelial surfaces (Walker and Isselbacher, 1977).

Nonimmunologic Defenses

A number of nonimmunologic factors, present either within the intestinal lumen or on the intestinal mucous surface, exist and are of importance as an adjunct to more classic host defense mechanisms of the gut (Walker, 1976). These nonspecific defenses help to control the proliferation of micro-organisms present in the gastrointestinal tract, aid in decreasing adherence of organisms to the gut surface, and are important in limiting the available antigen mass that may otherwise overwhelm local immunologic defense mechanisms and penetrate the mucosal barrier or enter the systemic circulation. Taken individually these factors contribute very little to the overall protection of epithelial surfaces. However, when all nonspecific defenses are operational, their combined contribution provides important additional protection.

Intestinal Secretions

Numerous factors exist in saliva and intestinal secretions that are of importance in preventing proliferation of specific organisms within the gut. Gibbons and van Houte (1975) have stressed the role of mucins (glycoproteins in mucus) and salivary polymers in controlling the adherence of streptococcal, staphylococcal and Lactobacillus organisms to the epithelial surface of the intestinal mucosa. If these organisms can be inhibited from adhering to an epithelial surface, their proliferation can also be controlled and they may be cleared from the mouth by the natural washing effect of saliva. When operational, this initial encounter with Gram positive organisms from the external environment provides an excellent means of minimizing the passage of these micro-organisms into the gastric reservoir. Glycoproteins and glycolipids present in the mucous coat lining epithelial surfaces (mucins) have a similar molecular structure as components of the epithelial cellular surface and act as receptors for micro-organisms. Mucins apparently interact with organisms migrating through the mucous coat and provide a competitive inhibition for the attachment of these flora to the epithelial surface. Without a specific receptor on the cellular surface, organisms can be readily removed from the intestinal cavity by mechanical means (peristalsis). These same mucins exist in secretions throughout the gastrointestinal tract and presumably function in a similar fashion to help control both bacterial and viral proliferation. In addition to microbial protection, mucins may also interact with

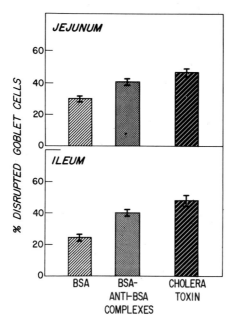

Fig. 2 The average percentage of disrupted goblet cells ($\pm$ S.E.) in 20 villi from each jejunal and ileal section of intestine from three groups of rats exposed to BSA, complexes of BSA with rat antibodies to BSA, or cholera toxin. A significant increase in the number of disrupted goblet cells was noted in rat jejunum and ileum exposed to immune complexes compared to those exposed to BSA alone ($P < 0.001$). The difference in percentage of disrupted goblet cells in intestine exposed to complexes or cholera toxin was not significant ($P < 0.1$). From Walker, W. A., Wu, M. and Bloch, K. J. (1977). *Science* **197**, 370.

allergens, enterotoxins, and other biologically active substances to prevent their penetration across the epithelium (Stombeck and Harrold, 1970). Recent work for this laboratory has shown that an enhancement of goblet cell mucus release occurs in association with immunologic reactions on the intestinal surface (Walker *et al.*, 1977) (Fig. 2).

Gastric Barrier

The concept of the gastric barrier to bacterial, viral, and antigen penetration of the small intestinal cavity is an important consideration in the nonimmunologic defense of the gut. Several studies have shown that achlorhydria may be associated with an increased proliferation of Gram positive micro-organisms within the small intestinal cavity and with an increased incidence of gastrointestinal infections (Goldstein *et al.*, 1962). In addition to intestinal flora, excessive quantities of ingested food antigens may gain access to the small intestine in the absence of a gastric barrier. Kraft *et al.* (1967) have reported an increased incidence of circulating antibovine serum albumin (BSA) antibodies in adults with achlorhydria, suggesting that BSA may not be degraded in the stomach and therefore may be present in greater concentrations for absorption by the small intestine. These studies suggest that the digestive effect of gastric acid and pepsin may provide an important limiting antigenic material into the intestinal tract.

Indigenous Intestinal Flora

In addition to nutrition *per se*, normal bacterial and viral populations in the gastrointestinal tract are valuable deterrents to the overgrowth of pathogens that may be of potential importance in infectious disease states. After birth, the newborn infant's intestine becomes rapidly colonized with a mixture or organisms which comprise the normal or indigenous microbial population of the gut. The nature of intestinal flora is determined by a number of factors including diet (Porter and Rettger, 1940) (nursing v. bottle-feeding) and competitive interactions with other organisms (Gorbach, 1971). Certain naturally occurring factors in the succus entericus may also limit the growth of intestinal micro-organisms.

Peristaltic Movement

Many investigators feel that the mechanical movement of the intestine as part of peristalsis provides the most important factor in controlling proliferation of bacteria within the small intestine (Back and Petran, 1934). The importance of normal peristaltic activity within the intestine is apparent when one considers the consequences of clinical states in which peristalsis has been disrupted. The serious disruption of gastrointestinal function and extensive proliferation of bacteria within the small intestine as a result of stagnation of intestinal contents are consistent components of the "blind loop syndrome" (Reilly and Kirsner, 1959). The differences in bacterial growth within the small and large intestine may be directly related to the mechanical movement of these two segments of intestine. In the small intestine, peristalsis is vigorous and frequent and bacterial growth is limited. In contrast, the large intestine is less mobile and peristaltic movement is episodic resulting in prolonged periods of stagnation of luminal contents. The outcome is extensive proliferation of bacterial flora. These observations underscore the importance of mechanical cleansing as a defense mechanism of the gut.

Hepatic Filtration

Approximately 30% of the total liver mass is composed of reticuloendothelial cells (Popper and Schnaffer, 1972). This organ, which receives the major component of serum filtrate from the gastrointestinal tract, has an enormous capacity to phagocytize noxious substances which may gain access to the portal circulation. Therefore, it is reasonable to consider the liver as a "second line of defense" against invasion of the biologically active substances from the external environment of the gut. Evidence exists that biologically active macromolecules (Alpert and Isselbacher, 1967) and endotoxins can traverse the small intestine and enter the portal circulation. Yet under usual physiologic circumstances no ill effects (disease states) are apparent. This observation suggests that the liver or, more specifically, Kupffer cells in the liver may act as a filter to deter substances absorbed from the gut from entering the systemic circulation. When the reticulo-endothelial system of the liver is blocked in experimental animals or malfunctioning in certain destructive liver disease states, this filter system is defective and endotoxins/antigens may cause symptoms of clinical disease (fever, autoimmunity) (Triger and Wright, 1973).

Miscellaneous Factors

Numerous substances with potential inhibitory properties against bacteria have been reported within the succus entericus and on mucus coating epithelial surfaces. These substances may also contribute to the control of bacterial growth within the intestinal cavity. Lysozyme has been isolated from the gastrointestinal tract and suggested to contribute to lysis of micro-organisms within the gut when combined with complement and specific secretory immunoglobulin A (SIgA) antibodies (Adinolfi et al., 1966). This observation suggests that the paucity of bacterial growth within the small intestine may in part be due to high concentrations of bile at that site. In addition to these substances, "natural antibodies" have been isolated from intestinal contents which have generalized inhibitory properties against a number of intestinal pathogens but not against indigenous flora.

Development of Intestinal Host Defences

From the brief review of intestinal protective mechanisms in the foregoing paragraphs, it is apparent that numerous immunologic and nonimmunologic processes must function together in order to provide mucosal surface protection against infection. At birth, these processes are not completely developed and therefore do not work effectively to protect the neonate. A lack of intra-uterine stimulation results in an underdeveloped local secretory antibody system at birth. Shortly after birth, however, the ingestion of food antigens and the colonization of the gut with indigenous flora provide sufficient antigenic stimulation to evoke a rapid SIgA response. Selner et al. (1975) have documented development of local immunity in newborns. They have shown that very little response occurs for two weeks *post partum*, but by 28 days almost 100% of infants studied have demonstratable salivary SIgA levels. In contrast to the rapid response of SIgA to antigenic stimulation, serum IgA does not reach adult levels until after several years of life suggesting that secretory antibodies are more important in neonatal host defense than is serum IgA. It is of importance to note that the local immune response in premature infants to oral antigen stimulation may not be as effective as that of full term infants (Reiger and Rothberg, 1975). The appearance of antibodies in intestinal secretions most likely lags behind that of full term infants making this group more vulnerable to adverse environmental factors. Although no studies have been reported that investigate local cellular mediated immunity in premature and newborn infants, Silverstein (1972) suggests that an intact and functioning cellular immune system may be operating *in utero* to prevent a possible graft-v.-host response of maternal leukocytes after gaining access to the fetal circulation. It is therefore, probable that local CMI develops in response to local antigenic stimuli during the newborn period.

Very little is known about the developmental aspects of other host defenses in the human gastrointestinal tract. However, experimental animal (Walker and Isselbacher, 1975, 1977) and human fetal studies have suggested that the small intestinal tract in utero and during initial extra-uterine premature existence remains underdeveloped. The intestinal epithelial cell lacks a well-defined brush border and retains a primitive transport mechanism for endocytosis of large molecular substances (Walker and Isselbacher, 1975, 1977). Under these conditions antigens present in the intestinal lumen and on the intestinal surface are engulfed more readily and transported to the intestinal interstitial space (lamina

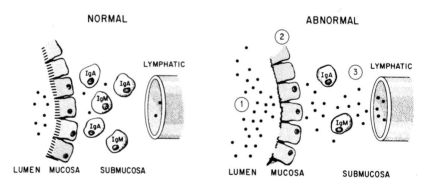

Fig. 3   Physiologic and pathologic transport of antigens across the intestinal mucosal barrier into the systemic circulation. Left, under normal conditions, factors within the intestinal lumen, on the surface of the epithelial cells and within the lamina propria combine to limit the access of antigens to the systemic circulation. Right, however, when these natural defenses are disrupted, excessive quantities of antigenic material may enter the circulation and contribute to clinical diseases. Factor contributing to pathologic absorption of antigens include (1) decreased intraluminal digestion, (2) disrupted mucosal barrier, or (3) decrease in IgA-producing plasma cells in the lamina proparia. From Walker, W. A. (1975). *Pediatric Clinics of North America* **22**, 731.

propria) or into the systemic circulation. Rothberg (1969) has actually measured circulating foreign antigens in serum samples from premature infants. After a short period of extra-uterine life (2 weeks), the capacity to engulf antigens and micro-organisms is less, presumably because of maturation of epithelial cellular function. It is likely that the absence of an established intestinal flora, the decrease in an effective gastric barrier, and lack of mucins or other antibacterial substances in the mucus coat of the small intestine contribute to the transient period of increased antigen penetration. Whatever the reason, the premature remains vulnerable for a transient period of extra-uterine existence. During this period, the infant may develop a life-threatening disease or become sensitized to disease states which may manifest themselves acutely or in later life. Furthermore, it has recently been reported (Widdowson *et al.*, 1976) that pathologic *E. coli* organisms can attract more readily to the immature small intestine than the intestine of the mature animal. This suggests an objective basis for increased infection potential during the period. The concept of *physiologic* and *pathologic* uptake of intestinal macromolecules in association with immunologic and nonimmunologic host defenses is shown in Fig. 3.

PASSIVE PROTECTIVE FUNCTION OF HUMAN MILK IN THE DEVELOPING INTESTINE

As stated in the foregoing discussion, newborn infants lack many specific and nonspecific intestinal features that are necessary to adequately protect them in the extra-uterine environment. Because of a functionally immature gastrointestinal tract, the perinatal period represents a time when increased susceptibility to development of clinical disease states may occur. Fortunately, "nature" has provided an excellent substitute to passively protect the vulnerable neonate during this critical period. This substitute, human milk, contains many factors which can compensate for processes lacking in the infant and at the same time stimulate the maturation of the gut towards independent function.

It is increasingly apparent that human milk contains not only important nutrients and protective factors for the newborn but also factors which can facilitate intestinal maturation. In recent studies, several investigators (Widdowson *et al.*, 1976; Heird and Hansen, 1977) have reported that the ingestion of colostrum can facilitate the maturation of mucosal epithelial cells, enhance absorption of digested foods and perhaps accelerate the development of an intact mucosal barrier. Widdowson *et al.* (1976) and others (Heird and Hansen, 1977) have shown that the gastrointestinal epithelium proliferates and matures more rapidly in experimental animals given maternal milk than those given isocaloric substitute formulas. Others (Heird and Hensen, 1977) have shown that brush border enzymes (lactase, sucrase, alkaline phosphatase) are enhanced after the ingestion of colostrum. These investigators have suggested that milk may contain a "mucosal growth factor" which facilitates the early maturation of the gut.

The implication of these observations with respect to intestinal host defences are obvious. As mentioned earlier, the premature infant because of an immature intestinal epithelial surface is more vulnerable to the adherence of bacteria and absorption of intestinal antigens. If the maturation of epithelial cells is accelerated, the period of vulnerability becomes shortened and the susceptibility to disease lessened.

Milk Antibodies

Nonhuman Mammalian Species

Intestinal uptake and transport of proteins has been most extensively studied in animals that acquire passive immunity either in part or entirely from the passage of maternal antibodies across the small intestinal tract (Walker and Isselbacher, 1975). Animals, such as ruminants, which receive all their maternal immunoglobulins in the *post partum* period have a short period of increased permeability to all macromolecules coming in contact with the intestinal mucosa. Maternal colostrum ingested during this period of increased permeability contains increased concentration of IgG antibodies, the predominant immunoglobulins present in serum. During this same period, γ-globulin levels in neonatal serum increase from virtually undetectable amounts to adult levels and marked proteinuria can be demonstrated to support this observation of enhanced macromolecular transport. After the period of enhanced uptake, which lasts only a few days, the intestinal tract quickly "closes' to prevent the further bulk passage of proteins. "Closure" is related to a morphological and functional maturation of small intestine epithelial cells. In contrast to the bulk transport of macromolecules in ruminants, animals such as rodents, which derive passive immunity in part from the intra-uterine transport of maternal antibodies and in part from the *post partum* intestinal uptake of immunoglobulins, have a prolonged period of selective transport of γ-globulins. The concept of selectivity in transport is supported by the observation that uptake and transport of γ-globulin proteins is much greater than the absorption of other proteins, such as albumin. The period of enhanced transport in rodents ceases abruptly at 20 days. Morphological studies during the period of enhanced absorption and afterwards demonstrate that the ultrastructural appearance of intestinal epithelial cells changes from a more primitive-appearing cell of the newborn (containing multiple membrane invaginations and vesicles in the apical cytoplasm) to the characteristic appearance of an adult intestinal epithelial cell (with its typical microtubular cytoplasmic network).

Human milk antibodies

In man, passive immunity is derived almost entirely from the intra-uterine transport of maternal antibodies (Walker and Isselbacher, 1975). Accordingly, there is very little absorption of γ-globulins across the intestinal tract. This is partly due to the nature of immunoglobulins in the ingested colostrum. Unlike the colostrum of ruminants and rodents, which contains IgG antibodies, the colostrum of man primarily contains secretory IgA antibodies (Lamm, 1976). This class of immunoglobulins cannot be readily transported across intestinal barriers because of the presence of secretory component on the γ-globulins molecule (Lamm, 1976). Although specific antibodies can be detected in the serum of newborn infants fed human colostrum compared to those on formula feedings, the antibody levels detected suggest a nonselective intestinal permeability to macromolecules rather than a selective transport of γ-globulins as demonstrated in the newborn rodent.

Additional protective factors

In addition to the immunologic factors demonstrated in human milk, several substances have been demonstrated to provide additional protection against systemic and gastrointestinal infection in newborn infants (Goldman and Smith, 1973). Lactoferrin, an iron-binding protein present in large concentrations, has been shown to possess inhibiting effects on the growth of *E. coli* and *Staphylococcus* by robbing these organisms of iron needed for their metabolism. However, the bacteriostatic effect is abolished by iron saturation. Lysozyme is found in significant amounts in the stools of breast fed infants and is known to possess powerful bacteriolytic properties. Its concentration in human breast milk is 300 × that of cow's milk. Growth factors contributing to *Lactobacillus bifidus* proliferation include nonspecific conditions such as the low buffering capacity of human milk and high lactose content which promoted an acid milieu within the colon and thereby prevents overgrowth of *Shigella*, *E. coli* and *Candida* organisms. In addition to these nonspecific factors, glycoproteins in milk are thought to promote the proliferation of these organisms. Other factors include an antistaphylococcal factor which helps control the low grade contamination present in all samples of human milk and prevent pathologic contamination of the small intestine. Complement components have also been demonstrated in human milk.

Many as yet undiscovered factors are undoubtedly present in human milk, particularly in colostrum, which maintain additional control over bacterial and viral proliferation in the gut. For example, mucin-like glycoproteins which interfere with bacterial attachment to the immature intestinal surface may be an effective control for the microbial environment. It is not inconceivable that adjuvants which promote local intestinal immunity may be discovered by future investigators. It would appear that "nature" has provided for the newborn a passive means of protecting itself from the environment. Virtually every deficiency or delay in maturation of host defenses is countered by a factor discovered in human milk which compensated for the deficiency.

REFERENCES

Adinolfi, M., Glynn, A. A., Lindsay, M. and Milne, C. M. (1966). Serological properties of IgA antibodies to *Escherichia coli* present in human colostrum. *Immunology* **10,** 517–524.

Alpert, D. H. and Isselbacher, K. J. (1967). Protein synthesis by the rat intestinal mucosa: The role of ribonuclease. *Journal of Biological Chemistry* **242,** 5617–5620.

Anderson, A. F., Schloss, O. M. and Meyers, C. (1925). The intestinal absorption of antigenic protein by normal infants. *Proceedings of the Society of Experimental Biology and Medicine* **23,** 180–187.

Back, G. M. and Petran, E. (1934). Bacterial activity in different levels of intestine and in isolated segments of small and large bowel in monkeys and in dogs. *Journal of Infectious Diseases* **54,** 204–215.

Bienenstock, J. (1975). The local immune response. *American Journal of Veteninary Research* **36,** 488–501.

Clark, S. L. (1959). The ingestion of proteins and colloidal materials by columnar epithelial cells of the small intestine in suckling rats and mice. *Journal of Biophysics and Biochemical Cytology* **5,** 41–61.

Gibbons, R. J. and van Houte, J. (1975). Bacterial adherence in oral microbial ecology. *American Review of Microbiology* **27,** 19–24.

Goldman, A. S. and Smith, C. W. (1973). Host resistance factors in human milk. *Journal of Pediatrics* **82,** 1082–1090.

Goldstein, F., Wirtis, C. W. and Josephs, L. (1962). Bacterial flora in small intestine. *Gastroenterology* **42,** 755–769.

Gorbach, S. L. (1971). Intestinal microflora. *Gastroenterology* **66,** 1110–1112.

Heird, W. C. and Hensen, I. H. (1977). Effect of colostrum on growth of intestinal mucosa. *Pediatric Research* **11,** 406–407.

Hirschberger, M., Mirelman, D. and Thaler, M. M. (1977). Mechanisms of attachment by a pathogenic strain of *E. coli* (0111/B4) to intestinal mucosa in pre and post weanling rats. *Pediatric Research* **11,** 500–507.

Katz, J., Spiro, H. M. and Herskovic, T. (1968). Milk precipitating substance in the stool in gastrointestinal milk sensitivity. *New England Journal of Medicine* **278,** 1191–1197.

Korenblat, R. E., Rothberg, R. M., Minden, P., *et al.* (1968). Immune response of human adults after oral and parenteral exposure to bovine serum albumin. *Journal of Allergy* **41,** 226–232.

Kraft, S. C., Rothberg, R. M., Kramer, C. M., *et al.* (1967). Gastric output and circulating antibovine serum albumin in adults. *Clinics in Experimental Immunology* **2,** 231–240.

Lamm, M. E. (1976). Cellular aspects of immunoglobulin A. *Advances in Immunology* **22,** 223–229.

Lev, R. and Orlic, D. (1973). Uptake of protein swallowed amniotic fluid by monkey fetal intestine in utero. *Gastroenterology* **65,** 60–65.

Moxey, P. C. and Trier, J. S. (1975). Structural features of the mucosa of human fetal small intestine. *Gastroenterology* **68,** 1002–1007.

Müller-Schoop, J. W. and Good, R. A. (1975). Functional studies of Peyer's patches: Evidence for their participation in intestinal immune responses. *Journal of Immunology* **114,** 1757–1763.

Popper, H. and Schaffner, F. (1972). "Progress in Liver Diseases", 201–220. Grune and Stratton, New York.

Porter, J. R. and Rettger, L. F. (1940). Influence of diet on distribution of bacteria in stomach, small intestine and cecum of white rat. *Journal of Infectious Diseases* **66,** 104–111.

Reilly, R. W. and Kirsner, J. B. (1959). Blind loop syndrome. *Gastroenterology* **37,** 491–501.

Reiger, C. H. L. and Rothberg, R. M. (1975). Development of the capacity to produce specific antibody to an ingested food antigen in the premature infant. *Journal of Pediatrics* **87**, 515–518.

Rothberg, R. M. (1969). Immunoglobulin and specific antibody synthesis during the first weeks of life of premature infants. *Journal of Pediatrics* **75**, 391–397.

Selner, J. C., Merrill, D. A. and Claman, H. N. (1975). Salivary immunoglobulin and albumin: Development during the neonatal period. *Journal of Pediatrics* **87**, 515–519.

Silverstein, A. M. (1972). Immunological maturation in the fetus: Modulation of the pathogenesis of congenital infection and disease. *In* "Ontogeny of Acquired Immunity", 17–20. CIBA Foundation Symposium. Elsevier, Amsterdam.

Stombeck, D. R. and Harrold, D. (1970). Binding of cholera toxin to mucins and inhibition by gastric mucin. *Infection and Immunology* **10**, 1266–1272.

Tomasi, T. B., Tau, E. M., Solomon, A., *et al.* (1965). Characteristics of an immune system common to certain external secretions. *Journal of Experimental Medicine* **121**, 101–111.

Triger, D. R. and Wright, R. (1973). Studies on hepatic uptake of antigen II. The effect of hepatotoxins in the immune response. *Immunology* **25**, 951–960.

Walker, W. A. (1975). Antigen absorption from the small intestine and gastrointestinal disease. *Pediatric Clinics of North America* **22**, 731–740.

Walker, W. A. (1976). Host defense mechanisms in the gastrointestinal tract. *Pediatrics* **57**, 901–916.

Walker, W. A. and Isselbacher, K. J. (1975). Uptake and transport of macromolecules by the intestine: Possible role in clinical disorders. *Gastroenterology* **67**, 531–550.

Walker, W. A. and Isselbacher, K. J. (1977). Intestinal antibodies. *New England Journal of Medicine* **297**, 767–773.

Walker, W. A., Isselbacher, K. J. and Bloch, K. J. (1972). Intestinal uptake of macromolecules: Effect of oral immunization. *Science* **177**, 608–610.

Walker, W. A., Wu, M. and Bloch, K. J. (1977). Stimulation by immune complexes of mucus release from goblet cells of the rat small intestine. *Science* **197**, 370–375.

Widdowson, E. M., Colombo, V. E. and Artavams, C. A. (1976). Changes in the organs of pigs in response to feeding for the first 24h after birth. II. The digestive tract. *Biology of the Neonate* **28**, 272–279.

Williams, R. C., Showalter, R. and Kern, F., Jr. (1975). *In vivo* effect of bile salts and cholesiramine on intestinal anaerobic bacteria. *Gastroenterology* **69**, 483–491.

Williams, R. C. and Gibbons, R. J. (1972). Inhibition of bacterial adherence by secretory immunoglobulin A: A mechanism of antigen disposal. *Science* **177**, 697–698.

Wilson, S. J. and Walzer, M. (1935). Absorption of undigested proteins in human beings. *American Journal of Diseases of Children* **50**, 49–57.

Wu, A. L. and Walker, W. A. (1976). Immunological control mechanism against cholera toxin: Interference with toxin binding to intestinal receptors. *Infection and Immunity* **14**, 1034–1042.

DISCUSSION

Bullen There is just one point I wanted to make. You left out the question of lactoferrin. Wherever you get secretory IgA you get lactoferrin. What I suggest is that the mucus contains large amounts of secretary IgA and lactoferrin, and this is probably the major protective mechanism in the gut. It is very interesting that you get a slow maturation of IgA synthesis in the child. Presumably breast milk compensates for this job because it contains both the IgA and the lactoferrin. You can imagine two systems interlocking quite well.

Walker I agree with your statement. My presentation has dealt with areas that I am most familiar with, rather than to be comprehensive. I assumed you would be commenting on this in your subsequent presentation. I agree with you that this is very important protective mechanism and should be discussed.

Another observation should be mentioned with respect to mucosal barrier protection is some evidence exists to suggest that under conditions of immature mucosal surface area there are increased numbers of receptors for bacteria and presumably for toxins. This may also be a contributory factor in newborns who preferentially develop bacterial infections, toxogenic diarrhoeas etc.

Soothill I think this is marvellous work. I think that we should consider the effect the feeding has on the flora, it may be relevant for immunopathology as well as gross infection, because, after all, for instance, *E. coli* endotoxin is a very powerful adjuvant. There is evidence to suggest this is so in the field of atopy, and that not all the infants are going to be the same from this standpoint. The common immunodeficiencies associated with the state of atopy may work in part by the mechanism you have been hearing about. There are numerous studies showing that these findings vary but Edwins, Swarbrick and Stokes in our Department have shown in detail how the three reactions to an ingested antigen—namely antibody response, immune exclusion and partial tolerance—are apparently genetically controlled, independently. So there is a very complex balanced response to the ingested antigenic material which will differ from individual to individual. We must therefore not assume that a method of control safe for the majority is safe for everyone. Environmental factors influence these things too, since nutrition effects the acquisition of tolerance to ingested antigens.

Hayward Do you know how the IgA reaches the gut? Is the enterohepatic circulation as important as in adults? Could you approach this by seeing whether breast feeding protects children who have bile duct disorders? Would you expect similar effects on antigen handling by newborns who had, say, either bile duct defects of ligated bile ducts?

Walker That is an excellent point. As you know, increasing evidence exists to suggest that IgA is not simply released across epithelial surfaces in contact with antigens as had been previous hypothesized but that IgA is also released by crossing the bile epithelium into bile secretion. I do not think anyone has looked at the biliary-atresia patient and increased infectivity. These patients have considerable postoperative problems with infection, but that is probably related to surgery rather than to bile duct ligation. Perhaps Dr John Walker-Smith has some information?

Walker-Smith I have no information on that point, but I would like to ask you about the extrusion zones. Philips *et al.*, 1979 have shown that extrusion zones may occur to some extent along the side of the villus as well as at the tip. Do you think that the extrusion zones, by providing a break in the integrity of the mucosal surface, might afford a significant site for entry of bacteria or viruses, or a food antigen.

Walker This process exists and may be significant as we showed in previous animal studies. In these studies we reported existence of trace protein enzymes in cell and between cells at the extrusion zones: presumably this process contributes to enhanced penetration of antigen. Whether or not this is an effective mechanism for bacterial penetration, remain to be demonstrated.

Adinolfi Do you agree that about 8% of the lymphocytes present, colostrum and milk are committed to the synthesis of anti *E. coli* antibodies. There seems to be a very strong selection in favour of this type of antibody producing cells.

Walker I am aware of that observation but cannot explain its significance unless antibodies are important to protection against *E. coli* in the newborn intestine and enter into colonization of the gut.

Allison There are interesting studies done on *Giardia lambia* in dogs. It happens that the dog is a host for the human organism and it is found that when the mother dogs are lactating the number of organisms in the intestine is enormously increased. One hypothesis is that you divert the IgA producing cells from the intestine to the milk, thereby decreasing protection. This would be an interesting possibility to look at as an example.

Denman Could I ask you some points relating to the manoeuvres which in experimental animals will interfere with the absorption of antigen. I ask this particularly with respect to the therapy based on the theory that increased antigen absorption in infancy predispostes to the subsequent development of allergic immune atopic reaction in the gut. Do you have data concerning the generation of immunity and immunological memory at sites distant from the gut and the classes of antibody which are generated as the result of manoeuvres which increase antigenic absorption?

Walker No, we do not. We are in the process of extending these initial observation of increased penetration of antigen across the infected gut. We have not determined specific antibody response to such antigen uptake.

Reeves Would you be prepared to comment on the finding by Ogra's group several years back, that some children who had died with a so-called sudden infant death syndrome and did possess secretory component, on immunofluorescent examination of the gut, seemed not to contain secretory component? Have you come across any other reason to suppose that some folk may be deficient in attaching secretory component to IgA?

Walker I am certainly aware of those studies. I have not seen anything subsequently published on this subject, however. I suspect that this was probably just a fortuitous observation. Secretory component is so ubiquitous in secretion that its deficiency seems unlikely. A case was reported in the *New England Journal of Medicine* by Dr Warren Strober *et al.* from National Institutes of Health, suggesting secretory component deficiency, but I do not think that the report was proven sufficiently to be sure of the observation. It is my contention, although it has not been demonstrated experimentally that one of the reasons why malnourished individuals have a decrease in secretory IgA, but increased serum IgA, is that the transport process for the dimeric IgA has been affected, altered by decreased levels of secretory component. However the contribution of SC deficiency to infant death syndrome may be a factor.

Walker-Smith   Would you like to comment on your experimental work on the role of gastroenteritis, particularly in the neonatal period, as a precursor for food allergies and so on?

Walker   We have shown that there is a direct correlation with disruption of the intestinal surface and enhanced penetration of antigenic material from the intestinal lumen across the mucosal surface into the circulation. Dr Walker-Smith has reported a clinical association between gastroenteritis and an increased tendency for atopic disease to occur when infants are exposed to milk proteins in the postinfected period. The increased uptake of intestinal antigen probably accounts for the clinical state, i.e. there is a transient disruption of the mucosal surface allowing for antigens to get across that might otherwise not penetrate resulting in an allergic response. Our laboratory is also interested in enhanced antigen with intestinal anaphylaxis because we believe that part of the ongoing pathogenesis of disease may be related to other immunologic processes occurring such as IgG-mediated complement fixing reaction and immune complex-mediated inflammation coincidental with the classic IgE reactions in the original intestinal anaphylaxis response.

Reiter   The question of maturation due to colostrum is fascinating to me at least. Would you tell me which animals you used for the study and also what relation it would have to the permeability of the gut during the first 24 to 36 hours of ungulates?

Walker   There have been several studies reported over the last few years. The animal model that we used is the rabbit. The reason that we used this model is that rabbit gut is morphologically similar to that of man and that the transmission of passive immunity to newborn is transplacental, as in man. We have noted that two newborns, delivered by Caesarian section, had decreased penetration of antigen if fed by mothers' milk than if fed by artificial means. We have yet to show whether or not this is because of antibody protection or because of enhanced maturation. We are in the process of studying the process described by Dr Elsie Widdowson, using the piglet as a model, and Dr William Hierd at Columbia, using the beagle puppy as a model, that ingestion of colostrum results in enhanced epithelial cell production and enhanced maturation of these cells. Presumably what is happening is that there is a trophic factor present in early colostrum which stimulates maturation.

This hypothesis is supported by a recent article in the PNAS showing that human colostrum can stimulate fibroblast turnover. The authors conclude that a trophic factor in milk facilitates this turnover process. There may also be a nonspecific protective process in milk such as the presence of antibodies which specifically interferes with *E. coli* organisms, *E. coli* toxins or a glycoprotein or some other substance.

Reiter   It is very important, because we always regard the first 24–36 hours as the most vulnerable period for microbial infection, due to the permeability of the gut.

Walker   I think this is true. Whether or not it matures that rapidly I do not know. However, you are talking specifically about the ungulate?

Reiter   Yes. The rabbit is a dangerous animal in another respect. The intestines are practically sterile. Although physiologically it is a good animal for the purposes of comparison, we have to remember that bacteriologically the rabbit is a unique animal.

Tyrrell   I have a simple question. You draw pictures which suggest they IgA is actually bound to the villi. Is this really so?

Walker   Yes, I think so. Several immunogists, including Dr John Bienenstock of McMaster University have suggested that there might be receptors within the glycocalyx compartment for IgA antibody. When I mention the glycocalyx I mean not only the surface of the microvillus but the mucous coat above that surface. I think that one of the reasons that secretory IgA is so effective is that it is maintained at that site rather than necessarily being washed down the intestine and therefore can effectively adhere to antigens as they interact with the intestinal surface.

Tyrrell   Is this another function of secretory component?

Walker   There is no evidence that the receptor attaches to secretory component; however, we know that the secretory component protects IgA against self-digestion by proteases.

Dewdney   You have obviously given us a lot of very important data with respect to the pathogenesis of food allergy. I want to be quite clear what you are saying you believe is. I have understood from what you have said that you think that the systemic consequences of food allergy, that is the nongut effects, are a consequence of antigen reaching the systemic circulation and stimulating IgE antibody in site distant from the gut. Is that your belief or do you feel that many of the systemic symptoms of food allergy might be due to adsorption of mediators, e.g. prostaglandins, histamine, and so on, from the gut into the systemic circulation, causing their own symptoms in the skin and in the lung?

Walker   My prejudice is that excessive antigen is taken up to cause allergy. I do not, unfortunately, have information to discern whether or not this process also affected by a mediator absorbed permeability allows for deposition of antigen at distant sites from the intestine leading to systemic disease suppression. There is some evidence to suggest kidney disease, liver disease, dermatitis etc., are mediated by the penetration of specific antigens such as milk proteins as demonstrated by immune complexes at these sites. I know of no study of intestinal production of mediators and their subsequent absorption into the circulation as a result of antigen exposure.

Chairman   Is this a terribly likely thing, because the amounts of histamine and so forth released locally is pretty small? If they given intravenously to an experimental animal would scarcely turn a hair.

Dewdney   What was in my mind was some work published from Guy's Hospital by, I think, Laurence Youlton, which was suggesting that prostaglandins were absorbed from food antigen antibody interactions in the gut, and going on to suggest that some of the anti-inflammatory drugs which inhibit prostaglandin synthetase might be useful drugs in the control of food allergy.

Chairman   You are talking about prostaglandins now?

Dewdney   Yes, and then extrapolating to other mediators.

Denman   Can we press Dr Walker a little more on this point? Can you distinguish between two situations? The first would be that the person is genetically predisposed to a particular form of hypersensitivity or allergy, and that the premature absorption of antigen following, say, gastroenteritis or premature withdrawal of breast feeding would precipitate allergy. The second one postulates that the premature absorption of antigen, either in qualitative or quantitative terms, precipitates an allergic or hypersensitivity state.

Walker   Your point is very well taken. I agree that vulnerable population is the genetically predisposed pateint. He is the one who most likely suffers from premature exposure to the antigen. I do not have any evidence to suggest that antigen exposure alone might result in an allergic reaction. It is possible, but I do not have any evidence to support this.

Cooper   I should like to go back to the role of IgA antibodies, particularly in the newborn, in protecting against entry of antigens and infectious agents. When the newborn is born, the gut up and down the lamina propria is virtually devoid of IgA-producing cells, but they are, as you point out, in Peyers' patches and in appendix, presumably all the clones of T and B cells that are needed, and when antigens come across from the gut, presumably via these specialized phagacytic or pinocytotic cells that Barkman first discovered, then cells are stimulated there, get into the lymphatics and then go around via the blood and then seed up and down the mucous surfaces throughout. Preferentially these are cells producing IgA 2, which is not susceptible to the proteolytic digestions of the IgA proteases and so forth that bacteria make. So, in essence, it takes a while, probably a week or so, before one can get this kind of response and get protective immunity via IgA antibodies.

Porter and his colleagues in this country especially have pointed out that if one gives to piglets bacteria in the feed you can prevent a lot of infections and that actually they grow better, and so forth. Is it worth reconsidering this kind of preventive measure to prevent certain kinds of infections in humans, and has work been done on that?

Walker I think your point is very important. This observation may be the reason why certain newborns develop infections which others do not and that the degree of bacterial exposure may control infectious disease. All newborns whether they are nursed or bottle fed, will have a certain degree of bacterial colonization, resulting in some antigenic exposure allowing plasma cells to be stimulated and migrate to the lamina propria. To illustrate this point, we know that the germ-free animal remains void of plasma cells, because of a lack of antigenic stimulus. The critical aspects of this process is the degree of exposure. The young infant that is overwhelmed with bacteria is the one that is more vulnerable to systemic sepsis and infection, both focally and systemically.

Smith You may know that there is one study by, I think, Robbins and his group from Bureau of Biologics in which they have attempted to immunize against haemophilus B by feeding children with live *E. coli* in which the capsular antigen is cross-reactive with the haemophilus B surface antigen. The reason we are doing this partly because the young baby responds very poorly to injected group B polysaccharide, and they were apparently able to induce an antibody response in a small number of babies. I think they were probably over the age of 6 months.

Walker-Smith Coming back to consider this time when there is little IgA about in the small intestine, it is interesting that the neonate leaves a germ free environment to enter a germ containing environment, and there is *pari passu* with this change quite a dramatic change small intestinal morphology from finger-like villi in the newborn to broader villi in the older infant.

This has been well demonstrated in animals. where it has been shown that there is, quite quickly, a change from slender finger-like villi to broad ridge-like villi. This quite dramatic morphological change is occurring at the same time when there is not much IgA to the small intestine around. Do you think that these observations may be related or what explanation is there for this change in small intestinal morphology in early infancy.

Walker I think they are related but I do not know why. There are striking changes in the intestinal tract of the germ free animal when it becomes conventionalized. I think this has to do with bacterial colonization, which somehow affects the intestinal epithelial turnover. I should like to raise another issue that has practical relevance, particularly pertinent as we deal with newborn infection. The increasing use of systemic alimentation in contrast to enteric alimentation. Several studies suggest that delivery of nutrients enterically is important for ongoing stimulation of gut maturation and turnover. It seems to me that infants treated solely by parental nutrition might potentially be more vulnerable than an infant that might other wise have been fed aseptically either from breast milk from breast milk bank, or an artifical containing formula. I wonder if there are any comments about that.

Reiter   I have a correction.

Chairman   You give the correction, and then we will have the last point.

Reiter   This feeding of antigen was for a while quite fashionable, but since the Hensen experiment people rely on the immunization of the mother animal intestinally to increase the IgA and specific IgA and they rely on the IgA milk to bridge the gap before the newborn animal can produce his own. I think the antigen feed which was produced by this firm has been withdrawn. I am not sure, but I think so.

Faulk   The human fetus recirculates amniotic fluid by swallowing, so the rather elegant system of lymphoid aggregates and phagocytic cells in the gut continuously bathed by amniotic fluid which is known to contain a number of maternal proteins. The child *in utero* is swallowing a great deal of maternal allotype antigens, yet when one examines gut lymphoid tissues such as Peyers' patches one does not find in the neonate evidence of antigen stimulation: This is only seen when the newborn starts swallowing environmental antigens. I wonder if this is a property of maternal allotypes as antigens or is it due to some peculiar property of the amniotic fluid? Also I would like to ask if one could cast some light on this particular problem by studying the gut of neonates who have sustained and intra-uterine infections?

Walker   Unfortunately there is very little information, in this area of research. Most of the studies deal with absorption from conception until 20 weeks' gestation or after stillborn delivery.

Therefore I do not know the answer to your question. It is generally accepted that bacterial colonization of the intestine causes rapid changes in the number of plasma cells that exist in the lamina propria in the *post partum* state in contrast to the sterile environment *in utero*. I am also aware that the intestine, bathed in amniotic fluid, is exposed to a number of foreign proteins which may be antigens. However, these substances are either low grade antigen or suppressed in their activity by intra-uterine suppressors such as α-feto protein which might interfere with the immunologic responsiveness. Whether or not this exists in man remains to be shown.

Development and Maturation
of Immunity in the Newborn

A. R. HAYWARD

Department of Pediatrics,
University of Colorado Medical Center,
Denver, Colorado, USA

INTRODUCTION

Evidence for the immunological immaturity of the newborn includes a susceptibility to overwhelming infection by a range of bacteria and a few viruses, and the difficulty of obtaining good antibody responses to some polysaccharide vaccines. In many other respects the fetus and newborn is mature as, for example, in accepting BCG and vaccinia immunization. Experience in patients with primary immunodeficiency syndromes suggests that the newborns' restricted range of susceptibility to infection could be due to defects of phagocytes, complement or antibody. Studies on newborn blood have demonstrated relative immaturity of each of these defence mechanisms. These include the relatively poor mobility and membrane deformability of newborn neutrophils (reviewed by Miller, 1979) and the presence of only about 80% of adult haemolytic complement activity. Although synthesis of most complement components starts well before birth, levels of C9 are significantly low in cord serum (reviewed Johnston, 1979). This review will concentrate on our observations relating to the perinatal development of lymphocyte responses in human newborns; the results of fetal studies are reviewed in greater detail by Hayward and Lydyard (1979).

DEVELOPMENT OF SPECIFIC IMMUNITY IN MAN

Most of the newborns' antibody protection is provided by maternal IgG and a lack of maternal antibody of appropriate specificity can contribute to devastating newborn group B streptococcal (Baker and Kasper, 1977) and varicella infections. The fetal response to intra-uterine infection by rubella, toxoplasmosis or syphilis is the strongest evidence for the prenatal acquisition of immunological competence and illustrates the restrictions under which early immune responses appear to operate. Cord serum IgM levels rise as a result of congenital infection and affected infants continue to make IgM antibodies to the infecting agent for several months after birth (Alford, 1965). In contrast, adults infected with the same organisms usually switch to making IgG antibodies in 2–3 weeks. Factors which could contribute to the prolonged IgM response of the newborn include the replicating nature of the antigen, slow immune elimination (especially for cytomegalovirus) and immune complex formation (Stagno et al., 1977) as well as possible intrinsic regulatory mechanisms. The predominance and persistence of IgM antibody in newborns immunized with *Salmonella* vaccine (Smith and Eitzman, 1964) and indirectly the results of *in vitro* studies described below, suggest that antigen replication is not solely responsible.

IN VITRO STUDIES

IgM is the predominant immunoglobulin class of plasma cells in pokeweed mitogen (PWM) stimulated cultures of newborn lymphocytes obtained from cord blood (Hayward and Lawton 1977). In these studies the response by newborn B cells was significantly less than by adult blood lymphocytes. The events which determine the amount of B cell differation into plasma cells (PC) in PWM stimulated cultures are complex, involving monocytes, helper and suppressor T cells and B cell proliferation (reviewed Fauci, 1979). Our recent studies have been directed towards the identification of the separate contributions of the newborns T and B lymphocytes.

T Cell Help

We found that newborn T cells were relatively inefficient helpers of PWM induced differentiation of adult as well as newborn B cells (Hayward and Lawton, 1977).

TABLE I.

Newborn T cells are less effective helpers than adult T cells for PWM induced B cell differentiation.

Mean number of PC $\times 10^{-3}$ generated by 5×10^4 B cells cultured with PWM and				
No T cells	Newborn T	Newborn T irrad.	Adult T	Adult T irrad.
1·5	17	47	68	180
±1·4*	17	29		41
			$P = <0·05$	

* ± Standard error.

The interpretation of these experiments was open to the objection that newborn suppressor cells might override any help which other newborn T cells might provide. We therefore irradiated newborn and adult T cells to abolish their suppressor activity and then compared the ability of these or unirradiated cells to help adult B cells differentiate in response to PWM. The results (Table I) indicated that newborn T cells remained poor helpers even when they no longer suppressed. We do not know why newborn T cells should be relatively poor helpers but it is not due to the lack of a subset of IgMFc receptor bearing (T_M) cells (Hayward and Lydyard, 1978).

T Cell Suppression

Lawler *et al.* (1975) and Olding and Oldstone (1976) showed that newborns T cells tended to suppress the division of their mothers' lymphocytes in mixed

TABLE II.

Effect of pharmacological agents on suppression by newborn T cells.*

Control PC number $\times 10^{-3}$	Newborn suppression	Newborn suppression in presence of		
		10^{-5} Hc	5 mM Li	5 µg ml^{-1} Indo
11·9	−87	+7·5	ND	−71
3·1	−77	+100	−45	ND
13	−94	−67	−83	−93
3·7	−87	−15	−41	−91
Mean	−86	+6	−56	−85
SE	4	34	11	8

* 5×10^4 adult blood lymphocytes were cultured for 6 days with PWM with or without 5×10^4 newborn cells and cortisol (Hc), Lithium chloride (Li), or indomethacin (Indo). The number of plasma cells per well was then determined and the results are expressed as % change from control without newborn cells, as in Hayward and Lydyard (1978).

TABLE III.

Suppression of PWM-induced PC differentiation of adult blood lymphocytes cultured with blood lymphocytes from premature infants.

| | PC number per well × 10^{-3} | | | |
| | | (weeks) | | |
Age	26	27	27	42
Control	13	13	6	3
Baby	0	0	0	1
Control + baby	2·5	0·6	1	0·6
% Change	−81	−95	−83	−81

lymphocyte culture. We found that newborn T cells suppressed PWM induced PC differentiation by unrelated adult lymphocytes (Hayward and Lawton, 1977). The suppressor cells had an Fc receptor for IgM and their activity was blocked by irradiation (Hayward and Lydyard, 1978). Subsequent experiments have indicated that suppression is also inhibited by 10^{-5} M cortisol and to a lesser extent by 5 mM lithium chloride (Table II). Indomethacin did not block suppressor activity. Suppressor activity was present in blood lymphocytes from premature infants of 26 weeks' gestation (Table III) and was also found in a single sample from a term baby of 13 days' age.

To determine the stability of newborn suppressor activity we have prepared T cell lines from cord blood in collaboration with Dr J. Kurnick. The cells were cultured in T cell growth factor from which the conditioning mitogen, PHA, had been removed by an anti-PHA immuno-absorbent. Lines were obtained from each sample of cord blood tested without further stimulation. Seventy five per cent of these lines had spontaneous suppressor activity (Table IV). Adult lymphocytes behave similarly provided that there is some mitogen remaining in the conditioned medium (Kurnick et al., 1976; Maca et al., 1979) and it does not appear that

TABLE IV.

Suppression of PWM-induced B cell differentiation of adult blood lymphocytes by newborn blood T cells after 10 days growth in conditioned medium.*

Sample	% Change
1	−59
2	−91
3	+62
4	−96

* 10^5 adult blood lymphocytes were cultured for 6 days with or without 10^5 T cells from continuous line cultures of newborn T cells. Per cent change is difference from control without T cells.

continuous culture selects in favour of either T_M or T_G cells (Pang and Booth, 1979).

B Cell Immaturity

Our own studies indicated that newborn B cells differentiated less well than adult B cells and that they made almost exclusively IgM, even when they were cultured with adult T cells to provide optimal T cell help. Although we have speculated in the past that the lack of B cell differentiation might reflect a commitment of newborn B cells to proliferation, recent studies have shown this to be false. Table V shows the frequency of dividing and interphase cells of male or female karyotype in mixtures of newborn and adult T and B cells. In each of three experiments fewer than 5% of the dividing cells were newborn B cells and there was a comparable deficiency of newborn B cells in interphase. Adult B cells, in contrast, accounted for about 50% of dividing cells after 6 days' incubation.

DISCUSSION

The success of neonatal vaccination against tuberculosis and smallpox, and the capacity of the newborn to reject foreign skin grafts, attest to the maturity of a range of T cell responses in the newborn. B cell responses, however, seem to be immature both as regards proliferation (Table V). and differentiation in response to PWM. B cell activation by PWM is obviously highly artificial so it is interesting that polyclonal triggering of newborn B cells with Epstein–Barr virus (EBV) also gives a predominantly IgM response (Bird and Britton, 1979). The response by adult cells to EBV is essentially T independent and yields IgG and IgA as well as IgM producing cells. The differences between the responses of adult and newborn

TABLE V.

Comparison of response to PWM of newborn and adult B cells cultured with adult T cells.*

	% of mitoses by B cells	% of interphase cells with B cell origin
Newborn	13 ± 4	6 ± 1
Adult	42 ± 7	24 ± 1

* 10^5 adult T cells were cultured with 10^5 T depleted cells from the cord blood of an infant of the opposite sex, or from an adult donor of the opposite sex. After 5 days' incubation the cultures were processed for karyotype analysis and stained with quinacrine hydrochloride. Mitoses were examined for the presence or absence of a fluorescent Y chromosome which would identify the cell as derived from the T or B cell source. In addition interphase cells were examined by Y fluorescence.

B cells would therefore appear to be determined at least in part by intrinsic characteristics. Perhaps the newborn predominance of IgM reflects the virgin nature of the B cell population but this is speculation. Recent observations by Pittard and Bill (1979) suggest that environment is also involved. They found that cord blood lymphocytes could be stimulated by PWM to make IgA in the presence of a protein isolated from human milk, with a molecular weight of over 50 000. IgA synthesis in their studies was measured by a double antibody radioimmunoassay so it is not known whether the cells which were making IgA were restricted to that isotype.

It is tempting to speculate that the spontaneous suppressor activity of newborn T cells has some functional significance. The suggestion that suppression is a defence against attack by maternal lymphocytes (Oldstone *et al.*, 1977) seems unlikely because T cell deficient infants can survive *in utero*. The temporal association between suppression and the intra-uterine environment in both humans and mice (Mosier *et al.*, 1977) could suggest that it arises in response to an environmental stimulus. One possible stimulus is maternal IgG. Deaggregated IgG is, under rather different experimental conditions, known to be able to elicit a suppressor response (Basten *et al.*, 1978) and the late anti-allotype responses which infants sometimes make (Speiser, 1966) indicates that maternal IgG can be recognized as foreign. It is conceivable that newborn suppressor activity serves to prevent responses by the newborn to the relatively weak antigenic stimulus of maternal idiotypes while permitting responses to stronger stimuli such as those in infection. The background to this reasoning is as follows.

Increasing importance is being attached to the possible role of anti-idiotype antibodies in the control of immune responses. As formulated in Jerne's network hypothesis (Jerne, 1974), contact with antigen stimulates clones of cells with appropriate receptors to mature into plasma cells secreting an antibody, A1. Just as the priming antigen was perceived as foreign, so also are the antigen binding sites of sites of the corresponding antibody, and the result is the production of another antibody A2 with specificity for the antigen binding site of A1. A2 is described as an anti-idiotype antibody for its specificity for idiotypic determinants rather than, for example, allotypic or isotypic determinants. Anti-idiotypic antibodies are most easily raised against homogeneous antibodies such as myeloma proteins, followed by antibodies of restricted heterogeneity. Examples of the latter are the antibody responses of inbred strains of mice to defined haptens such as phosphorylcholine (PhC). Observations on the anti-PhC response of mice provide experimental support for the network hypothesis (reviewed Köhler, 1975) under admittedly highly artificial circumstances. More recently anti-idiotype responses have been found in outbred animals (rabbits) following immunization with *Micrococcus lysodeikticus* (Wickler *et al.*, 1979).

The implications of anti-idiotype control are paradoxical as far as the fetus is concerned. Instead of encountering antigen first, making an antibody A1 and then using A2 to modulate A1, the fetus receives A1-n directly from its mother. If the fetus were to make anti-idiotype antibodies to A1 it is likely that long lasting immunosuppression would result. This is because immature animals are highly susceptible to tolerization by anti-idiotype antibodies (Accolla *et al.*, 1977), presumably because of the intrinsic immaturity of their B cells. There are clear similarities with anti-μ suppression in mice and anti-allotype suppression in rabbits (reviewed Lawton and Cooper, 1973; Mage, 1975), since each involves a long term alteration in the pattern of responsiveness as the result of an early receptor mediated inactivation. When, after birth, the environment provides antigen stimulus, it is possible that anti-idiotype responses could act to increase clonal diversity.

The interaction of maternal antibody and the animals developing immune systems could have important clinical implications for man. It is common observation that maternal IgG protects the newborn from pathogens to which antibody has been transmitted. However administration of antibody (such as zoster immune globulin) to a newborn at a critical time after suppression wanes but before the antigen was experienced could have different effects, such as the production of anti-idiotype antibodies.

ACKNOWLEDGEMENT

The author's current research is supported in part by a Biomedical Research Grant Program of the National Institutes of Health, BRSG RR-05357.

REFERENCES

Accolla, R. S., Gearhart, P. J., Sigal, M. H., Canceo, M. P. and Klinman, N. R. (1977). Idiotype specific neonatal suppression of phosphorylcholine responsive B cells. *European Journal of Immunology* **7,** 876.

Alford, C. A. (1965). Studies on antibody in congenital rubella infections. *American Journal of Diseases in Childhood* **110,** 455.

Baker, C. J. and Kasper, D. L. (1977). Immunological investigation of infants with septicemia or meningitis due to group B streptococcus. *Journal of Infectious Diseases* **136** Suppl. S, 98.

Basten, A., Miller, J. F. A. P., Loblay, R. *et al.* (1978). T cell-dependent suppression of antibody production. 1. Characteristics of suppressor T cells following tolerance induction. *European Journal of Immunology* **8,** 360.

Bird, A. G. and Britton, S. (1979). A new approach to the study of human B lymphocyte function using an indirect plaque assay and a direct B cell activator. *Immunology Review* **45,** 41–68.

Fauci, A. S. (1979). Human B cell function in a polyclonally induced plaque forming cell system. Cell triggering and immunoregulation. *Immunology Review* **45,** 93–116.

Hayward, A. R. and Lawton, A. R. (1977). Induction of plasma cell differentiation of human fetal lymphocytes: evidence for functional immaturity of T and B cells. *Journal of Immunology* **119,** 1213.

Hayward, A. R., Layward, C., Lydyard, P. M., Moretta, L., Dagg, M. and Lawton, A. R. (1978). Fc receptor heterogeneity of human suppressor T cells. *Journal of Immunology* **121**, 1.

Hayward, A. R. and Lydyard, P. M. (1978). Suppression of B lymphocyte differentiation by newborn T lymphocytes with an Fc receptor for IgM. *Clinical and Experimental Immunology* **34**, 374–378.

Hayward, A. R. and Lydyard, P. M. (1979). "B cell function in the newborn". *Pediatrics* **64**, 758.

Jerne, N. K. (1974). Towards a network theory of the immune system. *Annals of Immunology (Institut Pasteur)* **125c**, 373.

Johnston, R. B., Altenburger, K. M., Atkinson, A. W. and Curry, R. H. (1979). Complement in the newborn infant. *Pediatrics* **64**, 781.

Köhler, H. (1975). The response to phosphorylcholine: dissecting an immune response. *Transplantation Reviews* **27**, 24.

Kurnick, J. T., Bell, C. and Grey, H. M. (1976). PHA-induced activation of suppressor cells in normal human peripheral blood lymphocytes. *Scandinavian Journal of Immunology* **5**, 771.

Lawler, S. D., Ukaejiofo, E. O. and Reeves, B. R. (1975). Interaction of maternal and neonatal cells in mixed lymphocyte cultures. *Lancet* **ii**, 1185.

Lawton, A. R. and Cooper, M. D. (1973). Modifications of B lymphocyte differentiation by anti-immunoglobulins. *Contemporary Topics in Immunobiology* **3**, 193.

Maca, R. D., Bonnard, G. D. and Herberman, R. B. (1979). The suppression of mitogen and alloantigen stimulated peripheral blood lymphocytes by cultured human T lymphocytes. *Journal of Immunology* **123**, 246–251.

Mage, R. G. (1975). Allotype suppression in rabbits: effects of anti-allotype antisera upon expression of immunoglobulin genes. *Transplantation Reviews* **27**, 84.

Miller, M. E. (1979). Phagocyte function in the neonate: selected aspects. *Pediatrics* **64**, 709.

Mosier, D. E., Mathieson, B. J. and Campbell, P. S. (1977). Ly phenotype and mechanism of action of mouse neonatal suppressor T cells. *Journal of Experimental Medicine* **146**, 59.

Olding, L. B. and Oldstone, M. B. A. (1976). Thymus derived peripheral lympocytes from human newborns inhibit division of their mothers' lymphocytes. *Journal of Immunology* **116**, 682.

Oldstone, M. B. A., Tishon, A. and Moretta, L. (1977). Active thymus derived suppressor lymphocytes in human cord blood. *Nature, London* **269**, 333.

Pang, G. T. M. and Booth, R. J. (1979). The proliferative capacity of human T lymphocyte subpopulations in a continuous culture system. *European Journal of Immunology* **9**, 352.

Pittard, W. B. and Bill, K. (1979). Differentiation of cord blood lymphocytes into IgA-producing cells in response to breast milk stimulatory factor. *Clinical Immunology and Immunopathology* **13**, 430–434.

Stagno, S., Volanakis, J., Reynolds, D. W., Stroud, R. and Alford, C. A. (1977). Virus host interactions in perinatally acquired cytomegalovirus infections in man: comparative studies on antigenic load and immune complex formation. *In* "Development of Host Defenses" (Eds M. D. Cooper and D. H. Dayton) Raven Press, New York.

Smith, R. T. and Eitzman, D. U. (1964). The development of the immune response. Characterisation of the response of the human infant and adult to immunization with Salmonella vaccines. *Pediatrics* **33**, 163.

Speiser, P. (1966). New aspects of immunogenetic relations between child and mother. *Annals of Pediatrics* **207**, 20–35.

Wickler, M., Franssen, J. D., Collignon, C. *et al.* (1979). Idiotypic regulation of the immune system. Common idiotypic specificities between idiotypes and antibodies raised against anti-idiotypic antibodies in rabbits. *Journal of Experimental Medicine* **150**, 184.

DISCUSSION

Wood Could I ask whether the career of a T cell is immutable? If a T cell in the newborn is a suppressor cell, does it stay like that permanently, and do the T cells which have suppressor functions have different morphological characteristics from those which are helper cells or null cells?

Hayward If I can take the second part first, we do not know so far as newborns' T cells are concerned. If you identify Fc suppressor cells on the basis of their receptors, the answer is those with IgG receptors are morphologically different in that they have cytoplasmic granules, and those which have IgM receptors (which do not always participate in suppressor responses) are acid esterase positive. Perhaps the bulk of your question is: do the cells that suppress ever become capable of helping? Really we would have to draw on mice for the answer which is probably no, they do not. For instance, Con A suppressors in mice are always $Ly2^+3^+$ positive and there is really no evidence in mice that $Ly2^+3^+$ positive cells can ever turn into $Ly1^+$ positive cells which is the helper phenotype.

The difficulty really arises in the way in which the different T cell subpopulations in mice interact. It looks as though one needs a helper or amplifier population to persuade precursor cells which are $Ly1^+2^+3^+$ positive, to differentiate, to active suppressors. Although I did not say so earlier, we have some suggestion that newborn helper cells are relatively bad at helping suppressor precursors to turn into active suppressors. I do not think we entirely know the answer to your question.

Soothill I feel that for this discussion's point of view the way in which responses become more positive with birth, is especially interesting. We know that the balance between suppression and help experimentally can be importantly influenced by adjuvants. Is it possible that the transition that occurs results from the ingestion of adjuvantizing material such as *E. coli* endotoxin.

Hayward Yes, I am sure it is possible. It would be nice to speculate that antigen is one of the things responsible for turning off suppression, although we have no way of testing that at the moment.

Cooper I would like to comment briefly in response to Prof. Wood's question, can a suppressor cell change its spots and become a helper cell? It has been shown with regard to the T γ cells that have a suppressor capability that if they contact IgG immune complexes, then the Fc receptor for the γ change is not re-expressed. So that they become null with respect to their capacity to bind IgG immune complexes.

It has also been shown that they will then express more receptors for IgM Fc. Therefore, it is conceivable and is even proposed that a suppressor cell can in this way be induced to become a T μ cell and implied as being a helper cell. When you test the capacity of the converted T γ to T μ, if I can use that terminology, for help and suppression, as Moretta has done, you find that it has not changed its functional spots, it is still a suppressor and not a helper. It is conceivable that some of the newborn cells that one looks at have indeed contacted IgG immune complexes and are therefore T γ cells masquerading as T μ cells. That is why one sees this paradoxical suppression in the T μ sub population obtained from cord blood.

Hayward I agree, and we initially speculated that contact with immune complexes perhaps in the placenta would be important in triggering suppression by the IgG binding population. The difficulty of being sure that triggering through IgG Fc receptors is the only relevant stimulus is that we showed also that Con A activated IgM binding T cells could suppress very strongly and in mice anyway it is fairly well established that the Con A induced suppressor are $Ly2^+3^+$, whether they are Ly1 also has not really been excluded.

Denman Anthony, you started your very intriguing remarks by stating that a fetus which acquires a congenital infection can cope with it very well in terms of mounting an antibody response, and that prompts the suspicion that if you give the B cells of the newborn a tune they want to dance to, they will do it very satisfactorily. This makes one wonder about the relevance of the *in vitro* system you have been describing and whether one can really regard this as a proper counterpart of the kind of interaction that takes place *in vivo*. The mononuclear cell count of the newborn is high compared with older infants and these cells are more heterogenous in terms of cells spontaneously synthesizing DNA, stem cells and possibly cells of the monocyte macrophage series. Thus one wonders how homogeneous your mononuclear cell populations are, compared with those in older children. How sure can one be, that one does not have a mixture with other cell types which are in the blood of the newborn as part of their natural progress to other sites and which might not be found in the adult or the older child. Such patterns obviously could cause perturbations in terms of any mixing experiments one might do involving the culture of mixed cell population.

This is a technical question about the nature of your experiments, one also wonders about whether there is an *in vitro* situation which would persuade one that "suppressor" cells in the newborn perform functions that have physiological relevance. For example, if you took the cord blood lymphocytes of a child born to a mother with an auto immune disease such as auto-immune thyroiditis, one would expect that the mother's blood would contain B cells which would produce auto-antibodies specifically reacting with the thyroid, as has been demonstrated in this disease by Hall and his associates. We know that auto-antibodies appear transiently in the children born to such mothers, and one wonders whether the cord blood of the infant would specifically suppress auto-antibody production by the maternal B lymphocytes. In other words, can you envisage experiments which would persuade one that "suppressor T cells" from the newborn infant really could exhibit a suppressor function which is of physiological importance.

Hayward You would almost have to lead me step by step through them again.

Let me start off with the question of heterogeneity: we have no means of identifying unidentifiable cells, so I entirely concur that we do not necessarily know what we are looking for, and one must view things like even E rosetting with profound suspicion. These are not markers securely established as Ly antigens or TH² antigens. We can look for things like pre-B cells which are a precursor population and actually they are extremely difficult to find in newborn blood. There is obviously either something different in newborn blood, particularly in the non-T cell fraction, in that there are cells there with a very high spontaneous thymidine uptake.

We tried to construct our experiments to look at the responses of identifiable cells, and that was the sort of data that I was giving you. As far as the physiological relevance is concerned, something obviously has to turn off suppression and I have tried to suggest that it is antigen either in the form of congenital infection or antigen in the form of environmental antigen experienced after birth.

There is evidence in mice to suggest that that is the way in which other antigen such as BSA is handled; for instance, in mice deaggregated IgG gives rise to a population of suppressor cells, which other antigens like BSA do not induce. So, as far as my theoretical speculation is concerned, there is an animal precedent that suppression is related to response to immunoglobulin. I forget your final point, perhaps you could remind me.

Denman   I was asking whether you could show that suppressor cells would turn off an unwanted immune response.

Hayward   I do not know the answer.

Denman   I am interested in the control of antibody production.

Hayward   The problem with auto-antibody formation, of course, is that it takes place in the mother, and the maternal B cells are probably not accessible to foetal T cells. I would expect that if one could obtain large numbers of maternal cells, and it would obviously have to be B cells plus their helper cells and so on, one might well be able to turn off those responses with newborn T cells, but I would expect the effect to be antigen nonspecific way.

Allison   The thing that is important from the practical point of view is whether the immune responses in the newborn differ from those in the adults in a way which is important in controlling disease. A lot of basic information is missing. We know that when fetuses are exposed to some infections, e.g. lymphocytic choriomeningitis, they are able to make a little antibody that is, of course, the congenital infection which goes on to give rise to an immune complex disease later. In later infections to which you have already alluded, such as rubella, a lot of IgM antibody is produced and so this may be less able to control the infection than would a good high affinity IgG antibody such as you get in the adult. So clearly the switch mechanisms from IgM to IgG formation are of interest. I think the possibility of tolerance, or something like tolerance, emerges also in connection with the polysaccharide antigens that we have discussed today. We know that with

Pneumococcus polysaccharides that you can very easily induce tolerance, and that this is associated with T cell suppression as well as the nonresponse of the B cells. This has been carefully analysed by Philip Baker and others.

We need a lot more information about the nature of these differences between newborns and adults. Then I like Prof. Soothill's point, that if we are going to do anything about it we must try to improve the responses of mothers and newborns. One important question is whether one could use adjuvants of the kind which are now coming up such as the synthetic components of bacterial cell walls, muramyl dipeptides and derivatives which seem to be nontoxic in newborns. It would be interesting to do the kind of experiment that was indicated by John Soothill, comparing germ free mice with conventional mice to find out whether the suppressor population declines at different rates and whether you can manipulate this by adjuvants such as *E. coli* endotoxin or muramyl dipeptides. I should be interested to know whether you agree with this approach: in other words, first of all obtaining more ethical information and then, secondly ascertaining in what way it would be possible to increase the effectiveness of immune responses in the mothers and newborn.

Hayward Yes, we desperately need more data. I do not have germ free mice available and we were proposing to do experiments in sheep actually in order to see ways in which antibodies—since there is no transplacental passage of IgG in sheep—could modulate the immune response. As far as the effect of congenital virus infection is concerned, of course, Prof. Soothill has already done some studies relating to cytomegalovirus handling in congenital infection which suggests that the rate of excretion was at least temporarily altered by transfer factor. This led me to think that there was a possibly delayed switch or maturation of the immune response which might be contributing to the relatively slow elimination of that virus amongst others, and also therefore to its persistance and its capacity to cause serious brain damage. So I think the answer to your first question—which is really the most important one—is yes.

Adinolfi As to the physiological role, I wonder if we can clarify the important point about the receptor for the suppressor factor, because I understand from the work of Olding and collaborators (see Olding, 1979) that the suppressor cells present in newborn do not suppress cells from another newborn. This implies that the suppressor cells release a factor which acts as a receptor on adult cells. The receptor is present only in adult cells and not in fetal or newborn cells. If this is true during fetal life the suppressor cells do not have an autoregulatory function, because they do not have a receptor on which to act. Probably only during a critical period in perinatal life when the receptors start to be produced both suppressor cells and the receptors are active.

If this assumption is correct, suppressor cells will only damp the regulatory immune response during perinatal life, sometime after delivery. I say this, because you have mentioned the role that maternal IgG may have on the fetus and suggests that the suppressor cells may regulate the fetal response to maternal Ig idiotypes. It has been suggested that during fetal life the suppressor cells play a very important role in protecting the fetus against the maternal attack by "blocking" the maternal lymphocytes which have crossed the placenta. I find it difficult to believe that suppressor cells may have this function, because the fetuses with the Di George syndrome tolerate the maternal attack and yet they do not have T cells or suppressor cells. In a way I can see a function for the suppressor cells (Olding, 1979) during perinatal life when both suppressor cells and cells with a receptor for the suppressor are present, but I have no clear idea of their function during fetal life.

Hayward Your comment relates I believe mostly to the work of Olding and Oldstone, and in two fields. One is that suppression by newborn T cells protects against attack by mother. I completely concur with you that I would reject that argument for a number of reasons. There are mouse strain combinations that one can study in which, for instance, the fetus would not be able to reject maternal cells and there is no reason to believe that these animals do suffer from GVH disease. And as you rightly point out, rare children are born without T cells, again with no satisfactory evidence that they suffer from GVH disease.

The other question concerning the Fc receptor specificity of the newborn suppressor T cell and what it suppresses—our results actually differ from those of Mike Oldstone in that he finds the IgG binding T cells of human newborns to be particularly effective suppressors. However, his co-author on that particular paper has also shown that the Tg isolation system they used would be expected to produce the suppression they found. So the Tg results they obtained would be an expected artefact of the experimental system they used. The question is whether newborns will suppress each other or suppress mother.

In thymidine uptake experiments as Olding and Oldstone used, it is hard to distinguish between proliferation by suppressor cells and proliferation by other cells, which is why Peter Lydyard and I and others have used this extremely complicated assay looking for plasma cell production. T cells, whether helpers or suppressors, do not turn into plasma cells so we can distinguish between the response of the target cells which measure and the activity of the suppressor cell. However, T cells, helpers and suppressors, and B cells, may all divide and they may all take up tritiated thymidine. Therefore, combinations of suppressor cells may well both divide. If I remember rightly, the first experiments of Olding and Oldstone actually were done on the basis of mitoses, and under those combinations, again, there is no reason to suppose that the suppressor cells would directly suppress each other. In many mouse combinations and in my suppressor combinations the target of suppression is a helper cell or a B cell or a macrophage rather than the other suppressor cell.

Reeves I am pleased that Dr Hayward has raised this point about possible technical artefact giving rise to suppressor phenomena with particular regard to

the mode of purification of the lymphoid cells being used, because we have found
that one can get very marked variation in suppression seen in coculture with PHA
as mitogen, whether one is using cells purified from peripheral blood by a rouleau-
forming agent or whether one has used Ficol Hypaque purified cells. In passing I
would just like to ask what kind of mononuclear population he has been using in
these experiments, and also secondly, ask him whether he would be prepared to
comment on the possible significance of the phenomenon he has described, faced
up against the work of Waldman's group in America concerning the possibility
that patients with hypogammaglobulinaemia may be suffering from a similar kind
of problem, and work which I do not think has been entirely confirmed by
colleagues. Michael Denman may wish to comment on this.

Hayward I think as far as patients with common variable hypogammaglobulinaemia is concerned a proportion—and whether it is a third, a fifth or half does
not matter terribly—can be shown to have circulating T cells which will depress
the responses of other cells either in mitogen or antigen stimulated cultures or a
number of different assays. The argument hinges really about whether this is a
primary or secondary phenomenon. Perhaps the most informative observation by
Rebecca Buckley is of affected siblings in which one suppressed and one did not.
The third point, I suppose, is that antigen stimulated T cells from anyone,
whether antibody deficient or not, can suppress.

Coming back to the possible differences of cell separation methods, we have
actually used Ficoll–Triosil centrifugation to prepare the T cells and have gone
through a number of other manipulations like plastic adherence, treatment with
carbonyl iron, and so on to try and get rid of other cells which might be producing
suppression. The effect of lithium, irradiation, hyrocortisone and indomethocin
would all tend to go along with the idea that the cells that are responsible for the
suppression are T cells. We have, in conjunction with Jim Kurnick at the National
Jewish Hospital, tried to grow these T cells in continuous culture using
conditioned medium and, of four lines established from newborn blood, three
have suppressed and one has not.

Reeves Would you care to make a remark about how your data interrelate with
Waldmann's work?

Hayward That is what I was trying to do first. It is obviously possible that one
reason why patients might have hypogammaglobulinaemia is that their B cells
have failed to mature to a point at which they can behave like adult B cells. They
might go on behaving like newborn B cells so that they can make IgM but do not
switch on very well to make IgG or IgA. It is conceivable that persistent
suppression might cause antibody deficiency in children and adults if the
mechanism that normally turns off suppression fails to act. However, testing
lymphocytes from older patients with congenital antibody deficiency does not
really confirm that. A large number of them do not have suppressor cells. It might
be worth asking Max what the current results from his group are.

Cooper   I cannot do anything but agree with what you are saying. The bulk of evidence suggests that most immunodeficient patients who have B lymphocytes that are arrested in their further development failed to do so not because of excessive suppressive T cells, but because of inherent abnormality in them, the B lymphocytes. Even if one gives them normal T cells to help, most times they still do not go on to further differentiate, and moreover, their T cells often will provide helper factors for normal B lymphocytes. So I think it is unlikely to be a common cause. One possibility for the finding is that these patients are given γ globulin immune complexes, IgG immune complexes. That seems to be one of the triggering factors from pokeweed and thereby preferentially activate T γ cells.

Faulk   The idea of that GVH as a possibility during pregnancy carries with it the assumption that maternal lymphocytes enter the fetal circulation. I would like to say that at least in the human there is very little evidence to support that particular position. I do not think it would be very wise to hinge a physiological argument on dogma. We often fantasize about how these Di George syndromes in children with congenital immunodeficiencies actually get through their pregnancy if GVH is involved, but I do not think that this need trouble us a great deal because recent work has shown that a glycoprotein produced by the human syn-cytiotrophoblast is an extremely potent inhibitor of cell–cell interactions especially if the interactions are allogenic. This glycoprotein from the trophoblast stops only mixed lymphocyte culture reactions.

This is a relevant observation to human pregnancy, because human pregnancy is about the only situation which exists in nature where mixed lymphocyte culture reactions occur *in vivo*. That is why the MLC reaction is relevant to this discussion. Fetal cells enter the maternal circulation when they are coculture and this seems to be a usual concomitant of normal pregnancy.

The fetal cells that enter the mother can be found in the circulation six to eight years after the birth of a child. I do not know of any information from blood transfusions which show the existence of lymphocytes in a circulation six to eight years later, and it does suggest that the fetal lymphocyte are producing some inhibitor of maternal recognition. We come back to the problem cleft stick of why do you have this enormous amount of suppressor T cells in the fetus. One idea I favour comes from work that Tony Allison did several years ago showing the presence of antithyroid producing cells in the rabbit marrow. If we accept the biogenetic law that ontogeny recapitulates phylogenetically, then the embryo must pass through several different phases of plasma membrane antigens and we must then speculate about the possible mechanism which could cause the fetal immune system not to respond to self antigen. One fairly good way which would operate at a physiological level to prevent fetal recognition of these cells throughout pregnancy, would be suppressor T cells, and that might in part account for the high number of cells in cord blood.

REFERENCE

Olding, L. B. (1979). Interaction between maternal and fetal/neonatal lymphocytes. *In* "Current Topics in Pathology", (Eds E. Grundmann and W. H. Kiriten), Vol. 66, 83–104.

The Role of Milk and Gut Flora in Protection of the Newborn against Infection

J. J. BULLEN

National Institute for Medical Research,
Mill Hill, London, UK

From a bacteriological point of view the newly born infant is faced with a difficult problem. He or she must acquire the right flora for his or her alimentary tract. Failure to do so may lead to disaster in the shape of gastroenteritis, and many harmful bacteria are only too well equipped to colonize the intestinal tract if given the opportunity.

Under natural conditions the substrate for bacterial growth in the suckling infant consists of maternal milk or some modification of milk produced by digestion. In this respect it is worth emphasizing that before birth the human infant has the great advantage that the placentation *in utero* provides for direct transmission of maternal protective antibodies. Thus deprivation of maternal milk in man leads to loss of some protective mechanisms in the gut, but not to deprivation of maternal IgG which is so important in protection against bacterial invasion from the gut. In animals with epitheliochorial placentation, like the pig, deprivation of maternal milk leads to loss of protection in the gut and also to deprivation of maternal IgG which is normally absorbed from the colostrum during the first few hours of life. This is usually disastrous and may lead to losses from infection as high as 100%.

What are the protective mechanisms in the gut of the newly born infant? As already mentioned, circulating maternal IgG is a big safeguard. In the gut itself, however, the environment provided by maternal colostrum and milk is of paramount importance. The factors involved can be assessed partly by experiments *in vitro* and partly by studies on breast fed babies, compared with babies fed on various preparations of cows' milk. Circumstantial evidence from animal experiments is also useful.

THE UNIQUENESS OF HUMAN MILK

All mammalian milks differ significantly from each other and appear to be exactly tailored for the young of the individual species. For the present purpose we need to compare human milk with cows' milk since the composition of the milks has a direct effect on resistance and the bacterial flora of the gut.

Human colostrum contains about 5 mg of secretory IgA ml^{-1} and mature milk about 2 mg ml^{-1} (Rogers and Synge, 1978). Fairly constant levels of IgA (14 mg g^{-1} of milk protein) are reached by about 5 days *post partum* (Ogra and Ogra, 1978). IgM immunoglobulin is present in colostrum at approximately 29 mg g^{-1} milk protein but this declines to about 3–4 mg g^{-1} protein by the 120th day. IgG is present in only small amounts (1–5 mg g^{-1} milk protein) in both colostrum and milk (Ogra and Ogra, 1978). As far as antibodies are concerned, Gindrat *et al.* (1972) found high titres against O antigens of *Escherichia coli* representing the serogroups responsible for 31 out of 43 outbreaks of infection in the newborn. These antibodies are largely of the secretory IgA class (Hanson and Winberg, 1972). In the newborn infant little digestion of protein takes place in the stomach (Mason, 1962). The milk IgA is also resistant to digestion in the gut as a whole and can be detected in the faeces (Gindrat *et al.*, 1972).

Another major component of human milk is the iron binding protein, lactoferrin. In colostrum it is present in concentrations as high as 6 mg ml^{-1} but this falls to 2–3 mg ml^{-1} after 5 days. Transferrin is also present but only in small amounts (10–50 µg ml^{-1}) (Masson and Heremans, 1971). Both proteins are only partially saturated with iron (Bullen *et al.*, 1972).

As expected, cows' colostrum and milk contain immunoglobulins in quite different proportions to human milk. The most abundant immunoglobulin is IgG. The initial concentration of IgG may be as high as 60 mg ml^{-1} but in 7 days this has declined to less than 1·0 mg ml^{-1}. IgA starts at about 10 mg ml^{-1} and falls to about 0·5 mg ml^{-1}. The levels of IgM are approximately the same as the IgA (Porter, 1972). *Escherichia coli* antibodies are distributed among all three classes of immunoglobulin with the greatest concentration in IgM and IgG (Porter, 1972). Cows' milk contains 20–200 µg of lactoferrin ml^{-1} and the same amount of transferrin (Masson and Heremans, 1971).

In addition to immunoglobulins and the iron binding proteins other aspects of human milk have a direct bearing on bacterial growth in the gut. Mature human milk contains 6·9 g of lactose 100 ml^{-1}. This is approximately 1·4 × that in cows' milk. It contains 1·3 g 100 ml^{-1} of total protein, which is approximately 2·5 × less than that in cows' milk. Human milk also has a total phosphorus content of only 0·013 g 100 ml^{-1} which is about 10 × less than that in cows' milk. The relatively low concentrations of casein and phosphorus results in a relatively low buffering capacity of breast milk. To take the pH of cows' milk from 7·0 to 5·0 requires three times as much $N_{10}HCl$ as that required for human milk (C. L. Bullen and Willis, 1971).

THE INFLUENCE OF HUMAN MILK ON THE GUT FLORA

The Role of Specific Antibody and Iron Binding Proteins

Pathogenic *E. coli* capable of causing gastroenteritis must be capable of the following: (1) adherence to the mucosa of the small intestine; (2) production of enterotoxin; (3) rapid growth in the small intestine (Smith, 1976). Anti-adhesive effects of antibody have been demonstrated in the pig (Jones and Rutter, 1974; Rutter *et al.*, 1976). Similar effects may occur in the human infant (McNeish *et al.*, 1975). IgA in human milk appears to be responsible for inhibiting the effect of *E. coli* enterotoxin (Stoliar *et al.*, 1976), although anti-enterotoxic antibodies appear to be relatively unimportant in pigs (Smith, 1972).

One of the most important protective mechanisms in the small intestine is the suppression of bacterial growth by specific antibody. There is ample evidence for this. Smith (1972) showed that the viable counts of enteropathogenic *E. coli* in the small intestine of protected pigs could be 1000–10 000 × less than in unprotected controls. Equally good or better results were obtained by Köhler (1974). *In vitro*, both human and bovine milk have powerful bacteriostatic effects against pathogenic *E. coli* (J. J. Bullen *et al.*, 1972; Nagy *et al.*, 1976). Iron binding proteins are essential for this effect (J. J. Bullen *et al.*, 1972; 1978; Nagy *et al.*, 1976). J. J. Bullen *et al.*, (1972) showed that lactoferrin, only partially saturated with iron, produced a bacteriostatic effect identical to that of whole milk provided specific antibody was also present. The necessity for the iron binding capacity of the lactoferrin was shown by the abolition of bacteriostasis when the lactoferrin was saturated with iron. Griffiths and Humphries (1977) showed that bicarbonate was also essential for the effect. Rogers and Synge (1978) showed that purified IgA has a powerful bacteriostatic effect on *E. coli*, in the presence of lactoferrin, provided the antibody has the correct specificity for the corresponding *E. coli* serotype. These observations are particularly important since they demonstrate a real antibacterial role for IgA, probably for the first time.

Some workers, Jones and Rutter (1974) and Hill and Porter (1974) have suggested that porcine milk could have bactericidal effects against *E. coli*. However all tests made to show this property involve the addition of fresh rabbit serum (Hill and Porter, 1974) or fresh pig serum (Jones and Rutter, 1974) as sources of complement. There is little evidence that intestinal fluid contains complement and McNeish (1976) remarks that intestinal contents are usually "aggressively anticomplementary". The involvement of complement is particularly unlikely in the case of IgA. IgA antibody will not kill *Vibrio cholerae* in the presence of complement whereas IgM and IgG are highly active (Steele *et al.*, 1974). IgA is also a feeble opsonin (Steele *et al.*, 1974; Heddle and Rowley, 1975). However, IgA antibody is highly protective against *V. cholerae* infection in infant mice (Steel *et al.*, 1974). Since the intestinal fluid contains lactoferrin (Masson, 1970; Rogers and Synge, 1978) it seems highly probable that the IgA operates in concert with this iron binding protein in the gut. J. J. Bullen *et al.*, 1972 showed that the feeding of haematin to suckling guinea-pigs dosed with *E. coli* 0111 resulted in a 10 000-fold increase in the bacteria in the small intestine and a smaller though significant increase in the large intestine. This provides good evidence that the iron binding proteins are important in the gut in restricting bacterial growth since haematin can supply iron to *E. coli* in spite of the presence of lactoferrin. The latter does not bind haem compounds (J. J. Bullen *et al.*, 1978).

Development of an Anaerobic Lactobacillary Flora in the Large Intestine

At birth the human infant is probably exposed to all the organisms commonly found in the intestinal tract. However the breast fed infant may be more continuously exposed to anaerobic lactobacilli than bottle fed infants since these bacteria are found in the mouth, nose, vagina, and on the skin of the mother (Haenel *et al.*, 1958; C. L. Bullen *et al.*, 1973).

As already mentioned it is likely that the milk itself has a direct inhibitory effect on *E. coli* and other enteric bacteria in the small intestine. In the large intestine the situation is somewhat different. The total number of bacteria present is very much greater and the types of organism depend very much on whether the infant is breast fed or not. By and large the breast fed infant has a large population of *Lactobacillus bifidus* and a relatively small population of *E. coli* and other enteric bacteria. *Streptococcus faecium* is usually present in large numbers together with relatively small numbers of bacteroides, clostridia, and veillonellae (Mata and Urrutia, 1971; C. L. Bullen *et al.*, 1973). In the bottle fed baby *L. bifidus* is frequently absent altogether or present only in small numbers, while the counts of *Strep. faecium*, bacteroides and clostridia are greatly increased (C. L. Bullen *et al.*, 1973). In addition organisms such as *Clostridium paraputrificum*, *Proteus* spp., *Klebsiella* spp. and *Pseudomonas aeruginosa* are frequently encountered (Mata and Urrutia, 1971; C. L. Bullen *et al.*, 1976).

A characteristic feature of the faeces of the breast fed infant is the relatively low pH of 5·0–5·5 compared with a pH of 6·5–7·0 for bottle fed infants (Willis *et al.*, 1973). The faeces of breast fed infants also contain an acetate buffer which is absent from infants fed cows' milk (C. L. Bullen *et al.*, 1976). Acetate buffer at pH 5·0–5·5 is inhibitory to enteric bacteria but has no effect on the growth of *L. bifidus* or *Strep. faecium* (C. L. Bullen and Tearle, 1976). Thus the production of an acetate buffer acts as a selective mechanism for the encouragement of the characteristic bacteriological flora of the breast fed infant. This probably represents a protective mechanism of some importance.

As already mentioned human milk contains large amounts of lactose, little phosphate, is relatively low in protein, and is poorly buffered. Chromatographic analysis of metabolites produced *in vitro* by the saccharolytic organisms *E. coli*, *Strep. faecium* and *L. bifidus* commonly encountered in breast fed infants showed that acetic acid accumulates when these bacteria are grown in the presence of fermentable sugar (C. L. Bullen and Tearle, 1976). This finding suggests that the sequence of events in the large gut of breast fed infants is as follows. Initial contamination with *E. coli* leads to a fall in pH and the production of acid in the large gut. These conditions favour the growth of *L. bifidus* and a combination of *L. bifidus*, *E. coli* and *Strep. faecium* favour the rapid production of an anaerobic environment where the pH falls as acetic acid accumulates. All these conditions are favoured by the presence of abundant lactose in a poorly buffered milk. In these circumstances *L. bifidus* tends to dominate the environment (C. L. Bullen *et al.*, 1976).

Bottle fed infants receive a high protein, high phosphorus, low lactose diet. Most of the protein is caseinogen which would be expected to clot in the intestinal tract. The passage time though the small intestine of this relatively bulky material would provide ample time for the absorption of lactose and water. No acetic acid is produced by bacterial fermentation and the pH remains high in a well buffered medium. This discourages organisms like *L. bifidus* and encourages a putrefactive flora (C. L. Bullen and Willis, 1971; C. L. Bullen *et al.*, 1973).

THE BACTERIOLOGICAL CONSEQUENCE OF SUPPLEMENTARY FEEDING

It is a common practice, for the sake of convenience, to supplement breast feeding with occasional feeds of preparations based on cows' milk. The introduction of a different substrate into the gut would be expected to alter the bacterial flora, and this is precisely what happens. Breast fed infants given supplements still maintain a high faecal count of *L. bifidus* but tend to have higher counts of *E. coli* than those on breast milk alone, and a greater tendency to acquire organisms like *Proteus* spp. and *Pseudomonas aeruginosa* which are encountered in bottle fed babies. In addition, when supplements are given during the first 7 days of life the production of a strongly acidic faeces is delayed and never reaches its full potential (C. L. Bullen *et al.*, 1977).

CONCLUSIONS

The protective effect of human milk in the small intestine largely depends on the antibacterial effects of IgA antibodies, lactoferrin and bicarbonate. In the large intestine breast milk encourages the development of an anaerobic lactobacillary flora which is accompanied by acidic gut contents which are inhibitory to enteric bacteria. Bottle fed babies are deprived of these protective mechanisms in the gut and have a putrefactive flora in the large intestine, together with relatively high counts of *E. coli*.

REFERENCES

Bullen, C. L. and Tearle, P. V. (1976) Bifidobacteria in the intestinal tract of infants: an *in-vitro* study. *Journal of Medical Microbiology* **9**, 335–344.

Bullen, C. L. and Willis, A. T. (1971). Resistance of the breast fed infant to gastroenteritis. *British Medical Journal* **3**, 338–343.

Bullen, C. L., Willis, A. T. and Williams, K. (1973). The significance of bifidobacteria in the intestinal tract of infants. *In* "Actinomycetales: characteristics and practical importance" (Eds G. Sykes and F. A. Skinner), 311–325. Academic Press, London and New York.

Bullen, C. L., Tearle, P. V. and Willis, A. T., (1976). Bifidobacteria in the intestinal tract of infants: an *in-vivo* study. *Journal of Medical Microbiology* **9**, 325–333.

Bullen, C. L., Tearle, P. V. and Stewart, M. G. (1977). The effect of "humanised" milks and supplemented breast feeding on the faecal flora of infants. *Journal of Medical Microbiology* **10**, 403–413.

Bullen, J. J., Rogers, H. J. and Leigh, L. (1972). Iron-binding proteins in milk and resistance to *Escherichia coli* infection in infants. *British Medical Journal* **1**, 69–75.

Bullen, J. J., Rogers, H. J. and Griffiths, E. (1978). Role of iron in bacterial infection. *In* "Current Topics in Microbiology and Immunology", vol. 80, 1–35. Springer-Verlag, Berlin, Heidelberg.

Gindrat, J. J., Gothefors, L., Hanson, L. A. and Winberg, J. (1972). Antibodies in human milk against *E. coli* of the serogroups most commonly found in neonatal infections. *Acta Paediatrica Scandinavica* **61**, 587–590.

Griffiths, E. and Humphreys, J. (1977). Bacteriostatic effect of human milk and bovine colostrum on *Escherichia coli*: importance of bicarbonate. *Infection and Immunity* **15**, 396–401.

Haenel, H., Feldheim, G. and Müller-Beuthow, W. (1958). Zur Microbiologishen Okologic des Menschen. *Zentralblatt für Bakteriologie, Parasitenkunde Infektionskrankheiten und Hygiene Abt. 1* **172**, 73–93.

Hanson, L. A. and Winberg, J. (1972). Breast milk and defence against infection in the newborn. *Archives of Disease in Childhood* **47**, 845–848.

Heddle, R. J. and Rowley, D. (1975). Dog immunoglobulin. II. The antibacterial properties of dog IgA, IgM and IgG antibodies to *Vibrio cholerae*. *Immunology* **29**, 197–208.

Hill, I. R. and Porter, P. (1974). Studies of bactericidal activity to *Escherichia coli* of porcine serum and colostral immunoglobulins and the role of lysozyme with secretory IgA. *Immunology* **26,** 1239–1250.

Jones, G. W. and Rutter, J. M. (1974). Contribution of the K88 antigen of *Escherichia coli* to enteropathogenicity: protection against disease by neutralizing the adhesive properties of K88 antigen. *American Journal of Clinical Nutrition* **27,** 1441–1449.

Köhler, E. M. (1974). Protection of pigs against neonatal enteric colibacillosis with colostrum and milk from orally vaccinated sows. *American Journal of Veterinary Research* **35,** 331–338.

McNeish, A. S. (1976). Discussion. Agglutinating antibody response in the duodenum of infants with enteropathogenic *Escherichia coli* gastroenteritis. "Acute Diarrhoea in Childhood", 190–192. Ciba Symposium No. 42. Elsevier, Amsterdam.

McNeish, A. S., Fleming, J., Turner, P. and Evans, N. (1975). Mucosal adherence of human enteropathogenic *Escherichia coli*. *Lancet* ii, 946–948.

Mason, S. (1962). Some aspects of gastric function in the newborn. *Archives of Disease in Childhood* **37,** 387–391.

Masson, P. L. (1970). "La lactoferrine." Arscia, Brussels.

Masson, P. L., and Heremans, J. F. (1971). Lactoferrin in milk from different species. *Comparative Biochemistry and Physiology* **39B,** 119–129.

Mata, L. J., and Urrutia, J. J. (1971). Intestinal colonization of breast fed children in a rural area of low socioeconomic level. *Annals of the New York Academy of Science* **176,** 93–109.

Nagy, L. K., MacKenzie, T. and Bharucha, Z. (1976). *In vitro* studies on the antimicrobial effects of colostrum and milk from vaccinated and unvaccinated pigs on *Escherichia coli*. *Research in Veterinary Science* **21,** 132–140.

Ogra, S. S. and Ogra, P. L. (1978). Immunologic aspects of human colostrum and milk. *Journal of Pediatrics* **92,** 546–549.

Porter, P. (1972). Immunoglobulins in bovine mammary secretions. Quantitative changes in early lactation and absorption of the neonatal calf. *Immunology* **23,** 225–238.

Rogers, H. J. and Synge, C. (1978). Bacteriostatic effect of human milk on *Escherichia coli*: the role of IgA. *Immunology* **34,** 19–28.

Rutter, J. M., Jones, G. W., Brown, G. T. H., Burrows, M. R. and Luther, P. D. (1976). Antibacterial activity in colostrum and milk associated with protection of piglets against enteric disease caused by K88-positive *Escherichia coli*. *Infection and Immunity* **13,** 667–676.

Smith, H. W. (1972). The nature of the protective effect of antisera against *Escherichia coli* diarrhoea in piglets. *Journal of Medical Microbiology* **5,** 345–353.

Smith, H. W. (1976). Neonatal *Escherichia coli* infections in domestic mammals: transmissibility of pathogenic characteristics. "Acute Diarrhoea in Childhood", Ciba Symposium No. 42. 45–64. Elsevier, Amsterdam.

Steele, E. J., Chaicumpa, W. and Rowley, D. (1974). Isolation and biological properties of three classes of rabbit antibody to *Vibrio cholerae*. *Journal of Infectious Diseases* **130,** 93–103.

Stoliar, O. A., Pelley, R. P., Kaniecki-Green, Klaus, M. H. and Carpenter, C. C. J. (1976). Secretory IgA against enterotoxins in breast-milk. *Lancet* i, 1258–1261.

Willis, A. T., Bullen, C. L., Williams, K., Fagg, C. G., Bourne, A. and Vignon, M. (1973). Breast milk substitute: a bacteriological study. *British Medical Journal* **4,** 67–72.

DISCUSSION

Adinolfi   About the nonsense of the IgA antibodies, complement and the lysis of *E. coli*, several years ago Alan Glynn and I (Adinolfi *et al.*, 1966) showed that secretory IgA antibodies against *E. coli* were not lytic in the presence of complement, but if lysozyme was present in the *in vitro* test, lysis occurs. This observation has been confirmed by Porter, by Kaplan, by Tomasi and others. It has been shown that if the isolated components of the alternative pathway are added to certain strains of *E. coli*, lysis occurs only in the presence of lysozyme. This means that secretory IgA and anti *E coli* components of the alternative pathway interact, but they do not produce a "hole" big enough to induce lysis; if lysozyme is present it gets inside the cell, attacks the substrate and produced lysis. I think that it is not just a coincidence that the sites of synthesis of IgA and lysozyme are the same in colostrum saliva and Paneth cells.

Bullen   Yes, I agree that lysozyme might lyse certain bacteria. The only thing is, when talking about organisms like *E. coli*, the important thing is that if you add iron to the system you abolish the bactericidal effect. As far as I know, iron has no effect on lysozyme at all, or on complement. When you reverse the system with iron it is most unlikely that lysozyme is involved.

The trouble is, of course, that we have only done one experiment *in vivo*; Dr Reiter keeps mentioning this and I quite agree. More experiments should be done on the intact animal in the small intestine. But it is most unlikely that adding iron would interfere with the lysozyme system. Probably the main mechanism of control of *E. coli* in the small intestine is the lactoferrin and the IgA.

Sir Ashley   I should like to ask Dr Bullen about two points. He talked at the beginning about the protective effect of this system against infection. As we heard this morning, coliform infection is only a very small proportion of the horrors to which the infant is subjected and from which he dies. So this lactoferrin system appears to be limited not only to *E. coli* but to the few serotypes of *E. coli* with which you have done your very pretty experiments. Would it be fair to say that? Or have you found in milk a mass of different IgAs: IgAs of different specificities for different *E. coli* and other organisms?

Bullen   Yes, if you take different samples of human milk you will find that some will inhibit some strains of *E. coli*, but others will not. I suggest there is a wide spectrum of IgA with various serological specificities. If the iron binding protein and specific antibody is present, bacteriostasis occurs. On the other hand, with an organism like *Pseudomonas*, you do not get bacteriostasis with IgA and the lactoferrin, but you do get roughly a doubling of the generation time. This in itself is probably a protective mechanism. Of course, one need not postulate that this system is the be all and end all of protection. It obviously is not, especially because babies are protected by maternal IgG. Many babies must occasionally have large numbers of bacteria growing in their intestines, and they suffer from diarrhoea but do not die. If they were pigs, they probably would. On the whole, however, I think the IgA–lactoferrin system is probably very important.

Sir Ashley I think it is, but I am just trying to define the limits of its importance.

Bullen We do not know what the limits are. There is no proof, for example, that lactoferrin is involved in protection against *Vibrio cholerae*, but I am willing to bet it is. IgA is highly protective in the newborn mouse against *V. cholerae* and there has been no obvious explanation for this, as Steele and Rowley admit.

Sir Ashley I think that possibly the generally most important mechanism is not this one which goes only for a number of *E. coli* types, but the one that Philip Miller pointed out years and years ago, and Guy Meynell confirmed, namely, the low pH of the intestinal contents. I should have thought that was a much more general and valid protective mechanism against the variety of bacteria that infect the infant gut.

Bullen You mean in the large intestine?

Sir Ashley Yes.

Bullen Yes, I am sure it is a very important mechanism. But breast fed infants, for example, do not get cholera. So I would again be pretty certain that it is the maternal antibody. The trouble is that the experiments do not get done.

Reiter When we tested the bactericidal effect of bovine colostrum and postcolostral milk (Reiter and Brock, 1975) we thought to have "discovered" complement. However, complement was demonstrated as far back as 1907 by Pfandler and Moro. Undiluted colostrum is nonbactericidal because of its high immunoglobulin concentration–the well known Neisser-Wechsberg effect; on dilution, however, colostrum becomes bactericidal for Gram negative organisms because of the complement mediated bactericidal activity of specific antibodies. Complement can also be demonstrated in postcolostral milk up to ~ 14 days but not in mid-lactation milk. It appears again in the late lactation period and dry secretion.

The other point you made was the existence of anticomplementary factors in the intestine. However, I feel that the complement mediated antibody activity is so rapid that it can occur during suckling, or in the stomach, sensitizing and opsonizing bacteria, before they enter the intestines. Although complement is known to be extremely labile, it is little known that it is very acid resistant up to pH 2·4, but sensitive to trypsin and chymotrypsin (see Reiter, 1978).

You mentioned the lactobacilli: many years ago we had investigated the trace metal requirements of some lactic acid bacteria (Reiter and Oram, 1968). For some strains we were unable to show any iron requirements in media made up with "pure" distilled water and spectrographically pure metals unless we also incorporated an iron sequestering compound. The iron requirement of all the strains tested was extremely low.

Concerning Sir Charles's point, I suggest that it is not so much that those defence mechanisms must act against particular pathogens, but that after the neonate is born the intestine is immediately flooded by coliforms. What is needed is the suppression of the coliforms and endotoxins to allow the lactobacilli to emerge. It is not, therefore, only a matter of pathogens. The lactobacillary flora establishes itself very much faster when the neonates are suckled than when they are artificially fed. It is the balance of the flora that is important.

Bullen Taking your last point first, I entirely agree. The real issue is what actually causes the suppression of the *E. coli* in the intestine. We would suggest that it is the IgA antibody.

Reiter I agree.

Bullen Obviously the growth of the lactobacilli could follow on. Theoretically complement could have an effect but this has to be shown, which is a very different matter. If the intestinal contents are anticomplementary, one would not expect complement to work in the gut. As far as I can see, IgA has no bactericidal effect at all, even if the complement is added. Certainly this is true in the case of *Vibrio cholerae*. The point has been made that many samples of IgA have been contaminated with IgM and any bactericidal effect of the sample is a good indication of the degree of contamination with IgM.

Reiter I would like to stress that complement activated bactericidal activity, or at least the initiation of it, is very rapid, so we can assume that during attachment to the bacterial surface will take place. I do not think that anyone has shown that once bactericidal activity has been initiated, anticomplementary activity operates. I gave up the idea of lysozyme after it was disproven for so many years and I am now rather on the other side. Wherever there are high levels of lysozyme there are high levels of lactoferrin and high levels of IgA. In bovine milk it is quite the other way round.

Bullen There is no lysozyme either in bovine tears. Bovines are virtually deficient in lysozyme.

Reiter Yes, even the leukocytes are deficient in lysozyme. They go together and they are probably secreted together later in life.

Bullen I suspect that complement is probably a very efficient bactericidal agent against rough organisms. However, there are large numbers of bacteria against which it has very little effect unless there is specific IgG or IgM present.

Reiter Colostrum in milk is a multifactorial defence mechanism.

Tyrell It seems to me that one of the problems is that there have not been many investigations of real women producing real milk, watching what happens to their babies in relation to the organisms with which they are surrounded. I wonder whether I could get your opinion on whether it would be worth using specific methods for looking independently at specific antibodies against IgA found in milk. One could develop a test to look for that in relation to the serotypes of *E. coli* present in the mother's faeces.

Bullen That has been done; high titres of antibodies are found in human milk against 31 out of 43 strains of *E. coli* that commonly cause gastroenteritis.

Tyrell I am sorry, but you have missed my point. If we make generalizations we shall always be unable to decide whether the specific mother who provides the milk for the specific baby actually provides what that baby needs to control the infections with which it is surrounded. You were saying earlier that there was no evidence on this, that and the other, and I was trying to think of how one would get the sort of evidence that would clarify the matter. It seems to me that one must look at individuals.

Bullen One could certainly do that. If a mother was carrying a particular *E. coli* one could try to see whether or not the milk would inhibit that particular organism.

Tyrell I am sorry, but I am thinking of doing more than that, and dissecting that particular milk and asking whether it contains antibody or lysozyme or transferrin. Is it active as a biological mixture against the organism with which we know that child is being assaulted? Has that been done?

Bullen Not in individual cases, but human milk is active against large numbers of different strains of *E. coli*, although not necessarily against all *E. coli*. In human milk there is a very wide spectrum of IgA antibodies to many serotypes. I agree that any individual case would need to be looked at separately.

Walker-Smith Breast fed babies have far more lactose in their stools than have bottle fed babies. There is a physiological malabsorption of lactose. What do you think is the major reason for the acid pH of the colon of the breast fed baby?

Bullen One imagines this is entirely due to bacterial action. Once you get organisms like *E. coli*, *Strep. faecium* and *Lactobacillus bifidus* growing, they produce acid from the lactose. Eventually, an acetate buffer is produced.

Walker-Smith But do you think it is because of the mere presence of the unabsorbed lactose which has reached the large intestine which is the critical factor?

Bullen Yes, and I am sure this is one of the protective mechanisms. In the bottle fed baby, you cannot detect lactose in the faeces, whereas you can in the breast fed baby. In the bottle fed baby, there is no lactose present in the large intestine for the bacteria to ferment. Therefore, you do not get acetic acid produced, and what is more the buffering capacity of the milk is so high that you do not get a fall in pH.

Soothill In supporting what Dr Bullen has been saying, I should like to stress again that we need not only to kill pathogens but to establish a controlled flora, and for this bacteriostatic mechanisms are more likely to be appropriate than bactericidal ones. Though bactericidal systems are present in human milk, for example, the capacity for the fluid phase to opsonize for phagacytosis and killing by the cells that are in the milk, this process is absolutely swamped by the addition of iron. The question whether we get the right antibody there has been investigated by Hansen, when he fed *E. coli* to pregnant women and showed strain specific IgA-producing cells in their milk, and we know that lymphoid cells from the gut home to the mammary gland. Dr Bullen did not describe the mechanism of interaction of IgA and lactoferrin. I know he knows how this works, and I think it is the most exciting antibody action that has ever been described. He and his colleagues have shown the mechanism for this, and I should like to suggest that we ask him to tell us about it.

Bullen   I will if you like. The association constants for Fe of lactoferrin or transferrin, which are only partly saturated with iron, are so high that the amount of free ionic iron is 10^{-18} M. There is a very interesting evolutionary reason for this. Free ionic iron at concentrations greater than 10^{-18} M, precipitates as ferric hydroxide at neutral pH. Therefore it is a biological necessity that there is a mechanism for preventing ionic iron reaching higher concentrations, otherwise you would have a continuous precipitation of ferric hydroxide. An organism like *E. coli* has to get iron in order to live, and 10^{-18} M Fe is far too little for normal growth. It therefore secretes an iron-chelating agent, called enterochelin. This has roughly the same association constant for Fe as transferrin and can remove iron from unsaturated transferrin. We believe that antibody blocks the mechanism for the transport of enterochelin. Details of this have not been completely worked out yet, but it is suspected that the antibody prevents the secretion of the enterochelin by the organism.

If you by-pass the mechanism by saturating the serum with iron so there are large amounts of free ionic iron present, the bacteria are able to take it up. If haem compounds, like haematin, or haemoglobin, are present then the haem is taken up by the organism in spite of the presence of antibody. Iron binding proteins do not bind haem compounds. It is interesting that one of the most deadly combinations in the peritoneal cavity is *E. coli* and haemoglobin. Investigators found that the bacteria themselves were not very toxic, that the haemoglobin was not toxic, but when the two were mixed together they were very toxic indeed. The reason is that the organisms grow very fast in the presence of haem compounds.

Iron binding proteins cause metabolic alterations in bacteria, and work done by Dr Griffiths has shown that when *E. coli* are grown in an environment very low in iron, such as would occur in serum, they adapt themselves by producing iron-chelating agents. When the organisms are in a situation where there is very little iron, some of the tRNAs change slightly and this causes a shift in their elution pattern. This may be associated with the switching on of enterochelin production. In the case of the gonococci, freshly isolated strains are often resistant to the bactericidal effect of serum yet these become susceptible on cultivation *in vitro*. This bactericidal effect can be reversed by adding iron. It therefore seems likely that the freshly isolated *Gonococcus* has the ability to obtain iron from transferrin. In artificial medium, where plenty of iron is available, the mechanism for acquiring iron from transferrin is probably switched off.

To take another example, there has recently been a paper published by Yancey showing that a mutant of *Salmonella typhimurium* unable to produce enterochelin was not very pathogenic. Addition of enterochelin restored pathogenicity. This is yet another case where iron chelating agents in bacteria appear to be important.

Reiter   Before the "invention" of sIgA and before we knew about the homing to the mammary gland, a veterinarian, Petersen, and his collaborators from 1955 onwards (see Campbell and Petersen, 1963; Reiter, 1978) virtually fought for the acceptance of the mammary gland as an "exocrine endothelial gland"–needless to say with little success. Furthermore, when newborn calves and more recently newborn piglets (Salajka, 1975), were infected orally with *Salmonella pullorum* and *E. coli* respectively, the milk of the dams subsequently contained antibodies which had not been previously detected in the colostra or blood sera. This strongly suggested that the act of suckling infected the mammary glands which responded by producing specific antibodies. So perhaps that answers some of the questions: if the baby is infected with a strain of a serotype against which there are no antibodies in the milk normally, they could be produced on demand.

Chairman   You referred to the stabilizing effect of an acid colonic content in the infant's intestine. How does this stabilizing occur?

Bullen   As far as I know, it is the production of acetic acid from lactose, eventually producing an acetate buffer. As human milk is relatively unbuffered, you get a pH around 5·0–5·5. The lactose in the milk provides the substrate for the bacteria. So presumably they keep on manufacturing the buffer.

Chairman   I can see they will keep on doing it, but I wonder what good it does.

Bullen   If you have a pH of 5·0, you do not get growth of enteric bacteria.

Sir Ashley   It would be interesting to know something, in these investigations in the faecal bacteria, what is happening to the most common organism of them all which overtops *E. coli* a 100-fold or a 1000-fold. What is happening to all the *Bacteroides* organisms? And what is their part in colonization and stimulating or invading the baby?

Bullen   I am sorry I have left this out. I think I am right in saying that in the breast fed infant there are usually about 10 × less *Bacteroides* than in the bottle fed infant.

Sir Ashley   In the adult it is a 100 × more, there is a shattering difference.

Bullen   I am talking about the comparison between the bottle fed and the breast fed infant. The *Bacteroides* definitely are there, I forgot to mention that.

O'Grady   In your slide you were looking at the different IgAs and we were shown the bacteriostatic effect of the specific IgA. In fact, the growth rate of the organism was not altered for several hours and all that happened was that you shut off the size of the climax population.

Bullen   This is perfectly true.

O'Grady   What is the mechanism of that?

Bullen   We assume that what happens is that the organisms have a certain amount of iron when you put them into the medium and they just use it up. The bacteriostatic effect takes a little while to develop.

Sir Ashley   What happens if you use iron starved bacteria as your inoculant? Because then they ought to go straight, flat.

Bullen   I think this has been done and that is what happened, but I cannot swear to it.

Reiter   Schade has done it, with staphylococci. You cannot inhibit staphylococci by transferrin unless you grow them for several generations in an iron limiting medium.

Bullen   Are you talking about *Staph. aureus*?

Reiter   Yes, and Schade did it with transferrin.

Bullen   I think you have to be rather careful with the staphylococci. Most strains of *Staph. albus* are inhibited by serum transferrin, but most strains of *Staph. aureus* are not.

Reiter   He published several papers on this.

Bullen   Yes. But *Staph. aureus* obviously has a very efficient means of acquiring iron from transferrin. This is a very large subject. If you take sickle cell anaemia, for example, you get a much higher incidence of infection. But this is not often linked to the importance of iron binding proteins, and the real point is this. The presence of free haemoglobin in the blood does not interfere with the bactericidal effect of polymorphs. It is only when you put iron into the polymorphs themselves and neutralize the iron binding capacity of lactoferrin there that you get a complete collapse of the protective system. Patients with sickle cell anaemia are more susceptible to various infections, presumably because the presence of free haemoglobin interferes with the ability of the plasma to control extracellular bacterial growth. The polymorphs and the macrophages are quite untouched. However, there are instances where the availability of iron, either as iron salts, or as haem compounds, does have a catastrophic effect. One example, already mentioned, is the presence of haemoglobin in the peritoneal cavity with *E. coli*. Another is the giving of iron dextran to newly born Maori children who were thought to be deficient in iron. In this case the incidence of neonatal sepsis increased by more than tenfold.

Marshall   Infection with *Yersinia enterocolitica* is not uncommon in patients with thalassaemia major (Butzler *et al.*, 1978), whether they have been splenectomized or not. On the other hand infections in general are not excessively prevalent in children with this condition in London.

Bullen   Is this septicaemia?

Marshall   Yes.

Bullen   I am afraid I know nothing about that.

Chairman   This is the very frequently transfused children?

Marshall   Yes.

Bullen   I do not know anything about it.

Faulk   In children with thalassaemia who have received many transfusions one often finds antibodies to transferrin. I was curious to know if these antibodies might interfere in some way with the system that Dr Bullen is telling us about.

Marshall   I am intrigued by this organism, and that it does not necessarily seem to apply to other bacteria. Is there anything unusual about this particular host and this particular bacterium?

Sir Ashley I think John would agree with me in this. The point about haemachromatosis is wrong, I think, because people with haemachromatosis as such with a lot of iron stuffed away in cells are not particularly susceptible to infection. Those who are susceptible are those who suffer from haemolytic anaemias of various sorts. The trouble with investigating their effect is that in malaria and *Bartonella* the bursts of haemolysis come so frequently that you really cannot correlate them with the sudden attacks of salmonellosis of various sorts from which these patients suffer. But in sickle cell anaemias you have haemolytic crises at larger intervals and the fact is, unfortunately for the belief that the haemoglobin in the circulation predisposes to all the nasty things these children die of, these infective episodes have no relation whatsoever to the haemolytic crises. So we have to think very hard about the validity of this notion.

Bullen You would think, in fact, that they probably have got some relationship.

Sir Ashley I think it is perfectly valid thing to use the notion that the free haemoglobin in the plasma would predispose to infection. The trouble with the sickle cell example is that the episodes of infection do not coincide with the crises. By the time the infections come, the haem iron in the plasma has been cleaned up and popped into the liver or wherever it is stuffed.

Chairman Thank you very much. We started with some puzzles and we are left finally with one at the end.

REFERENCES

Adinolfi, M., Glynn, A. H., Lindsa, M. and Milne, C. M. (1966). *Immunology* **10**, 517–526.

Butzler, J. P., Segers, A. A., Cremer, N. and Blum, D. (1978). *Journal of Pediatrics* **93**, 619–621.

Campbell, B. and Petersen, W. E. (1963). *Dairy Science Abstracts* **25**, 345–358.

Reiter, B. (1978). *Journal of Dairy Research* **45**, 131–147.

Reiter, B. and Brock, J. H. (1975). *Immunology* **28**, 71–82.

Reiter, B. and Oran, J. D. (1968). *Journal of Dairy Research* **35**, 67.

Salajka, E., Cernohoks, J. and Sarmanova, Z. (1975). *Documento Veterinaria, Brno* **8**, 43.

Humoral and Cellular Immunities Transmitted by Breastmilk

L. MELLANDER, B. CARLSSON, U. DAHLGREN and L. Å. HANSON

Department of Clinical Immunology,
Institute of Medical Microbiology and Department of
Pediatrics, University of Göteborg, Göteborg, Sweden

In the multifactorial defence system against infections supplied to the neonate via breastmilk, the immunoglobulins play an important role, together with cells and unspecific factors. These include lactoferrin, lysozyme, complement factors, B-12 binding protein, lactoperoxidase and antistaphylococcal and "bifidus" factors (Hanson and Winberg, 1972). In contrast to serum the dominating immunoglobulin class is IgA, with a ratio between milk and serum antibodies against *Escherichia coli* O and K antigens which always exceeds 1. The mean ratios for antibodies of IgG and IgM classes seldom attain 1 (Table I). This indicates a local production of IgA antibodies while the IgG and IgM levels seem to be the result of transfer from serum or at least a very limited local production. The fact that these IgA antibodies almost exclusively belong to the secretory IgA type (SIgA) also

TABLE I.

Mean ratio for antibody levels in milk v. serum in samples from day 5 after parturition. (Range in brackets.)

	Antibodies against			
	Pool of 8 O antigens	Homologous O antigen	5 K antigens (mean)	K1 antigen
IgA	16·46	16·71	4·29	4·56
	(2·0–90·0)	(1·1–120·0)	(0·5–19·6)	(0·7–19·6)
IgG	0·22	0·23	0·39	0·34
	(0·0–0·5)	(0·0–0·9)	(0·0–2·0)	(0·0–1·5)
IgM	0·56	0·55	0·34	0·34
	(0·0–1·6)	(0·0–3·0)	(0·0–1·1)	(0·0–0·73)
Number	29	29	23	23

suggests local production (Hanson, 1961; Tomasi and Bienenstock, 1968). SIgA is composed of two IgA monomers stabilized by two polypeptide chains, the J chain and the secretory component. SIgA seems to be common to all mucous membranes and the molecule is specially resistant to variations in pH or degradation of enzymes (Tomasi and Bienenstock, 1968; Lindh, 1975) which is of importance for providing efficient local immunity in the variable milieux of secretions and mucous membranes, e.g. in the respiratory, gastrointestinal or genitourinary tract.

MILK ANTIBODIES RELATE TO INTESTINAL EXPOSURE

The milk SIgA antibodies are directed against several different structures on, for example, Gram negative bacteria. Thus there are antibodies against *E. coli* O and K antigens, *Salmonella, Shigella* and *Vibrio cholerae* O antigens and also against enterotoxins of *E. coli* and *V. cholerae* (Kenny *et al.*, 1967; Gindrat *et al.*, 1972, Holmgren *et al.*, 1976; Carlsson *et al.*, 1976 b; 1979 a, b). The consistent finding of antibodies in human milk against enterobacterial antigens is difficult to explain unless there is a link between the gut and the mammary gland. Swedish mothers, who are less exposed to "enteropathogenic" *E. coli* have significantly lower levels of milk antibodies to O antigens of such strains than Pakistani women (Ahlstedt *et al.*, 1977). The same is true for antibodies against enterotoxins from *E. coli* and *V. cholerae* (Holmgren *et al.*, 1976). The milk also contains antibodies against viruses such as rotavirus (Simhon and Mata, 1978) and poliovirus (Hodes *et al.*, 1964). Recently it was shown that there are also antibodies in human milk against parasites. Thus in samples from Ethiopia, Pakistan and Bangladesh, SIgA antibodies were detected utilizing the enzyme linked immunosorbent assay, (ELISA), against membrane as well as somatic antigens from *Entamoeba histolytica* Antibodies to *Giardia lamblia* were also detected in these samples by immunofluorescense and the whole parasite as antigen. Milk samples from Guatemala never contained amoeba antibodies and few were positive for *Giardia* (G. Huldt, 1979, pers. comm.).

Not only antigens from micro-organisms in the gut influence the milk antibody levels. We have found significantly lower SIgA milk antibody levels to cows' milk proteins in milk from mothers in Guatemala belonging to a social group which does not include cows' milk in their daily diet as compared to the more affluent Guatemala women who do. Mothers who could afford a regular cows' milk intake had higher levels of antibodies to cows' milk proteins.

A more definite proof of a link between antigenic stimulation in the intestine and the presence of milk antibodies was obtained in our studies, when women in late pregnancy were colonized with a harmless *E. coli* 083 strain. A few days later IgA plaque-forming elements appeared in the milk with specificity for the O antigen of the colonizing strain. There was no simultaneous serum antibody response (Goldblum *et al.*, 1975). Similar results were obtained using a live oral *Shigella* vaccine (Carlsson *et al.*, 1979 c), where IgA plaque forming cells were detected in milk from 6 out of 15 mothers without any influence on the serum antibody levels.

Oral immunization of rabbits (Montgomery *et al.*, 1974) and swine (Bohl and Saif, 1975) also resulted in the appearance of antibodies in their milk. Allardyce *et al.* (1974) showed that *Salmonella typhimurium* infection in humans during lactation resulted in antibodies in the milk.

MILK ANTIBODIES CAN BE USED AS AN EPIDEMIOLOGICAL TOOL

It is obvious that the breast fed babies get considerable amounts of SIgA antibodies directed against a variety of micro-organisms which are prevalent in their surroundings. Thus women living in countries where various *Salmonella* and *Shigella* are common have higher milk antibody levels against these pathogens than less exposed Swedish women (Table II). Preliminary observations in Pakistan suggest that severely undernourished women produce extremely low milk volumes, which will diminish their total output of antibodies but the relative antibody levels are high and at the same level as in a Swedish population (Carlsson *et al.*, 1976 a). Studies of chronically malnourished mothers in Guatemala showed that their ability to produce SIgA antibodies in response to an antigenic challenge is not impaired since the highest levels of antibodies to *Salmonella* C were found

TABLE II.

The enteromammaric link seems to give epidemiological information. Means of IgA antibody levels in milk samples from 1 month after delivery measured with the ELISA and expressed in % of a reference serum.

Micro-organism	Milk samples from						
	Sweden $n=16$ $*n=5$	Pakistan under nourished $n=13$	Guatemala			Ethiopia	
			rural $n=19$	urban poor $n=21$	urban elite $n=20$	urban poor $n=7$	urban elite $n=5$
E. coli (8 common strains)	72		14	17	37	15	34
E. coli (enteropathogenic)	6	19					
Salmonella							
C1	9		12	21	31	17	27
E1	4		16	21	27	11	31
Shigella sonnei (D)	16*		15	59	58		
flexneri (B6)	71*		102	124	118		

concomitantly with the lowest concentration of total SIgA (Hanson *et al.*, 1979 b). The influence of undernutrition on milk volumes, however, needs to be further investigated.

ANTIGENIC EXPOSURE CAN RESULT IN ANTIBODY FORMATION AT DISTANT SITES

Different mechanisms can be considered to explain the appearance of antibodies in milk after antigenic exposure on various mucosal sites. Transport of antigen from the gastrointestinal tract, stimulating immunocompetent cells in the mammary gland, is possible, but no serum antibody response has been observed in experiments where intestinal immunization has resulted in a milk antibody response (Montgomery *et al.*, 1974; Goldblum *et al.*, 1975). Since it has been shown that hepatocytes have the capacity to specifically pick up IgA from serum (Lemaître-Coelho *et al.*, 1977) the question arose whether a similar mechanism could account for the secretory IgA antibodies found in the milk. We have tried to study this possibility in rats immunized perorally with *E. coli* 06 bacteria, which resulted in milk antibody levels higher than in serum. After blocking the passage of bile from the liver to the intestine, an increase was shown in serum IgA levels against the 06 bacteria used for the vaccination. No increase was noted in the milk, so uptake of IgA from serum into the secreted milk appears unlikely.

A more probable explanation is that specific IgA-producing cells home to the mammary gland after they have been exposed to antigens from the intestinal content in the Peyer's patches (PP). This may be part of a generalized homing process of IgA-producing cells to mucous membranes and exocrine glands from the PP.

IgA-producing cells from mucous membranes in the intestine as well as the respiratory tract can be provided by cells from the PP, or from bronchus associated lymphoid tissue (BALT). (Craig and Cebra, 1971; Rudzik *et al.*, 1975). It has also been shown that antigenic stimulation in the gut is followed by migration of specialized lymphoid cells from the PP via the mesenteric lymph nodes to other parts of the gut mucosa where they produce IgA antibodies (Robertsson and Cebra, 1976; Pierce, 1978). The secretory IgA response is not only transferred from PP in the intestine to the mammary gland but also to the intestine, the lacrymal and salivary glands and possibly also the urinary and respiratory tracts (Hanson and Brandtzaeg, 1980). Milk taken from rats with experimental *E. coli* pyelonephritis shows an increase in IgA antibodies against the infecting strain. The respiratory tract also showed on IgA antibody response against the pyelonephritis causing bacteria, but no IgA antibodies were detected in serum (Hanson *et al.*, 1979 b).

The migration of IgA-producing cells from PP has been proposed to be directed by a specific mechanism. There are indications that the homing to the mammary gland is dependent on hormonal factors. The number of plasma cells found intra-epithelially increased during late pregnancy and the beginning of lactation. This increase of IgA-producing cells was parallel to the proliferation of the glandular epithelium (Weisz-Carrington *et al.*, 1977). The same cellular effects seen during lactation could be induced by treating virgin animals with progesterone, oestrogen and prolactin (Weisz-Carrington *et al.*, 1978). Studies by Klareskog *et al.* (1979) suggest that Ia antigens on epithelial cells of exocrine glands might direct the homing. These Ia antigens could be detected on epithelial cells in the mammary gland of lactating animals but were absent in virgin animals and could be induced by lactogenic hormones.

Elson *et al.* (1979) have proposed a somewhat different model for the mechanisms underlying the IgA cell traffic. When IgA B cells are induced by antigen in the PP, they leave and drain into the mesenteric lymph node from where they randomly distribute throughout the body. Terminally they differentiate and lodge in sites where there is sufficient specific IgA T helper cells. The ratio for helper to suppressor activities of these IgA specific T cells varies for different tissues. Peyer's patches T cells were found to contain particularly high levels of IgA T cell helper activity as compared to that of peripheral lymph nodes or spleen. It is likely that an antigenic stimulation in the PP could induce a strong IgA response at the same time as the IgG and IgM responses are suppressed. Pittard and Bill (1979) have shown that when the supernatant from incubated early milk cells was added to peripheral blood lymphocytes IgA synthesis was significantly increased but no effect was shown on the IgG or IgM synthesis. This effect was absent when supernatant from more mature milk cells was used.

EFFECTS OF VACCINATION ON MILK SIgA

It has been demonstrated that immunity against, e.g. cholera in mice is primarily due to secretory IgA antibodies against the bacteria and its enterotoxin (Lange and Holmgren, 1978). Studies have shown that parenteral cholera vaccination in previously nonvaccinated women living in endemic areas results in boosting of serum antibodies as well as milk and saliva SIgA antibodies. Previously parenterally vaccinated women in nonendemic areas respond only with serum antibodies without any or very slight temporary increase in their milk and saliva antibody levels after parenteral boosting. The same increase in milk antibody level was seen after parenteral polio vaccination of women in endemic areas. Surprisingly milk antibodies decreased if the booster was given perorally with live polio vaccine (Svennerholm *et al.*, 1979).

The results indicate that it is possible to improve the passive immunity transferred to the baby via breastmilk after vaccination. If peroral vaccination with live polio vaccine in endemic areas diminishes the SIgA response and so decreases intestinal protection this can be of clinical and epidemiological importance. The interpretation of these findings is not yet apparent but they could be explained by recent observations that immunological unresponsiveness may be detected at local sites as well as in the serum after intestinal antigen exposure. This unresponsiveness seems to be mediated by T suppressor lymphocytes from the spleen (Richman, 1979; Mattingly and Waksman, 1978).

THE CELLULAR IMMUNE RESPONSE

Large numbers of leukocytes are present in human milk during late pregnancy and the first weeks of lactation. Colostrum has the highest cell count varying from $1 \cdot 1 \times 10^5$–$1 \cdot 2 \times 10^7$ cells ml^{-1} (Mestecky *et al.*, 1979). At the end of the first week after delivery the cell count has decreased to about 10^5 cells ml^{-1}. Macrophages constitute 30–80% of the total cell count, the remaining cells are neutrophil granulocytes and T and B lymphocytes.

Little information is available about the function and role of the macrophages in breast milk. The proportion of phagocytic cells shows great variations between different individuals. Macrophages in colostrum and milk are presumably involved in the defence against infections both in the breast and in the neonatal gut. The phagocytic capacity of colostral cells is comparable to that of peripheral blood cells and the proportion of phagocytic cells is even higher than in blood. Fresh human colostral cells can ingest and to some extent also kill organisms like *Candida albicans* and *E. coli* (Ho and Lawton, 1978). The killing of bacteria like *E. coli* takes place after opsonization utilizing the classical pathway for complement activation (Robinson *et al.*, 1978). Macrophages might also play a role in the defence against micro-organisms in the infant's gut via their content of IgA, lysozyme, C4 and transferrin (Pittard *et al.*, 1977). The cytoplasm of macrophages contains SIgA antibodies and it is suggested that these cells can function as a transport vehicle or storage for immunoglobulins in the breast milk (Pittard *et al.*, 1977). Some data also indicate that the macrophages amplify the T cell reactivity either by direct cellular co-operation or by processing the antigen (Ogra and Ogra, 1979).

About 50% of the lymphocytes in colostrum or milk are recognized as T lymphocytes (Diaz-Jouanen and Williams, 1974; Smith and Goldman, 1978). These cells have lately been examined for reactivity to mitogens and antigens and their response to a number of microbial antigens, such as *Candida albicans*, tetanus toxoid and streptokinase is surprisingly low compared to peripheral blood lymphocytes from the same donors. Colostral cells, however, respond to other antigens like mumps as well as blood lymphocytes do (Parmely *et al.*, 1977). These data suggests that the milk T lymphocytes represent a selected cell population different from peripheral blood lymphocytes. Some studies have shown that unseparated milk cell populations respond to a lower degree to stimulation with PHA than purified T cells, which means that there might be a specific mechanism suppressing T cell reactivity. Cell free supernatants from colostrum and milk can also suppress the proliferation of milk cells after stimulation with PHA. The mechanisms behind this suppression are not yet determined (Ogra and Ogra, 1979).

Information about the immunological benefits for the newborn transmitted by the ingested immunocompetent cells is still relatively deficient. There is some evidence that a cell mediated local immunity is transferred to the baby since tuberculin positivity has been demonstrated in babies after breast feeding (Mohr, 1972; Schlesinger and Covelli, 1977). It has also been suggested that partly digested cells or smaller molecules transported by the T cells, like transfer factor or migration inhibitory factor can be transferred to the breast fed baby (Diaz-Jouanen and Williams, 1974). Recent studies in experimental animals (Head *et al.*, 1977) have also provided some evidence that the suckling can passively provide resistance to a syngeneic tumour through the milk of resistant mothers.

Most B lymphocytes in colostrum or milk bear surface IgA (Diaz-Jouanen and Williams, 1974) and are also thought to produce IgA antibodies (Murillo and Goldman, 1970). This is in variance with the findings of Pittard *et al.*, (1977) who found no active synthesis of IgA. The same authors proposed that the immunoglobulins in milk originate from colostral macrophages which may be passive transport vehicles for IgA. These discrepancies might be explained by the findings which show that IgA synthesis by B cells to be regulated by a separate set of T cells (Elson *et al.*, 1979). Pittard and Bill (1979) have lately demonstrated that colostral cells in culture produce a soluble factor which serves as a regulator of B lymphocyte differentiation. Cell free media from colostral cells stimulates IgA synthesis in peripheral blood cells, while IgG and IgM synthesis is not affected. This factor may also play a role in the maturation of immune response in the gastrointestinal tract of the newborn. Several difficulties are, however, still involved in separation and characterization of the milk cells.

The most recent studies have just started to elucidate the selective mechanisms involved in the mammary gland to enrich colostrum and milk with immunoglobulins and cellular components. The role of the ingested lymphocytes in the intestine of the newborn has yet to be fully explained.

SUMMARY

Human milk provides the breast fed baby with various defence factors of humoral and cellular character. Immunoglobulins, especially SIgA with specificity for many enterobacteria, viruses or parasites play an important role together with other factors like lactoferrin, lysozyme and complement. There seems to be a close link between antigenic stimulation in the intestine and the occurrence of specific antibodies in the breast milk. This means that milk antibodies can possibly provide epidemiological information and it has also been shown that an existing mammary gland response can be boosted by vaccination. There are also a large number of leukocytes present in milk as macrophages, neutrophil granulocytes, and T and B lymphocytes.

REFERENCES

Ahlstedt, S., Carlsson, B., Fällström, S. P., Hanson, L. Å., Holmgren, J., Lidin Janson, G., Lindblad, B. S., Jodal, U., Kaijser, B., Sohl Åkerlund, A. and Wadsworth, C. (1977). "Immunology of the gut", 115–134. Ciba Foundation Symposium No. 46 (new series). Elsevier, Exerpta Medica, North-Holland.

Allardyce, R. A., Shearman, D. J. C., McClelland, D. B. L., Marwick, K., Simpson, A. J. and Laidlaw, R. B. (1974). Appearance of specific colostrum antibodies after clinical infection with *Salmonella typhimurium*. *British Medical Journal* **3**, 307–309.

Bohl, E. H. and Saif, L. J. (1975). Passive immunity in transmittable gastroenteritis of swine: Immunoglobulin characteristics of antibodies in milk after inoculating virus by different routes. *Infection and Immunity* **11**, 23–32.

Carlsson, B., Ahlstedt, S., Hanson, L. Å., Lidin-Jansson, G., Lindblad, B. S. and Sultana, R. (1976 a). *Escherichia coli* O antibody content in milk from healthy Swedish mothers and mothers from a very low socio-economic group of a developing country. *Acta Paediatrica Scandinavica* **65**, 417–423.

Carlsson, B., Gothefors, L., Ahlstedt, S., Hanson, L. Å. and Winberg, J. (1976 b). Studies of *Escherichia coli* O antigen specific antibodies in human milk, maternal serum and cord blood. *Acta Paediatrica Scandinavica* **65**, 216–224.

Carlsson, B., Cruz, J. R., Garcia, B., Hanson, L. Å. and Urrutia, J. J. (1979 a). "Nutrition and metabolism of the fetus and infant", 263–273. Nutricia Symposium V. Martinus Nijhoff, North-Holland.

Carlsson, B., Kaijser, B., Ahlstedt, S., Gothefors, L. and Hanson, L. Å. (1979 b). Antibodies against *Escherichia coli* capsular K antigens in human milk and serum. Their relation to the *E. coli* gut flora of the mother and neonate. *Acta Paediatrica Scandinavica* in press.

Carlsson, B., Meitert, T., Garon, E., Cogulescu, L. and Hanson, L. Å. (1979 c). Antibody response in breast milk after oral immunization of pregnant women with a live *Shigella* vaccine. In preparation.

Crago, S. S., Prince, T. G., Pretlow, J. R., McGhee, J. R. and Mestecky, J. (1979). Human colostral cells. I. Separation and characterization. *Clinical Experimental Immunology*. Submitted for publication.

Craig, S. W. and Cebra, J. J. (1971). Peyer's patches: An enriched source of precursors for IgA-producing immunocytes in the rabbit. *Journal of Experimental Medicine* **134**, 188–200.

Diaz-Jouanen, E. and Williams Jr., R. C. (1974). T and B lymphocytes in human colostrum. *Clinical Immunology and Immunopathology* **3**, 248–255.

Elson, C. O., Heck, J. A. and Strober, W. (1979). T cell regulation of murine IgA synthesis. *Journal of Experimental Medicine* **149**, 632–643.

Gindrat, J.-J., Gothefors, L., Hanson, L. Å. and Winberg, J. (1972). Antibodies in human milk against *E. coli* of the serogroups most commonly found in neonatal infections. *Acta Paediatrica Scandinavia* **61**, 587–590.

Goldblum, R. M., Ahlstedt, S., Carlsson, B., Hanson, L. Å., Jodal, U., Lidin-Janson, G., Sohl Åkerlund, A. (1975). Antibody-forming cells in human colostrum after oral immunization. *Nature* **257**, 797–799.

Hanson, L. Å. (1961). Comparative immunological studies of the immune globulins of human milk and of blood serum. *International Archives of Allergy* **18**, 241–267.

Hanson, L. Å. and Brandtzaeg, P. (1980). Mucosal defence system. *In* "Immunologic Disorders in Infants and Children", 2nd edn (Eds. E. R. Stiehm and W. A. Fulginiti) 137–164. Saunders, Philadelphia.

Hanson, L. Å. and Winberg, J. (1972). Breast milk and defence against infection in the newborn. *Archives of Disease in Childhood* **47**, 845–848.

Hanson, L. Å., Andersson, B., Carlsson, B., Cruz, J. R., Dahlgren, U., Mattsby Baltzer, I. and Svanborg Edén, C. (1979). The secretory IgA system and mucosal defence. *Scandinavian Journal of Infectious Diseases*. In press.

Hanson, L. Å., Carlsson, B., Cruz, J. R., Garcia, B., Holmgren, J., Khan, S. R., Lindblad, B. S., Svennerholm, A.-M., Svennerholm, B. and Urrutia, J. (1979 b). The immune response in the mammary gland. National Institute of Child Health and Human Development Conference on the Immunology of Breast Milk. In press.

Head, J. R., Beer, A. E. and Billingham, R. E. (1977). Significance of the cellular component of the maternal immunologic endowment in milk. *Transplantation Proceedings* **9**, 1465–1471.

Ho, P. C. and Lawton, J. W. M. (1978). Human colostral cells: Phagocytosis and killing of *E. coli* and *C. albicans*. *Journal of Pediatrics* **93**, 910–915.

Hodes, H. L., Berger, R., Ainbender, E., Hevizy, M. M., Zepp, H. D. and Kochwa, S. (1964). Proof that colostrum polio antibody is different from serum antibody. *Journal of Pediatrics* **65**, 1017–1018.

Holmgren, J., Hanson, L. Å., Carlsson, B., Lindblad, B. S. and Rahimtoola, J. (1976). Neutralizing antibodies against *E. coli* and *V. cholerae* enterotoxins in human milk from a developing country. *Scandinavian Journal of Immunology* **5**, 867–871.

Kenny, J. F., Boesman, M. I. and Michaels, R. H. (1967). Bacterial and viral coproantibodies in breast-fed infants. *Pediatrics* **39**, 202–213.

Klareskog, L., Forsum, U. and Peterson, P. A. (1979). Hormonal regulation of the expression of Ia-antigens on mammary gland epithelium. In preparation.

Lange, S. and Holmgren, J. (1978). Protective antitoxic cholera immunity in mice: Influence of route and number of immunications and mode of action of protective antibodies. *Acta Pathologica et Microbiologica Scandinavica Section C* **86**, 145–152.

Lemaître-Coelho, I., Jackson, G. D. F. and Vaerman, J. P. (1977). Rat bile is a convenient source of secretory IgA and free secretory component. *European Journal of Immunology* **8**, 588–590.

Lindh, E. (1975). Increased resistance of immunoglobulin A dimers to proteolytic degradation after binding of secretory component. *Journal of Immunology* **114**, 284–286.

Mattingly, J. A. and Waksman, B. H. (1978). Immunologic suppression after oral administration of antigen. I. Specific suppressor cells formed in rat Peyer's patches after oral administration of sheep erythrocytes and their systemic migration. *Journal of Immunology* **121**, 1878–1883.

Mohr, J. A. (1972). Lymphocyte sensitization passed to the child from the mother. *Lancet* **i**, 688–689.

Mohr, J. A., Leu, R. and Mabry, W. (1970). Colostral leucocytes, *Journal of Surgical and Oncology* **2**, 163–167.

Montgomery, P. C., Rosner, B. R. and Cohn, J. (1974). The secretory antibody response. Anti-DNP antibodies induced by dinitrophenylated type III pneumococcus. *Immunological Communications* **3**, 143–156.

Murillo, G. J. and Goldman, A. S. (1970). The cells of human colostrum. II. Synthesis of IgA and β1 c. *Pediatric Research* **4**, 71–75.

Ogra, S. S. and Ogra, P. L. (1979). Components of immunologic reactivity in human colostrum and milk. National Institute of Child Health and Human Development Conference on the Immunology of Breast Milk. In press.

Parmely, M. J., Beer, A. E. and Billingham, R. E. (1977). In vitro studies on the T-lymphocyte population of human milk. *Journal of Experimental Medicine* **144**, 358–370.

Pierce, N. F. (1978). The role of antigen form and function in the primary and secondary intestinal immune response to cholera toxin and toxoid in rats. *Journal of Experimental Medicine* **148**, 195–206.

Pittard, W. B. and Bill, K. (1979). Immunoregulation by breast milk cells. *Cellular Immunity* **42**, 437–441.

Pittard, W. B., Polmar, S. H. and Fanaroff, A. A. (1977). The breast milk macrophage: a potential vehicle for immunoglobulin transport. *Journal of Reticuloendothelial Society* **22**, 597–603.

Richman, L. K. (1979). Immunological unresponsiveness after enteric administration of protein antigens. National Institute of Child Health and Human Development Conference on the Immunology of Breast Milk. In press.

Robertsson, S. M. and Cebra, J. J. (1976). A model for local immunity. *Ric. Clin. Lab.* **6**, (Suppl. 3), 105.

Robinson, J. E., Harvey, B. A. and Soothill, J. F. (1978). Phagocytosis and killing of bacteria and yeast by human milk cells after opsonisation in aqueous phase of milk. *British Medical Journal* **1,** 1443–1445.

Rudzik, O., Clancy, R., Perey, D., Dry, R. and Bienenstock, J. (1975). Repopulation with IgA containing cells of bronchial and intestinal lamina propria after transfer of homologous Peyer's patches and bronchial lymphocytes. *Journal of Immunology* **114,** 1599–1604.

Schlesinger, J. J. and Covelli, H. D. (1977). Evidence for transmission of lymphocyte responses to tuberculin by breast-feeding. *Lancet* **ii,** 529–532.

Simhon, A. and Mata, L. J. (1978). Anti-rotavirus antibody in human colostrum. *Lancet* **i,** 39–40.

Smith, C. W. and Goldman, A. S. (1978). The cells of human colostrum. I. *In vitro* studies of morphology and functions. *Pediatric Research* **2,** 103–109.

Svennerholm, A.-M., Hanson, L. Å., Holmgren, J., Lindblad, B. S., Kahn, S., Nilsson, A., and Svennerholm, B. (1980). Milk antibody responses to live and killed polio vaccines in Pakistani and Swedish women. *Journal of Infectious Diseases*, in press.

Tomasi, T. B. and Bienenstock, J. (1968). Secretory immunoglobulins. "Advances in Immunology", Vol. 9, 1–96. Academic Press, New York.

Weisz-Carrington, P., Roux, M. E. and Lamm, M. E. (1978). Plasma cells and epithelial immunoglobulins in the mouse gland during pregnancy and lactation. *Journal of Immunology* **119,** 1306–1309.

DISCUSSION

Allinson   Do you think that it could be a feasible proposition in Africa or some other continent to feed women deliberately with killed strains of *E. coli* which are known to be pathogenic to increase and broaden the specificity of this type of protection?

Mellander   We think so, and we are working on finding out more about it, especially just before weaning when we know the child will have a hard time. Maybe just before weaning you could vaccinate the mother against what is at that moment prevalent, and then we would try to see how that affects the growth of the child.

Walker   The work with which I am familiar from your laboratory and from other studies is that functioning of the enteromammary immune system requires a hormonal environment that exists during the third trimester of pregnancy. I am asking if oral immunization during active nursing is as effective as that occurring in the third trimester of pregnancy.

Mellander   We do not know this yet. In Pakistan we are doing vaccination trials at different times. Also, you can see that on the *E. coli* 083 trial we did not get any milk antibodies because it was too early. We have to find an optimum time. But I think in an urban setting in a developing country there is the problem that they stop breast feeding very early because they have to.

Walker The other question I have is that generally speaking cholera toxin is an excellent adjuvant and you showed that there is a decrease in poliovirus antibodies when polio vaccine was used in conjunction with the cholera vaccine. Is it possible that there is some competition for immune responsiveness between the two vaccines?

Mellander It has been described also for yellow fever vaccine together with cholera vaccine.

Walker Cholera vaccine *per se* produces a highly positive antibody response. I do not have a good explanation for it and I just wondered if you had an alternate explanation.

Hayward You would expect in part that the most dangerous organisms for the infant would be those most likely to infect the mother, and so you would expect her in part perhaps already to be primed. And attempts to immunize her against less prevalent organisms which might improve her antibody response against those organisms might be less useful to the baby since the baby would be less likely to meet them. What I actually wanted to ask you was that since selective IgA deficiency is quite common, what happens to the babies of mothers with selective IgA deficiency?

Mellander We have only seen one case. Maybe somebody else knows.

Chairman Does anybody know?

Soothill Which of these antibodies in milk interfere with immunization? Is it still accepted that high levels of anti-polio antibody interfere with immunization with oral polio vaccine? Does this occur with other vaccines?

Faulk I should like to ask your opinion about a study done at a Nutritional Institute in India. They set out to test the hypothesis that breast fed babies would absorb the IgA from the mother's milk and that the serum IgA in the baby would thus be higher. What they in fact found was that all immunoglobulins in the breast fed infants were higher, and these were higher even in those infants whose mother's milk did not contain immunoglobulin. This implies the most intriguing concept that breast milk perhaps contained adjuvant or something as yet ill defined that switches on the child's immunoglobulin synthesis. Has this been followed up, and what are your ideas on that study?

Mellander I do not know if I am in line with your question, but it was reported that IgA from saliva and nasal secretion in newborn babies showed quicker and higher responses in those who were breast fed than those who were bottle fed.

Faulk That is true, but is there any evidence that breast milk contains a substance which causes breast fed infants to synthesize more immunoglobulins?

Mellander We have no data on that.

Soothill One example has been described; when piglets were fed milk from mothers who were immunized to an antigen which had antibody, the response to parenteral immunization of the offspring was greater than in those which had not received such antibody. If we assume that piglets absorb IgA through the gut, we have got the surprising finding that if you give an antigen with IgA antibody to it, the response is greater than if you give the antigen alone. This is a specific effect but, of course, if you had a wide diversity of IgA antibodies to intestinal antigens being absorbed it could explain the phenomenon; unfortunately I do not think that humans absorb IgA.

Walker I am not sure that that is entirely accurate, that SIgA can be absorbed from the gut of newborn piglets because Dr P. Porter reported several years ago that secretory component present on dimeric IgA blocked uptake of this antibody from the gut.

Soothill Such an effect could result from the proportions of the IgA which is monomer.

Reeves I wonder if you would expand on the statement in your abstract about the fact that homing of the lymphoid cells from Peyers patches to the mammary gland is directed by Ia antigens which are under hormonal control. Are you referring to Ia antigens on the lymphoid cells, on the epithelial cells, or both, and could you say a little more about the hormonal control.

Mellander There are indications that Ia antigens on the epithelial cells are under hormonal control.

Walker Dr Michael Lamm in an experimental animal model (mouse) has shown that in nonpregnant mice, hormones of pregnancy can effect the homing of lymphocytes to breast tissues, so this suggests the homing phenomenon is under hormonal influence.

Marshall Cytomegalovirus is excreted in breast milk, and it has been suggested that this may be the source of infection for some infants. Is it known whether there is also antibody to CMV in the milk?

Mellander Yes, there is.

Tyrrell I want to return to the table in which you showed that there were specific plaque-forming cells, and often in milk in which there was no detectable antibody, if I understood the table correctly. Could you tell us whether you think these cells are important in mediating immunity? What evidence is there that this may be so?

Mellander You mean the cells produced or carried the IgA?

Tyrrell I understood that they are found in the milk and therefore will get to the baby. The question is: can they protect, and if so, how?

Mellander There has been discussion on which kind of cell we have found, if this is a B cell producing antibodies or if it is a macrophage carrying the IgA. The cell is not properly identified, but we believe that most are IgA producing cells as such a specific antibody was produced and a macrophage should not carry such specific antibodies but more of a mixture. If it is a macrophage carrying these antibodies into the gut, we do not know its effect.

Tyrrell You have no experimental or observational data as to whether it protects or not?

Mellander No.

Smith What proportion of the secretory IgA in the milk is absorbed?

Reiter Only minimal amounts, (Ogra and Ogra, 1979).

Walker How can you show that degree of transport of secretory IgA? There have been several papers showing that there has been no or very little transport.

Smith There is some epidemiological evidence from Philip Gardner's work that breast feeding may protect against respiratory syncytial virus infection. I just wonder what mechanism you envisage might be responsible.

Mellander It has been discussed, that if the milk contains RS antibodies and is inhaled it is protecting the mucosa.

Denman Whilst we are on the subject of transport, what mechanisms have been shown to exist whereby cells or the products of cells obtained through the milk by the infant can be absorbed from the gastrointestinal tract and can reach functional lymphoid cells or sites of lymphoid cell proliferation in the newborn baby?

Mellander I do not know any good study, but I think there are other people here who know more about it.

Soothill Infants with severe combined immunodeficiency breast fed by their mothers do not die of GVH, so the number of lymphoid cells getting in must be small.

Adinolfi Beer and Billingham claim that the T cells present in colostrum can produce graft v. host reaction in newborn rats and mice. These are complex experiments, but in certain maternofetal combinations, they have shown GVH in the newborn following lactation.

Denman What is the cell doing to protect itself against digestion whilst it is waiting to be absorbed?

Adinolfi Why they are not digested, you mean?

Denman Yes, we are all familiar with the idea that large lymphocytes are excreted from the lumen of the gastrointestinal tract into the lumen as the final end stage of that cell's traffic pattern, but for it to go into reverse stretches credulity a little.

Walker There is some indirect evidence that cellular immunity can be transmitted from mother to infant. I do not think there is any evidence that it is via cell transport as opposed to cell breakdown products.

Hayward Obviously there are a lot of red herrings in milk, and I assume that antigen is transferred that way too, and that could be responsible for the transfer of some cell mediated immunity to babies occasionally.

Walker That is true. There is evidence that cow's milk protein can be transmitted into human milk. Also I have a comment about cytomegalovirus; Beer has shown that tissue cultured lymphoid cells from human milk release cytomegalovirus, and so presumably the virus in some way is attached to the lymphoid cell or in the extracellular fluid that has been separated, so presumably CMV can also be transmitted via human milk to the offspring.

Chairman Do you know about antibodies in milk to CMV? That is the question that Dr Marshall asked earlier on, do you know the answer to that, whether antibody to CMV is found in milk? Is it in saliva, do you know?

Walker I do not know.

Wood I have read a report somewhere which I would have thought ought to be confirmed, but there are reasons why it may be difficult to do so, to suggest that infants born to mothers who are tuberculin positive may show some reactivity to tuberculin injected into them, whereas this is not so to mothers who are tuberculin negative. Dr Hayward's comments about antigen transfer in breast milk may also apply to that in that there may be protein from tubercle bacillus in breast milk, but I would have thought that the amount was likely to be very small.

Hayward It is a study by Leikin Wang and Oppenheim, is it not? Dr Walker, are you associated with Gill? They showed antigen transfer.

Walker Yes.

Faulk That is an interesting point because there is another route through which the child might receive antigen and that, of course, is through the placenta. There is a rather nice study by Thomas Gill where he showed in an animal model that the offspring of mothers immunized with a particular antigen, when immunized with the same antigen, gave a secondary rather than a primary response. So there could be a lot going on in addition to transmission of antigen through breast milk.

Wood There are two human reports of a similar kind. One is concerned with delayed hypersensitivity to mumps antigen in an Eskimo isolate. That sounds a bit unlikely, but I think it is true. It relates to the detection of positives in the offspring of mothers who were involved in a mumps epidemic some time before they were pregnant. Now was that a transmission of immunity, or of antigens? Field and Caspary more recently drew attention to the fact that *in vitro* you could show that the lymphocytes of infants born to tuberculin positive mothers were reactive to tuberculin. That is not a matter of breast milk; it sounds like some transplacental thing.

Cooper Dr Mellander, I should like to ask if there has been any work on the necessity for local antigenic stimulation to get the greatest antibody response in milk. Cebra showed that the clones of IgA precursor B cells were initially stimulated in Peyers patches and then seeded to the lamina propria of the rest of the gut. But if he did not repeat the antigenic stimulation locally, the antibody response was fairly shortlived and was not of great magnitude. One would think that the same requirement for local antigenic boost for a heightened and prolonged IgA antibody response would exist for the breast as well. Is there evidence for that?

Mellander Presumably not since specific IgA milk antibody titres stay high all through lactation.

Chairman What was the local stimulus? I did not quite follow that.

Cooper The basic principle is that an antigen entering at a random site in the gut will probably not encounter the clones necessary to respond to it, whereas antigen entering through the Peyer's patches will stimulate appropriate clones which then escape from there, go around the circulation, and then home to the lamina propria. Now the same antigen will find the appropriate clone regardless of its entry site along the gut epithelium. This second step of local antigen stimulation seems to be required for the most optimal response. One would think that the second step would be important in gaining higher levels of IgA antibody in milk.

Chairman   Yes, it seems relevant.

Allison   How do you propose to introduce antigen into the breast?

Cooper   I think that that is constantly done by the feeding baby. As a matter of fact, I think there is a term for it–diathelial immunization.

Reiter   In fact, there was a pilgrimage to Göteborg by all the pig people to try to find the best ways of oral vaccination and the most important point which has come out is that you can only vaccinate effectively with live vaccine, not just feeding antigens.

Wood   There was talk about Peyer's patches just now, and Max Cooper was referring to the importance of that organ. I wonder if he or Dr Mellander would spare a thought for the much neglected tonsil as a possible source for antigen entry in this context, or even as a place for maternal cells to home to on the way down.

Chairman   Are there any comments on the tonsil?

Cooper   I think they probably are important, judging from Ogra's studies, in seeding IgA-producing cells along the nasopharynx, but I do not believe there is evidence that they are important in seeding cells elsewhere.

Soothill   I should like to comment on the interpretation of Ogra's studies on tonsillectomized children. He did not study the same children before and after tonsillectomy. Since relative IgA deficiency is an important cause of recurrent sore throats I believe that the difference he was describing may have resulted from the underlying immunodeficiency leading to the tonsilectomy and not the effect of the tonsillectomy. I have discussed this with him and he agrees; he cannot refute this interpretation of his data.

The Contribution of Milk

to Resistance to Intestinal Infection

in the Newborn

BRUNO REITER

National Institute for Research in Dairying,
Shinfield, Reading, UK

Although the antibacterial activity of milk became known about the same time as that of blood—at the end of the last century—it attracted only intermittent attention (for reviews see Reiter and Oram, 1967; Hanson and Winberg, 1972; Goldman and Smith, 1973; Reiter, 1967, 1976, 1978a, b; Braun, 1976; McClelland et al., 1978).

Epidemiologists wondered why "scarlet fever" streptococci were not spread through the consumption of milk, largely not heat treated at that time; some veterinarians investigated the role of milk antibacterial factors in relation to infection of the mammary gland. Other workers discovered that ungulates are born without immunoglobulins in their blood and depend on the ingestion of colostrum for protective antibodies; these are absorbed into the blood through the gut wall, which remains permeable 24–36 h after birth. For a long time these findings seemed irrelevant for the human neonate which is born with immunoglobulins transmitted through the placenta. The situation changed drastically with the discovery of sIgA. Subsequently, colostrum and milk became recognized as playing a protective role in the gastrointestinal tract (GI) of the newborn, as had been evident for animals even before the discovery of sIgA. It can now be accepted that colostrum and milk bridge the immunological gap of the newborn against intestinal infections until its own defences are built up.

Besides immunoglobulins, complement and leukocytes, colostrum and milk also contain nonantibody factors, mainly lysozyme, lactoferrin and/or transferrin, lactoperoxidase and other, as yet, little investigated factors. These components are proteins; they occur in the colostrum and milk of all species but in different concentrations, like the classes of Igs.

At the NIRD, research has been concerned with bovine milk and with the calf as an experimental animal. The advantages are: availability of bovine milk for large scale isolation of components, and purification of the proteins for the study of their mode of action. Calves can be removed from the dam immediately after birth and fed colostrum and milk unaltered or with additives, thus avoiding digestive and nutritional complications. Calves are monogastric as long as they have no access to roughage for the development of their rumen, are easy to cannulate in the GI tract, and can be used for prolonged periods because of their slow growth. A disadvantage is the calf's unique digestive system in which the high casein milk is clotted by rennin. Furthermore bovine milk contains little lactoferrin or lysozyme but high concentration of lactoperoxidases. The calf is therefore suitable for the study of the lactoperoxidase system but not for the other two nonantibody components of milk. Although the latter two proteins can be isolated from bovine milk, smaller animals such as piglets or guinea pigs would be more suitable for their study because of the technical difficulties in isolating these proteins on a large scale from bovine milk.

This paper re-examines the possible role of lysozyme and lactoferrin and deals in greater detail with the lactoperoxidase system which readily kills Gram negative organisms *in vitro* and *in vivo*. It briefly describes also other factors which may have protective properties.

LYSOZYME (*N*-ACETYL MURAMYL HYDROLASE, E.C.3.2.1.17.) (L)

When Fleming (1922) discovered this bactericidal and lytic enzyme it appeared to fulfill the characteristics of a naturally occurring bactericidal substance—"to be selectively more lethal to bacteria than the host cells". In spite of the ubiquitous distribution of lysozyme (L), the narrow bactericidal spectrum appeared to exclude any protective role *in vivo*. Since then, L has become a tool in biophysics, chemistry, physiology and clinical medicine (see Osserman *et al.*, 1974). However, its biological role may now warrant a new appraisal.

Lysozyme irrespective of its source (egg albumin, milk or tears, bacteriophage), hydrolyses the peptidoglycan in the cell wall or outer membrane of bacteria. *Micrococcus lysodeikticus* is a suitable organism for the assay of albumin L because of the high content of peptidoglycan in its cell wall. The susceptibility of an organism to L is influenced by the presence of O-acetyl groups (e.g. the development of resistance to L in *M. lysodeikticus*), substitution with teichoic acid, the occurrence of free amino groups in the peptide chain, high degree of peptide cross linking and high content of N-unacetylated glucosamine residues in the peptidoglycan (Osserman et al., 1974). Some Gram positive organisms which cannot be lysed by albumin L can be rapidly lysed by highly specific bacteriophage lysins: group C streptococcal bacteriophage lysin only lyses groups C and A (Krause, 1958) and group N phage lysin only groups N and D (Oram and Reiter, 1965), Moreover, in the case of Gram negative organisms albumin L only attacks the peptidoglycan after treatment with EDTA or chloroform but specific phage lysins again are strongly lytic (Weidel, 1951).

The rate of lysis and the lytic spectrum depend therefore on the composition and structure of the cell wall (or outer membrane) *and* the characteristics of the enzyme itself.

Biological Significance

It has been known for a long time that L is important in determining the rate of lysis of Gram negative organisms killed by the complement mediated antibody system (e.g. Wardlaw, 1962). Adinolfi et al. (1966) demonstrated that in contrast to IgM and IgG, sIgA (isolated from human colostrum) bound complement only in the presence of L, thus killing and lysing a complement–antibody susecptible strain of *E. coli*. This finding has been confirmed (Hill and Porter, 1974) but also disputed (Heddle et al., 1975).

TABLE I.

The lytic effect of bovine milk, human milk and egg white lysozyme on live *Micrococcus lysodeikticus*.

Source of lysozyme	Rate of lysis $\Delta\%$ T min^{-1} * (buffer)
Bovine milk	1·82
Human milk	1·70
Egg white	0·63

* Determined in spectrophotometer at 540 μm.
Buffer: phosphate buffer pH 6·2.
Compiled from Vakil et al. (1969).

TABLE II.

Sensitivity of different bacteria to bovine or human milk lysozyme under different conditions.

	Rate of lysis $\Delta\%$ T min^{-1}	
Organisms	Bovine buffer	Human buffer
Streptococcus lactis	0·2	0·00
Staphylococcus aureus	0·03	0·05
Sarcina lutea	0·08	0·04
Streptococcus faecalis	0·17	0·04
Bacillus cereus	0·10	0·23
Escherichia coli	0·12	0·10
Serratia marcescens	0·10	0·00
Proteus vulgaris	0·06	0·00
Pseudomonas fluorescens	0·08	0·08
Pseudomonas aeruginosa	0·30	0·21

Compiled from Vakil *et al.* (1969).

Irrespective of this "new role" it has long been established, although largely neglected, that the bactericidal spectrum of L isolated from milk is different from that of L from albumin. Vakil, *et al.*, (1969) compared L from albumin and from human and bovine milk (Table I) and found that *M. lysodeikticus* is nearly three times more susceptible to the milk L that to the albumin L. Also, the lytic spectrum of milk L is far wider (Table II).

Yet another aspect of L activity seems to have been neglected. Nakamura (1923) followed the L work of Fleming and largely confirmed its distribution, heat resistance and similarity and dissimilarity to bacteriophage (at the time phage lysin was not yet known). He used both albumin and tear L and discovered that there is an optimal NaCl concentration for the activity of the enzyme; in this way it behaved like phage, optimal absorption depending on the electrolyte concentration (Reiter and Oram, 1962). Nakamura noted the difference between L of egg white and of tears but also discovered that organisms which were not lysed at neutral pH, could be lysed after exposure to L at pH 3·5 and transfer to alkaline conditions, pH 9·8. Peterson and Hartsnell (1955) extended these observations using albumin L and demonstrated lysis of a large number of Gram negative bacteria *in vitro*; lysis was partly due to the enzyme itself but was very much increased according to the technique of Nakamura (Fig. 1).

To my knowledge these findings do not appear to be mentioned in recent literature on the possible intestinal role of L. However, considering the low pH in the stomach, although buffered by milk, the higher pH in the large intestine may

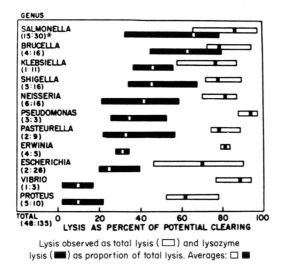

GENUS

Lysis observed as total lysis (□) and lysozyme
lysis (■) as proportion of total lysis. Averages: □ ■

Fig. 1   Lysis of Gram negative genera.
*Numbers in brackets are the species and strains screened, respectively. Peterson and Hartsnell (1955).

activate the milk L. Obviously this phenomen deserves further consideration and
investigation.

Diagnostic role

Other interests in L were associated with the diagnosis of ulcerative conditions of
the intestine (Peterson and Hartsell, 1955) but the diagnostic value seems now to
be disproven. Falchuk et al., (1975), for instance, reported that the mean levels in
the sera of controls, and of patients with ulcerative colitis and bacterial and
nonbacterial enteritis, were not significantly different ($P < 0.001$) but appreciably
elevated in Crohn's disease. In the case of enteritis, however, increased levels of L
would surely occur in the intestine and be reflected in the faeces, but not in the
blood. There are indeed several reports that in the case of acute diarrhoea of
infants, the L increases in the faeces (e.g. Krawczuk et al., 1978) and declines with
the improvement of the clinical symptoms. The authors ascribe the increase to
cellular elements of the intestinal wall caused by inflammatory infiltration (Ballamy
and Nielson, 1974). This may well be so but McClelland and van Furth (1975)
studied the incorporation of ^{14}C labelled amino acids into L and demonstrated that
the enzyme was synthesized in vitro in the mucosa of the GI (and respiratory) tract.
It is therefore possible that inflammatory conditions lead to increased L synthesis
per se. Korhonen (1973) found that the L level in milk increased after infection and
inflammation of the bovine udder. Although the leukocytes increased at the same

time, the L cannot be derived from the cells because bovine leukocytes do not contain it (Padgett and Hirsch, 1967). The increase of L is therefore due either to passage from the blood or to local synthesis. L now appears to be indentical with the blood β lysin, once considered the primary bactericidin active against Gram positive organisms and independent of the complement–antibody system against Gram negative organisms (Fodov, 1887; Donaldson *et al.*, 1974; Selsted and Martinez, 1978).

Evaluation

It is interesting that Selsted and Martinez (1978) conclude their paper with the sentence " . . . . that many microorganisms can be defined as saprophytes or potential pathogens may, therefore, be a consequence of the selective nature of non-specific serum microbicidal factors such as those we have evaluated (L)". Fleming is reported to have given a similar answer to critics of the L system " . . . but how many organisms would be pathogens if they were not lysed by L".

Can we from the foregoing come to any conclusion on the possible role of L in the GI of the infant? Since the mucosal tissue is capable of synthesizing L it can be postulated that the intake of human milk bridges the L gap. However we have no evidence of any beneficial effects because unfortunately milk L tends to be equated with albumin L and feeding babies with the latter enzyme does not seem to bring any advantage (e.g. Hanneberg and Finne, 1974). Meaningful trials could be made with L of milk origin using large scale chromatographic separations.

LACTOFERRIN (LF)

Since the original demonstration of the bacteriostatic activity of LF *in vitro* (Masson *et al.*, 1966; Oram and Reiter, 1966, 1968) the distribution, chemical characteristics and mode of action have been extensively reviewed (e.g. Masson, 1970; Bullen *et al.*, 1978). An *in vivo* effect of LF, however, has been investigated only once: Bullen *et al.* (1972) demonstrated that suckling guinea-piglets dosed with haematin showed a dramatic increase in their intestinal coliforms compared with the control animals. The results of this work have rightly been extensively cited in the paediatric literature as proof that LF suppresses coliforms because human milk, like that of guinea-pigs, contains high concentrations of LF. It is, however, regrettable that this work has not been repeated by other workers up to date. There is a need to test the role of LF not only by feeding haematin as an alternative source of iron but also by comparing iron-saturated and unsaturated LF; this will be discussed in a later section.

Since Dr Bullen has dealt with LF, this section will only be concerned with some aspects not touched upon.

The Role of Bicarbonate and Citrate

The iron binding capacity of LF is directly related to the bicarbonate level—mole for mole—(Masson, 1970) but inversely related to the citrate concentration (Table III) (Reiter *et al*, 1975; Bishop *et al.*, 1976; Griffith and Humphrey, 1977; Dolby *et al.*, 1977b). Citrate can exchange iron from LF (and conalbumin—Aisen and Leibman, 1968) and the iron citrate formed can then be actively taken up by the organisms.

It so happens, however, that there exists an *in vivo* situation which illustrates the role of bicarbonate/citrate (Reiter and Bramley, 1975; Reiter, 1976). Cows are usually impregnated during their lactation period but milking is stopped 2–3 months before calving. During this drying off period, milk proteins are reabsorbed and blood proteins diffuse into the dry udder. Since citrate is also reabsorbed and bicarbonate diffuses into the udder, optimal conditions for bacterial inhibition by LF appear to be created, particularly as the LF can rise in the "dry secretion" to ~ 50 mg ml^{-1}. Such dry secretions were found to be inhibitory for *E. coli in vitro* and the inhibition was reversed by the addition of iron. Shortly before parturition when the colostrum begins to be formed, citrate increases again and bicarbonate decreases. Peaker and Linzell (1975) called citrate the "harbinger of parturition". The high concentration of citrate and low concentration of bicarbonate abolish the inhibitory effect of LF, and "dormant" coliforms can multiply and cause mastitis. (The possible implication for the calf ingesting mastitic coliforms has so far not been considered.) Indeed, it is very rare to detect coliform infection in the dry udder, but after parturition, mastitis due to coliforms does occur. To test this hypothesis bovine quarters were infused with a strain of *E. coli* (~ 200 cfu ml^{-1}) known to produce mastitis. In 14/14 lactating quarters mastitis became established but in none of the dry quarters (0/14; 2 days prior to parturition, 2/2 quarters, however, became infected after infusion of *E. coli* (Reiter and Bramley, 1975).

TABLE III.

Effect of citrate and bicarbonate on the bacteriostatic activity of dialysed colostrum.

HCO$_3^-$ (μm ml^{-1})	Citrate (μm ml^{-1})			
	0	0·1	1	10
0	0·7*	1·9	2·6	2·4
0·7	0·7	0·9	2·5	2·5
7·0	1·1	1·1	1·1	2·4
70·0	1·0	0·7	0·7	0·8

* Increase in log$_{10}$ viable count after 6 h incubation.
From Reiter *et al.* (1975).

When two dry quarters were infused with iron prior to the inoculation with the coliform organisms, both quarters became mastitic (unpublished). This experiment indicated, but did not prove, that the LF in the dry secretion became saturated with iron—the LF was not purified from these quarters to assay the degree of saturation.

It would therefore be of some interest to investigate the fate of iron bound to LF in the intestine. Since the main intestinal buffer is bicarbonate, does it offset the citrate in the milk, is it made available for bacterial multiplication or even absorbed as iron citrate in the intestine? Since the milk of different species contains different levels of LF *and* citrate, this question requires detailed investigation.

The Role of Immunoglobulins (Igs)

Bullen *et al.* (1972) first suggested that LF had little bacteriostatic activity in colostrum or milk unless specific antibodies were also present. They demonstrated that an inoculum of 2×10^2 ml^{-1} of *E. coli* increased in about 8 h to just below 10^7 ml^{-1} in the absence of either LF or Igs; it increased in the presence of LF to only $\sim 10^5$ ml^{-1} and to about 5×10^3 after addition of Igs. The addition of Igs, in the form of specific IgG, had therefore a spectacular effect but the reduction with LF alone of nearly $2 \times \log_{10}$ viable count is also appreciable ($\sim 99\%$ reduction).

Rogers (1976) and Rogers and Synge (1978) reported that the bacteriostatic mechansim of transferrin (TF) required IgG, and LF requires IgA. Both classes of immunoglobulins inhibit either the synthesis or secretion of a bacterial iron binding substance, enterochelin, which can reverse the bacteriostatic activity of LF or TF.

Spik *et al.* (1978) also reported that IgA isolated from human milk increased bacteriostasis by LF with a "milk sensitive" strain (Dolby *et al.*, 1977a) in inactivated milk (heated at 100°C) but less so when IgA and LF were added to peptone water. The authors suggested that milk may stabilize in some manner the bacteriostatic activity; IgG$_1$ isolated from bovine colostrum had a role similar to human IgA. More recently, however, Samson *et al.* (1979) examined the effect of LF in hypogammaglobulinaemic human milk, deficient in sIgA. The pattern of inhibition, reversible by iron, was the same as when sIgA was added, irrespective of whether the sIgA contained specific antibodies or not. The authors came to the conclusion that IgA did not enhance the bacteriostatic activity of LT. Dr J. M. Dolby, CRC, Harrow (pers. comm.) recently tested 2 samples of bovine LF and 7 batches of human purified LF in a synthetic medium and found that purified human LF at a concentration of 2 mg ml^{-1} had a similar inhibitory effect to that found by Bullen *et al.* (1972). In contrast, bovine LF at the same and lower concentrations had a considerably more marked bacteriostatic effect. Addition of IgA antibody to all LF's considerably increased bacteriostatic activity for bacteriostatic strains but not commensals.

TABLE IV.

Bacteriostatic activity of bovine colostrum after adjustment of pH to 7·4 with bicarbonate against enteropathogenic (EPEC) and nonenteropathogenic isolates (NEPEC) of E. coli from baby faeces.

Isolates	No. of strains tested	Bacteriostasis*	
		< 10-fold	> 10-fold
EPEC	50	34	16
NEPEC	50	39	11

* Average increase of inoculum after 6 h incubation at 37°C.
Average increase after saturation with iron ov. 400-fold: (200–850).
From Reiter (1978b).

Purified bovine LF was also found to be bacteriostatic against both a serum sensitive and serum resistant strain (Law and Reiter, 1977) and bovine colostra inhibited 50 enteropathogenic and 50 nonenteropathogenic isolates of E. coli from baby faeces. The addition of iron reversed the inhibition (Reiter, 1978b). This indicated that specific antibodies were not required for the inhibition of human serotypes by bovine colostrum (Table IV). Furthermore 24/50 enteropathogenic and 10/50 nonenteropathogenic isolates were killed by bovine colostrum after addition of complement. Since the complement mediated bactericidal activity of antibodies is highly specific, it appears that the bovine colostrum contains antibodies against human strains or, alternatively, there exists a considerable cross-reaction between bovine and human strains (Table V) (Reiter and Brock, 1975).

TABLE V.

Bactericidal effect of bovine colostrum diluted 1:8 in complement containing milk, against enteropathogenic (EPEC) and nonenteropathogenic (NEPEC) isolates of E. coli from baby faeces.

Isolates	No. of strains tested	Bactericidal*	Growth†
EPEC	50	24	26
NEPEC	50	10	40

* Bactericidal: $\dfrac{\text{Inoculum cfu}}{\text{cfu after incubation at 37°C}} < 1$

† Growth: as above > 1.
From Reiter (1978b).

Notwithstanding such speculation specific antibodies against all 100 strains could not have been present in the bovine colostrum.

Susceptibility to Digestion

Any *in vivo* activity presumes that LF resists the digestive process. Purified LF has been shown to be susceptible to tryptic digestion. LF yielded up to five different fragments with molecular weights ranging from 25 000 to 52 700. The apoform of LF was found to be extremely labile and its bacteriostatic activity was rapidly lost (Brock *et al.*, 1976; Brock *et al.*, 1978).

McClelland (pers. comm.) submitted human colostrum and milk instead of purified LF to peptic acid and tryptic digestion. Peptic digestion released the iron from milk and abolished the bacteriostatic effect. The same results were obtained with low pH alone. However in our experience purified LF kept at 37° for 1 h at pH 5·0 or 3·0 lost 25 and 90% respectively of its original iron-binding capacity but recovered almost all of it after 4 h incubation at pH 7·4 at 37° (Law and Reiter, 1977). Tryptic digestion of human milk (McClelland, pers. comm.) did not affect the iron binding or bacteriostatic activity of LF.

Considering the increase of gastric pH in the infant's stomach, from 2·5 to 6·5 after feeding of milk, the slow drop of pH in 2 h to 5·2 (Mason, 1962) and the passage of most of the milk undigested directly into the duodenum (Henderson, 1942) it can be assumed that LF remains undigested in the stomach and reaches the duodenum largely intact.

THE LACTOPEROXIDASE SYSTEM (LPS)

The complete LPS was first demonstrated in bovine milk and consists of lactoperoxidase (E.C.1.11.1.7) (LP), thiocyanate (SCN^-) and H_2O_2 (Reiter *et al.*, 1963; Reiter *et al.*, 1964). It has been shown to inhibit pathogenic and nonpathogenic streptococci but only temporarily. Staphylococci and Gram negative organisms such as coliforms, pseudomonads, salmonellas, shigellas etc. are inhibited at pH near neutral but killed at lower pH (Reiter *et al.*, 1973/1974; Björck, *et al.*, 1975; Reiter *et al.*, 1976). *Mycobacterium tuberculosis* is not affected at all (Jackett *et al.*, 1978). LP and H_2O_2 can also react with other substances in milk such as indican or iodide but they become inhibitory only at unphysiological concentrations (Reiter *et al.*, 1964).

Distribution of Lactoperoxidase (LP) in Bovine Milk

LP occurs in the milk of all animal species tested so far—bovine, porcine, caprine, murine and human; it is also present in other biological secretions, e.g. saliva, tears, cervical mucus (Reiter and Gibbons, 1964; Reiter and Oram, 1967; Klebanoff and Smith, 1970; Schindler et al., 1976). In bovine milk, its concentration, expressed as protein is high c. 30 μg ml^{-1}, but expressed as units of activity, the values given by different authors are difficult to compare. The assay of LP depends on the oxidation of a hydrogen acceptor in the presence of H_2O_2 in a given time at a given wavelength. Since different H^+ acceptors have been used, the units expressed vary greatly.

Korhonen (1973) tested mid-lactation milk of 146 animals and arrived at an average value of 456 mu ml^{-1} (316–600) independently of the leukocyte content. The values reported by Kiermeier and Kayser (1960) were much higher, av. 10 000 mu ml^{-1}, and they made the interesting observation that the postparturition level in the colostrum is relatively low (450–800 mu ml^{-1}) and rises to 16 000–24 000 mu ml^{-1} in the first week, gradually declines in the next week and remains at an approximate constant value of about 10 000 mu ml^{-1} throughout the lactation period. It appears therefore that the LP concentrations actually increases after parturition while concentrations of other protective proteins such as sIgA, IgM, IgG complements, lactoferrin and lysozyme decrease.

Distribution in Human Milk and Saliva

Human milk was first analysed for LP by Gothefors and Markland (1975); they estimated the LP level at about 5% that of bovine milk. Using the new and very sensitive assay by Schindler and Bardsley (1975); Stephens et al. (1977) reported average values of 226 mu ml^{-1} with a range of 26–519 in 9 samples, 1–69 days post partum. Using the same assay methods, we determined the LP values in a number of milk samples.

Sixty milk samples from Gambian mothers, 1–9 months post partum, gave an average value of 230 mu ml^{-1} of LP with a range of 4–922 mu ml^{-1}. Since 20 mu ml^{-1} LP is about the limit for bactericidal activity (see later) only 7 out of 60 samples fell below this level. Quite a different picture emerged when a smaller number of milk samples was assayed for LP in the UK. Four colostral samples, 1 day post partum, contained the highest concentration of LP, average 700, (519–970); 21 samples up to 10 days post partum contained an average of 314 mu ml^{-1} (60–970) but a surprising number of samples from 10 days post partum onwards were negative, 10 out of 18. Neglecting the negative sample the average of the positive samples was only 88 mu ml^{-1} (21–207) (unpublished). In contrast to the bovine colostrum, human colostrum appears to contain the highest concentration of LP, but this declines rapidly.

Although LP levels are lower in human milk than in bovine milk it is important to remember that the human baby is born with LP in its saliva but not the calf (Morrison and Steele, 1968; Gothefors and Marklund, 1975). The distribution of

LP in the saliva of different animals differs (Morrison and Allen, 1963; Thomson and Morell, 1967). Only in the guinea-pig is LP secreted by all three salivary glands—submaxillary, paratoid and sublingual. All other animals tested secrete it in either one or both of the submaxillary and paratoid glands. In mice Osugi (1977) demonstrated LP peroxidative activity of the submandibular gland on the seventeenth day *in utero*; adult mice showed this activity in both the submandibulary and parotid but not sublingual gland. In man only the submandibular has any activity (Saji *et al.*, 1967; cited by Osugi). In man the LP activity—notwithstanding the difference in the assay methods—is roughly about 10 times as high in the saliva as in bovine milk.

Resistance to Digestion and Low pH

LP was shown very early on to be resistant to proteolysis, used in the first step in purification of the enzyme from milk or whey (Morrison *et al.*, 1967). More recently it has been shown that LP remains active in human gastric juice (Gothefors and Marklund, 1975). Abomasal samples withdrawn from cannulated calves showed that before feeding (intervals of 12–18 h) only traces of LP were present (Table VI) but after feeding raw milk the level of LP rises sharply (Reiter *et al.*, 1979). Since the saliva can enter the abomasum only during feeding, salivary LP in the older calf is diverted into the rumen between feeding. In the human baby, however, we can expect that the stomach always contains LP.

It has been previously shown that LP is resistant to low pH, up to 3. (Wright and Tramer, 1958). The time exposure to low pH was however only 30 min and it was recently found that longer exposure at pH 4·0, 3–6 h) inactivates LP (unpublished). This could be of considerable interest because the survival of LP in the baby's stomach would depend on the frequency of feeding.

LP has also been detected in the intestine. Stelmaszyńska and Zgliczyński (1971)

TABLE VI.

Concentration of LP in calf abomasal fluid before and after feeding raw milk.

Time of sampling	Before feeding	After feeding		
		30 min	60 min	120 min
LP concentration (u ml^{-1})	$0·009 \pm 0·004$	$1·4 \pm 0·97$	$1·14 \pm 0·88$	$1·09 \pm 0·68$
No. of samples assayed	75	20	18	19

Mean values with standard deviations are shown. Four calves were sampled over a period of 50 days.
At 5 h, no LP was detected in the abomasal fluid.
Note: the milk feeds contained $1·9 \pm 0·85$ u ml^{-1} ($n = 11$).
From Reiter *et al.* (in press).

isolated a peroxidase from the mucosa of the hog intestines which was identical to LP. It has not yet been decided whether the enzyme is synthesized like sIgA, lysozymes and lactoferrin intestinally, derived from saliva or from eosinophils which are packed with LP.

Source and Distribution of Thiocyanate (SCN⁻)

SCN^- is an ubiquitous anion in animal tissue and secretion. It occurs in the mammary, salivary and thyroid gland, stomach, kidney, and fluids such as synovial, cerebral, spinal, lymph and plasma. The concentration of SCN^- in body fluids is related to the diet and to habits such as smoking. It is partly derived endogenously during the detoxification reaction between thiosulphates and cyanide, catalysed by rhodanse. Principally, however, it is derived after ingestion of the anion, its esters and other precursor compounds such as nitriles and isothianates. Many plants are rich in glucosinolates which after hydrolysis by myrosinase yield SCN^- and/or isothiocynates and nitriles; tobacco smoke is a common source of cyanide. Some plants such as cassava, sweet potatoes, millet or sugar cane are particularly rich in cyanogenic glycosides which on hydrolysis release cyanide. Excessive amounts of ingested SCN^- are rapidly excreted, its half-life being 2–5 days (Wood, 1975).

At first we had assumed that in the calf milk would be the main source of SCN^-, the saliva being diverted between feeding. However, it was found (Reiter *et al.*, 1980) that the SCN^- concentration in the abomasum of cannulated calves was far higher between feeding than in the milk and was actually diluted after feeding (Table VII). It appears, therefore, that SCN^- is actively secreted in the calf's stomach confirming the earlier results obtained with mice, rats, guinea-pigs and hamsters (Logothetopoulos and Myant, 1956). Our observations were made with calves between 5 and 13 days because of the time lag between surgery and sampling. It is therefore possible that the SCN^- of the milk is important shortly after birth when the calf does not secrete HCl (in contrast to the human newborn).

TABLE VII.

Concentration of SCN^- in calf abomasal fluid before and after feeding raw milk.

Time of sampling	Before feeding	After feeding		
		30 min	60 min	120 min
SCN^- concentration (mM)	0.45 ± 0.14	0.15 ± 0.08	0.15 ± 0.08	0.20 ± 0.09
No. of samples assayed	17	30	37	38

Mean values with standard deviations are shown. Four calves were sampled over a period of 50 days. From Reiter *et al.* (1980).

In the human, it has been thought that the SCN^- concentration of the stomach was derived from the saliva (Ruddel *et al.*, 1977) but it now appears that the SCN^- is actively secreted (by the parietal cells which secrete HCL?) as it was shown that in patients who are stimulated by insulin and histamine the SCN^- concentration in the stomach exceeded the salivary SCN^- concentration (Boulos *et al.*, 1977). (Incidentally the data in *Documenta Geigy* (1973) wrongly state that gastric juice is devoid of SCN^-).

Source of H_2O_2

It is generally assumed that H_2O_2 is absent from milk; this is difficult to understand considering the very high metabolic activity of the secretory tissue. Indeed, we detected trace amounts of H_2O_2 in freshly drawn milk but only recently did we employ a sensitive enough assay to detect nm of H_2O_2 when we measured the H_2O_2 extracellularly generated by polymorphonuclear leukocytes in milk; sodium azide had to be used to inactivate both catalase and LP of the milk to detect trace amounts of H_2O_2 (Korhonen and Reiter, unpublished). This possibly also explains the observation that freshly drawn milk is bactericidal for a few hours (C. M. Cousins, NIRD, pers. comm.).

In vivo lactic acid bacteria have always been found to be a source of H_2O_2; these organisms rapidly colonize the GI and in the calf up to 80% were found to be H_2O_2 producing (Marshall, 1978; Reiter *et al.*, 1980).

Mode of Action

LP complexes with H_2O_2 and oxidizes SCN^- to an intermediary oxidation product which was first thought to be $S(CN)_2$ (Oram and Reiter, 1966b) but now almost certainly is $OSCN^-$, a structurally related oxidation product (Hogg and Jago, 1970a, b; Hoogendoorn *et al.*, 1977; Aune and Thomas, 1977). The end products of the oxidation process — CO_2, NH_4^+, SO_4^{++} — are noninhibitory (Oram and Reiter, 1966b).

(1) $$SCN^- + H_2O_2 \xrightarrow{\text{LP}} (SCN)_2 + H_2O$$

$$(SCN)_2 + H_2O \longrightarrow HO\,SCN + SCN^-\,H^+$$

$$HO\,SCN^- \rightleftharpoons H^+ + OSCN^-$$

or

(2) $$SCN^- + H_2O_2 \xrightarrow{\text{LP}} OSCN^- + H_2O$$

In streptococci and lactobacilli some of the glycolytic enzymes were found to be inhibited by the LPS but only temporarily. Streptococci of many serogroups are

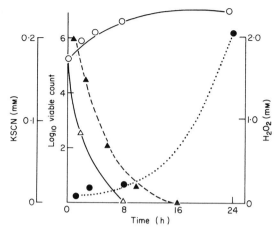

Fig. 2 Bactericidal effect against *E. coli* 0111 of LP (1·5 μg ml⁻¹), SCN⁻ (0·225) mM), and GO (0·1 μg ml⁻¹) in a synthetic medium. Control, growth in medium only (○); bactericidal system decrease in viable count (△); oxidation of SCN⁻ (▲); H₂O₂ level (●). Reiter *et al.* (1976).

inhibited by the LPS—including group A (*Str. pyogenes*), group B (*Str. agalactiae*) and group D (*Str. bovis*). These organisms are self inhibitory, in that being catalase negative they endogenously produce H_2O_2 (Reiter *et al.*, 1964; Oram and Reiter, 1966a).

Gram negative, catalase positive organisms such as coliforms, salmonellas, shigellas and pseudomonads and multiple antibiotic strains of *E. coli* are not only inhibited but also killed at a pH below 7·0, but H_2O_2 must be exogenously supplied. In Fig. 2 the H_2O_2 is generated by glucose oxidase/glucose; as long as SCN^- is present, H_2O_2 is used up for the oxidation and none or very little free H_2O_2 can be detected. The low levels of H_2O_2 are non inhibitory but once all the SCN^- is oxidized they rise to bactericidal levels.

While metabolic activities such as glucose uptake and amino acid are interrupted within minutes of exposure to the system, death occurs only after 1–2 h and is followed by lysis (Fig. 3). The target of $OSCN^-$ is now known to the inner membrane of the bacteria, indicated by the immediate leakage of potassium (Marshall and Reiter, 1976; Marshall, 1978; Reiter, 1978) and is very likely due to a de-energizing effect of the inner membrane (Law and Reiter, unpublished), the "power house" of bacteria. Two further results indicate that the target of the $OSCN^-$ is in the membrane: mycoplasma do not possess an outer membrane but only a cholesterol containing single membrane and were also found to be killed by the LPS (unpublished). However, *Sarcina lutea*, which has a carotenoid pigmented inner membrane, was not killed by the LP but only inhibited. White mutants of the same strain were killed (Reiter, 1978b, 1979). Since carotenoids are well known quenchers of singlet oxygen, free radicals may be involved in the disorientation of

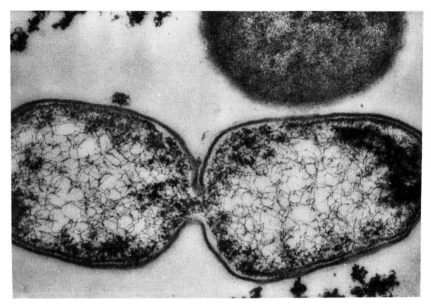

Fig. 3   **Damage and lysis to** *E. coli* 9703 after exposure to LP system, 1·5 h, × 57 600. Cells were collected on a Millipore filter (0·22 mm pore size), covered with a thin layer of agar and fixed to 1 h in 0·2 M cacodylate-HCl buffered 3% gluteraldehyde. The filter was washed in buffer, fixed for 1 h in 1% osmium tetroxide *en bloc* stained with 1% uranyl acetate for 0·5 h. After dehydration in a graded series of alcohol–water mixtures, it was embedded in araldite. (By courtesy of B. E. Brooker and D. E. Hobbs, NIRD).

the inner membrane. These results are similar to those obtained by Krinsky (1974) who demonstrated that only the white mutants of *S. lutea* were killed intracellularly by polymorphonuclear leukocytes.

In vitro bovine milk or whey kills Gram negative organisms provided all three components of the LPS are present. Thus human milk becomes bactericidal (Fig. 4) after addition of a source of H_2O_2 plus SCN^- (unpublished); the latter would be provided by the milk of saliva of the newborn or by secretion in the stomach—an assumption as yet unverified.

Biological Activity of the LPS

For some time now it has been recognized that enteropathogenic strains of *Escherichia coli* (and other intestinal pathogens) associate intimately with the epithelial surface of the intestine. This attachement favours proliferation of the organisms and reduces their removal in the lumen by peristalsis; subsequently, the enterotoxins produced by the attached organisms evoke disease symptoms.

Certain plasmid controlled surface antigens such as K_{88} or K_{99} in *E. coli* are

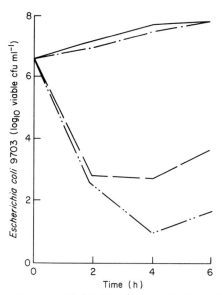

Fig. 4   Bactericidal effect of human milk (10 days after parturition) containing 20 mu ml^{-1} LP. Control, ——. Additions: (1) SCN (0·225 mM) and H$_2$O$_2$ (0·222 mM), — —; (2) as (1) plus 200 mu ml^{-1} LP, —··—; (3) as (2) plus 1 mM Na$_2$S$_2$O$_4$, —·—.

responsible for the attachment and pathogenesis in the piglet and calf respectively (e.g. Ørskov *et al.*, 1975; Ørskov *et al.*, 1961; Jones, 1977) and plasmid controlled colonization factors have also been discovered in *E. coli* from the human gut (Evans *et al.*, 1975; Evans and Evans Jr., 1978). In the case of *Vibrio cholerae*, chemotaxis and motility have also been shown to be essential, enabling the organisms to traverse the continuous mucous blanket covering the intestinal villi and to become attached (Allweiss *et al.*, 1977).

A useful method to study attachment was developed by Sellwood, *et al* (1975). They used brush border cells isolated from pig intestines and observed the attachment of the enteropathogenic strain of *E. coli* possessing K$_{88}$ antigen. The addition of specific sIgA to *E. coli* possessing the K$_{88}$ antigen largely prevented attachment. A similar phenomenon was observed when porcine and bovine pathogenic coliforms were exposed to the LPS, attachment being appreciably inhibited (Fig. 5). Counting the numbers of bacteria attached, the control showed an average of 14·6 bacteria cell^{-1} and 2·9 respectively. Such results were obtained both with *E. coli* possessing K$_{88}$ or K$_{99}$ antigen using porcine and bovine brush border cells (Reiter *et al.*, unpublished; Reiter, 1978).

In Vivo Bacerticidal Activity of the LPS

The direct bactericidal activity of the LPS was observed in cannulated calves

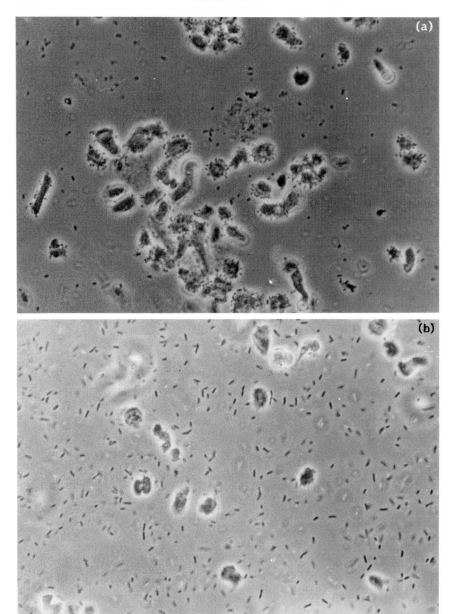

Fig. 5   Attachement of *E. coli* 0149 K_{88} a,c to isolated brush border cells. (a) Attachment of *E. coli*. (b)
Reduced attachment of *E. coli* after exposure to LP system. Porcine brush border cells were washed by
centrifugation and resuspended at approx. 10^6 ml^{-1} in phosphate buffered saline (PBS). A K_{88}-positive
strain of *E. coli* (0149: K91 (B), K88ac (L): H10) was grown on Nutrient Agar at 37°C overnight,
harvested in 5 ml PBS, washed and resuspended at approx. 10_8 ml^{-1}. Two 0·5 ml aliquots of the K_{88}

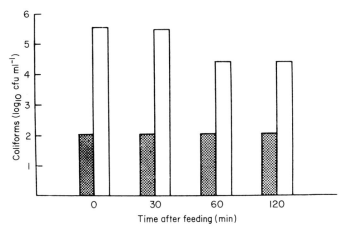

Fig. 6   Bactericidal activity of abomasal fluid on addition of glucose oxidase. Abomasal fluid was inoculated with *E. coli* 9703 (10^6 cfu ml^{-1}) and glucose (0.3%) and glucose oxidase (0.1 *u* ml^{-1}) added (solid columns), or glucose (0.3%) glucose oxidase (0.1 *u* ml^{-1}) and $Na_2S_2O_4$ (1 mM) added (open columns).

(Reiter and Marshall, 1975/76; Reiter *et al.*, 1980). Calves were fed *E. coli* in 200 ml of heated milk which was then followed by 2 litres of raw milk containing the native LP and a source of H_2O_2. Figures 6 and 7 showed that both glucose oxidase/glucose and lactobacilli were equally effective in activating the LPS to eliminate *E. coli* from the abomasum, the coli numbers being reduced from 10^6 ml^{-1} to less than 10^2 ml^{-1}. When a reducing agent such as dithionite was added, most of the coliform organisms were recovered, proving that the LPS was responsible for the bactericidal activity, since the OSCN$^-$ is reduced to SCN$^-$ by dithionite (or other reducing agents), thus reversing the bactericidal activity of the LPS (Reiter *et al.*, 1976).

When heated milk was fed to calves infected as above, the coliform organisms were recovered in the abomasum. When raw milk was fed some reduction in the number of organisms occurred which could also be reversed by a reducing agent, thus indicating that the LPS has operated *in vivo* even in the absence of an exogenous source of H_2O_2, presumably because the colonizing lactobacilli provided the H_2O_2. The addition of an exogenous source of H_2O_2, e.g. glucose oxidase/glucose reduced the number of coliforms to less than 10^2 cfu ml^{-1} as in the previous experiment.

positive *E. coli* were taken and to one was added the complete LP system. Both were left standing at 37°C with occasional stirring for 30 min. The samples were then centrifuged and resuspended in 0.5 ml PBS. 0.5 ml of brush borders were now added to each, and the tubes mixed and allowed to stand for a further 15 min at 37°C with occasional stirring. 0.5 ml of each was then mounted under a cover slip on a glass slide and photographed under phase-contrast condition. (Reiter *et al.* unpublished.) × 800.

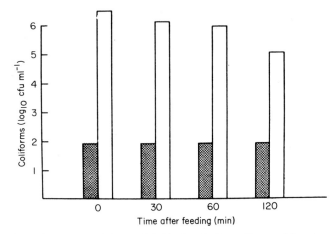

Fig. 7   Bactericidal activity of abomasal fluid after feeding milk containing *Lactobacillus lactis* ($10^6 \sim$ cfu ml^{-1}) and *E. coli* ($\sim 10^6$ cfu ml^{-1}). For details see legend of Fig. 4.

THE BACTERIOSTATIC AND BACTERICIDAL ACTIVITY OF GUINEA PIG MILK (GPM) MEDIATED BY LACTOFERRIN AND THE LACTOPEROXIDASE SYSTEM

Bullen *et al.* (1972) ascribed the inhibition of *E. coli* in the intestines of suckled guinea pigs to the high levels of lactoferrin in GPM. Recent assays (Stephens *et al.*, 1979) of lactoperoxidases in GPM and previous assays on guinea-pig saliva (Thomson and Morell, 1967) showed the highest concentration of lactoperoxidase of any species (average 22000 mu ml^{-1} range 4569–54500). The results of experiments to separate the effect of LF by the addition of iron and the effect of lactoperoxidase by the addition of a reducing agent (Stephens *et al.*, 1979) are unfortunately difficult to interpret because the authors assumed that the contaminating bacterial flora such as *Str. faecalis* supplied H_2O_2 to activate the LPS. (pasturization did not eliminate the inhibitory effect, which is not surprising, since *Str. faecalis* is known to be heat resistant). We tested a single sample of GPM and can confirm its high LP concentration (6600 mu ml^{-1}); we also found the highest concentration of SCN$^-$ recorded for any type of milk, 30 p.p.m. (unpublished). Stephens *et al.* (1979) found that, as in bovine milk, the LP increased *post partum* and attributed this to the increasing oestrogen levels. LP is therefore also in GPM the only "protective" protein which rises in the post colostral stages instead of declining like Igs, LF and L.

Although some of the results obtained were not consistent, the most "favourable" results showed that GPM, 7 days *post partum*, containing 6800 mu ml^{-1} of LP inhibited *E. coli* after 3 h incubation at 37°C. This inhibition was not reserved by iron but only by a reducing agent (penicillamine or cysteine), when the count of viable bacteria increased 50-fold. Some of the samples were not only bacteriostatic but also showed bactericidal activity, which was reversed by a reducing agent. Sometimes, partial reversal was obtained by the addition of iron, but this could also have been caused by the direct effect of iron on the trace amounts of H_2O_2 (Gladstone and Walton, 1971; Kaplan et al., 1975).

Unfortunately this newly gained knowledge cannot be combined with the results obtained in vivo by Bullen and coworkers because their experiments were terminated 3 days after birth and the only GPM sample at 3 days tested by Stephens et al. (1979) contained 8600 mu ml^{-1} of LP and permitted a 23-fold increase in viable organisms, increased 65-fold after addition of iron, but the reversal effect with a reducing agent was not tested for. Returning to the guinea-pig experiments by Bullen and coworkers it is possible that the haematin in the dosed guinea-piglets not only acted as an alternative source of iron for the coliforms but also catalytically decompose H_2O_2 produced by the lactic acid bacteria colonizing the intestines. Previously this effect on H_2O_2 has been shown only with iron salts (Haber and Weiss, 1934) but Fig. 6 shows that haematin rapidly decomposes H_2O_2 generated by glucose oxidase/glucose.

The guinea-pig experiments remain of great interest because we now have an animal model in which the milk contains both high concentrations of iron binding protein and lactoperoxidase. It may even be that LF is most important immediately after birth, and the LPS when the LF concentration declines and the LP increases.

Phagocytosis by Milk Leukocytes

The role of leukocytes does not strictly fall under the title of this paper but it is possible that extracellular killing by macrophage does occur; in this case the LPS may be involved hence its inclusion in this section.

Pitt (1974) and Pitt et al (1977) reported that suckling rats exposed to daily hypoxia survived oral infection with Klebsiella pneumoniae while rats artificially fed or fed frozen rat milk succumbed (100 and 90% respectively). The addition of milk leukocytes to the formula feed or to frozen rat milk largely protected the rats, indicating that protection was due to phagocytosis. The composition of the milk leukocytes was 80–90% macrophages, 1–10% polymorphonuclear neutrophils and 5–10% lymphocytes. In vitro experiments demonstrated the bactericidal activity of the leukocytes in formula feed or frozen milk, the former allowing proliferation of the organisms, the latter having only bacteriostatic activity in the absence of the leukocytes.

It is of some interest to note (a) the milk macrophages in the experiments described were found to be adhesive, i.e. activated; (b) the leukocytes removed from the stomach of the rats died after 15 min as judged by the staining reaction with neutral red; and (c) less than 50% of the bacteria were cell associated, suggesting that killing was partly extracellular; (d) no bactericidal activity occurred in stationary tubes; to kill the bacteria it was necessary to tumble the test tubes, apparently to supply the O_2 requirements.

Respiratory Burst Generating H_2O_2

Like neutrophils, phagocytosis macrophages undergo a "respiratory burst"; the consumed O_2 is not used in oxidative phosphorylation but rather in the formation of superoxide anion (O_2^-) and H_2O_2. These O_2 metabolites and possibly the product of their interaction—hydroxyl radical (^-OH) and singlet oxygen ($^-O_2$) are now regarded as bactericidal both intracellularly and extracellularly (e.g. Johnston et al., 1975; Johnston et al., 1978; Nathan et al., 1979a). The latter authors lysed P_{388} lymphoma cells with activated macrophages but only under aerobic conditions and in the presence of a minimal concentration of glucose (0·03 mM), and not in the presence of galactose. Catalase abolished the cytoxicity, indicating that H_2O_2 was responsible for the effect, while superoxide dismutase reduced the cytotoxicity only marginally. Quenchers of singlet oxygen, hydroxyl radical, sodium azide or cynanide were without effect. Starch particles with covalently bound glucose oxidase, which produce only H_2O_2, lysed the lymphoma cells; hence H_2O_2 rather than O_2^- appears to be responsible for the extracellular lysis by macrophages. Nathan et al. (1979b) showed that Trypanosoma cruzi was killed by activated macrophages which they ascribed entirely to H_2O_2 production. They estimated that 10^6 cells released about 30 nM H_2O_2; thus the calculated concentration within the cytoplasm would be ~ 76 nM H_2O_2 or over LD_{100}s. They now support the early hypothesis that the variation in virulence of macrophange-parasitizing bacteria such as Mycobacterium tuberculosis hominis, Pasteurella pestis, Brucella is positively correlated with their catalase activity.

More recently in vitro experiments (Korhonen and Reiter, unpublished) have shown that bovine PMN, for instance, generate large amounts of extracellular H_2O_2 when exposed to casein, and appreciable amounts when triggered by IgG_1 and IgG_2, but not sIgA. The strong effect of casein is not surprising, considering that casein is strongly chemotactic for polymorphonuclear neutrophils (Wilkinson, 1972) and they were shown to ingest casein avidly and fat globules in unheated milk containing opsonins, but it impaired their capacity to kill staphylococci intracellularly (Russel and Reiter, 1975; Russel et al., 1976, 1977; Paape and Guidry, 1977).

How relevant is the foregoing to the results obtained with Klebsiella aerogenes (Pitt et al., 1977), and with Staphylococcus aureus, Escherichia coli and Candida albicans? (Robinson et al., 1979). O_2 appears to be required. We can therefore assume that the rat activated leukocytes also generate bactericidal concentrations of O_2^- or H_2O_2 intracellularly for ingested bacteria and extracellularly for the "non-associated" or free bacteria. However rat milk plus leukocytes proved to be more bactericidal than formula feed plus leukocytes. This can mean either that the feed reduced some of the H_2O_2 effect or that the rat milk increased it. The latter interpretation is supported by the results obtained by Nathan et al. (1979a) obtained with lymphoma cells. It has been known for a long time that in biological systems H_2O_2 can oxidize halogens and other oxidizable substances in the presence of lacteroxidase (Reiter et al., 1964). Klebanoff (1967) suggested that lactoperoxidase or myeloperoxidase (the peroxidative enzyme of neutrophils) can iodinate bacteria and kill them. Nathan et al. (1979a) thought, therefore, to increase the toxicity of the extracellular H_2O_2 generated by the macrophages by adding lactoperoxidase and iodide. Surprisingly there was no increase, contrary to previous results obtained by Edelson and Cohn (1973): a dramatic reduction of the toxic effects occurred. Nathan and collaborators attributed the reduction in toxicity to the protein content of the foetal calf serum which would have become iodinated thus interfering with the effect on the target cells. This interpretation is supported by the results of Russell and Reiter (1975), Russel et al. (1976, 1977). In buffer at pH 7·0 5·0 the lactoperoxidase/iodide/H_2O_2 system killed over 99% of *Staph. aureus* but only 50 and 80% respectively in the presence of 2% of milk or casein.

Involvement of the lactoperoxidase system?

Milk, like other biological secretions, contains lactoperoxidase but the oxidizable substance is thiocyanate and not iodide which only becomes bactericidal at nonphysiological concentrations (Reiter, Pickering and Oram, 1964). Mouse milk was found to contain high concentrations of lactoperoxidase (unpublished) and if we can extrapolate to rat milk, the difference in bactericidal activities in rat milk compared with formula feed (Pitt, 1974; Barlow and Heird, 1977) could be attributed to the activity of the LPS, provided that, as can be expected, thiocyanate is also present in the rat milk. Proteins do not interfere with the bactericidal effect of oxidized thiocyanate, unlike iodide, since it is equally active in buffer or milk. Robinson et al. (1979) demonstrated *in vitro* that azide reduced the bactericidal effect of the leukocyte preparation isolated from human milk. Azide is known to inhibit lactoperoxidase and myeloperoxidase, (Klebanoff et al., 1966) the latter occurring in neutrophils. Since the leukocyte preparations contained varying proportions of neutrophils, the azide would inhibit their bactericidal activity but not that of the macrophages which are devoid of myeloxidase. Human milk, in spite of the presence of leukocytes proved to be only bacteriostatic for *E. coli* (Robinson et al., 1979) and not bactericidal as was rat milk. This could be due to lack of O_2, lack of glucose, or lack of activation of the macrophages. The authors suggested that the reversal of bacteriostasis by iron was due to saturation of the milk lactoferrin but iron is also known to have a direct effect on the neutrophils because it has been shown (Kaplan *et al.*, 1975) to impair their microbicidal activity by the removal of H_2O_2.

Survival of Leukocytes in the GI Tract

For macrophages or neutrophils to have any antibacterial effect, they must withstand ingestion by the neonate. Paxson and Cress (1979) exposed human milk leukocytes *in vitro* to changes in osmolality, pH and temperature. They confirmed that, like rat cells (Pitt *et al.*, 1977), only about 50% of the leukocytes removed from the stomach were alive and they were killed by freezing; the cells survived 24 h at $-5°C$, heating to $56°C$ (time not stated) and a pH range of 3–7. The heat resistance is in the same range as determined by other workers on the immunoglobulins and other protective proteins of human milk (Ford *et al.*, 1977; Raptopoulou-Gigi *et al.*, 1977; Evans *et al.*, 1978; Eyres *et al.*, 1978).

OTHER NON-ANTIBODY INHIBITORS

Properdin, conglutinin and basic (antibacterial) proteins have been reported in the literature but not sufficiently investigated to form a judgement of their possible importance for the neonate (discussed in Reiter, 1976).

Fatty Acids

György (1971) reported on an antistaphylococcal factor in human milk which protected mice against staphylococcal infections. He attributed this effect to higher unsaturated fatty acids, possibly $C_{18:2}$. In this context it is interesting that the intestines of the suckling rabbit are almost sterile, and although rabbit milk itself is not antibacterial, the chyme in the stomach of the suckling rabbit becomes highly bactericidal due to the production free *n*-deanoic and *n*-octonoic acid (Smith, 1966; Cañes-Rodiguez and Smith, 1966).

Xanthine Oxidase

This enzyme occurs at a high concentration of $120\ \mu g\ ml^{-1}$ in milk (Groves, 1971), is associated with the fat globule membrane and is known to generate H_2O_2 from substrates such as xanthine or hypoxanthine (Green and Pauli, 1943). However, milk contains only low concentrations of oxidizable substrates and it is therefore unlikely that enough H_2O_2 is produced for any bactericidal or bacteriostatic activity. It was, however, suggested that the H_2O_2 is utilized in the LP catalysed oxidation of thiocyatate (Reiter and Oram, 1967). The latter suggestion was indeed confirmed (Klebanoff, 1974).

Vitamin B$_{12}$ and Folate Proteins

The binding capacities of these proteins has attracted considerable attention because only the free vitamin and folic acid can be taken up by bacterial species which colonize the GI. Theoretically therefore bacteria which cannot synthesize these substances should be suppressed in the GI. Witholding these binding substances could therefore have a similar effect on the bacterial ecology in the GI tract as the iron sequestering lactoferrin (or transferrin) (Gullberg, 1973, 1974; Ford, 1974). Recently McClelland (Edinburgh) (pers. comm.) studied the possible role of B$_{12}$-binding proteins on the bacterial flora of the human GI using "representative" intestinal organisms (coliforms, bacteroides, bifidobacteria and clostridia). They were found to take up free but not bound B$_{12}$; trypsin slightly reduced the molecular size of the protein but without releasing vitamin B$_{12}$ or affecting the bacteriostatic effect on B$_{12}$ dependent organisms. Thus McClelland does not support an *in vitro* bacteriostatic role for the vitamin B$_{12}$ binding protein.

ATTACHMENT OF *E. COLI* TO MILK FAT GLOBULE

The milk fat globule (FG) is surrounded by a true cell membrane, This can be shown by electron microscopy (unit membranes) and is supported by the serological cross reaction between FG and their membranes (FGM) and they are also agglutinated by the cold agglutinins present in blood *and* milk (Reiter, 1967). More recently it was found that the agglutination of RBC by *E. coli* possessing K$_{88}$ or K$_{99}$ antigens is inhibited by FG or FCM. The receptor destroying enzyme of *Vibrio cholerae* which is known to destroy RC receptor on the RBC for the *Vibrio* also destroyed the receptor on the FG and FGM for the coliforms (Reiter and Brown, 1976).

The agglutination of RBC however is nonspecific in the sense that RBC of any species, in this case of guinea-pigs, can be used for agglutination. It was therefore investigated whether *E. coli* can directly attach to FG or FGM, postulating that the FGM as a true cell membrane may possess the same specific receptors as brush borders. Indeed it was found that enteropathogenic bovine strains of *E. coli* possessing K$_{99}$ antigen only attached to bovine FGM, porcine enteropathogenic strains possessing K$_{88}$ antigen only to porcine FGM, while human entero-pathogenic strains possessing so-called colonization factors (Evans *et al.*, 1975; Evans and Evans, 1978) attached to human FGM but there was also a low attachment rate to porcine FGM by these strains (Fig. 8). The bovine and porcine

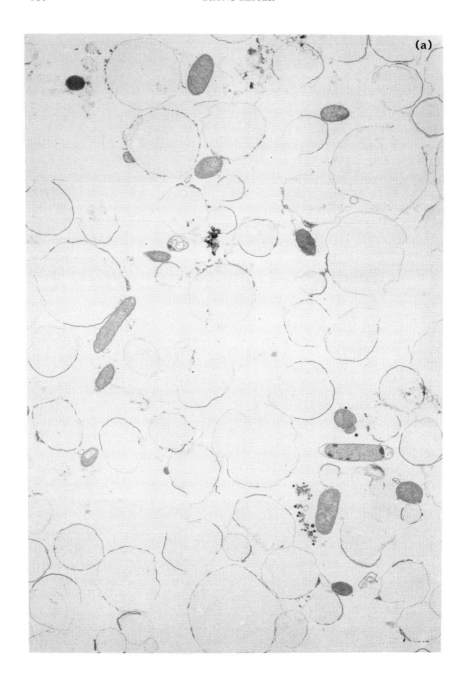

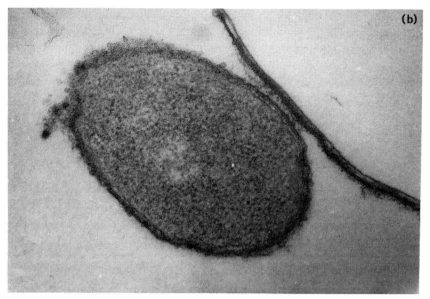

Fig. 8   (See Fig. 5).   The milk was fixed by addition of an equal volume of 6% gluteraldehyde in 0.2 M cacodylate-HCl buffer (pH 7·2). After 20 min the milk was centrifuged at 1000 **g** for 5 min and the cream layer removed and broken into small pieces. They were washed several times in 0·2 M cacodylate-HCl buffer (pH 7·2) and postfixed for 1 h in 1% osmium tetroxide in 0·1 M cacodylate buffer. Samples were then washed in distilled water, treated with 1% aqueous uranyl acetate for 0·5 h, dehydrated in dimethoxypropane and embedded in Araldite. Sections were cut using a Reichert Om U2 ultramicrotome, stained with lead citrate and examined in a Hitachi HU–11E electron microscope. (a) ×6360 (b) ×54 000. (Reiter *et al.*, unpublished).

strains failed to attach to FGM after exposure to the lactoperoxidase system while the human strains remain unaffected. The latter strains which are mannose sensitive (fail to attach to RBC in the presence of mannose) were also inhibited by mannose from attaching to FGM. Clearly the mode of attachment between these strains differs (Reiter *et al.*, unpublished). These experiments raise the question whether this attachment is so strong that it hinders the attachment to the intestinal wall *in vivo*.

GASTRIC ACIDITY

It is generally accepted that the gastric acid secretion is an important, or even most important "bactericidal barrier" against enteric infections (reviewed by Gianella *et al.*, 1973). Although abundant experimental and indirect evidence exists that enteric infections are promoted in achlorhydric patients, or by ingestion of bicarbonate prior to infusion with salmonellas, shigellas or choleras, the effect of the neutralization of the gastric hydrochloric acid by ingestion of milk seems to have been largely neglected.

Human milk has a lower buffering effect than bovine milk, yet, Maffei and Nóbrega (1975) found that the pH in bottle fed babies was lower than in breast fed babies. This apparent contradiction could be explained if we assume that the bottle fed baby is stimulated to secrete more HCl than the breast fed one. It is interesting that Maffei and Nóbrega (1975) also observed that infants with chronic diarrhoea and protein-calorie malnutrition has high pH values and bacterial overgrowth, essentially of Gram negative bacteria (Enterobacteraceae and Pseudomonads). Since infants with acute diarrhoea did not show such changes, the authors suggest that the gastric overgrowth occurs during the development of the disease to the chronic state. Although the breast fed infants had a gastric pH similar to those with chronic diarrhoea but without overgrowth, Maffei and Nóbrega suggest that *other factors*, besides pH, regulate bacterial growth in the gastric content of breast fed babies.

A CASE FOR NATURAL FEEDING OF THE NEWBORN

It is now generally recognized that colostrum and milk contain a multifactorial antibacterial system for the protection of the newborn until its own defence system is sufficiently developed to withstand the environmental challenge. Since the classes of immunoglobulins and the proportion of the nonantibody factors vary according to animal species, it is logical to conclude that suckling by the dam or feeding the host specific milk without any heat treatment, is most likely to fulfil such a defensive role. At this stage of our understanding, the relative importance of each of the antibacterial (and antiviral, not dealt with in this paper) factors occurring in milk is difficult to assess. Probably the total protective effect is greater than the sum of the individual factors.

The Igs and possibly also lactoferrin, have specific activities; that means the mother needs to have had an antigenic "experience" against the organisms to produce the specific Igs in the mammary gland for the protection of the newborn (Goldblum *et al.*, 1975). According to a much older suggestion, the mammary gland may even produce antibodies "on demand". The evidence is scant but of some interest. Petersen and his collaborators fought from 1955 onwards (before the discovery of IgA) for the acceptance of their thesis (reviewed by Campbell and Petersen, 1963) that the mammary gland was an "exocrine endothelial gland" capable of producing antibodies against bacteria and viruses. They suggested a direct stimulus of the mammary gland by the suckling young which was recently confirmed. When newborn calves (Campbell *et al*, 1957) or piglets (Salajka *et al.*, 1975) were infected with *Salmonella pullorum* and a pathogenic strain of *E. coli* respectively, the milk of the dams subsequently contained antibodies which had not been previously detected in the colostra or blood sera. This strongly auggested that the act of suckling infected the mammary glands which responded by producing specific antibodies. Petersen and his collaborators called this route of immunization for the benefit of the suckling offspring "diathelic"—through the duct.

It is generally accepted that sIgA is the most important class of Igs for the protection of the newborn because it is resistant to proteolysis. However, other classes of Igs seem also to survive the passage in the GI tract to some degree. Michael *et al.* (1973) added complement to faecal extracts of babies from 1–14 days old; they detected high bactericidal titres, corresponding to the Ig levels of the colostrum and post colostrum milk feed. Although the classes of the faecal Igs were not determined, it is likely that IgM was involved because it is the most efficient class of Igs for complement activated bactericidal activity. All the 3 classes of Igs—and lactoferrin, lysozyme and lactoperoxidase—are absorbed by bacteria. The question arises therefore whether these absorbed proteins are as susceptible to proteolysis as by themselves. Chaicumpa and Rowley (1972) exposed *Vibrio cholerea* to complement inactivated antiseum *in vitro*, and then orally infected 5-day-old suckling mice; the organisms failed to kill the mice because they were efficiently phagocyted and eliminated from the blood. These experiments show that the opsonizing activity of the Igs, almost certain to be IgG in a hyperimmune serum, remained unimpaired in the GI of the mice. IgG appears to sensitize bacteria for phagocytosis because it increases the hydrophobic interaction; sIgA makes bacteria less sensitive because the bacteria became less negatively charged and less liable to hydrophobic interaction (Stjernström *et al.*, 1977; Magnusson *et al.*, 1978).

It would be of some interest to investigate the susceptibility to proteolysis of the Igs when attached to bacteria—this includes not only the proteins derived from colostrum and milk but also those from saliva, including lactoferrin, lysozyme and lactoperoxidase. During suckling, contaminated organisms could be coated by salivary proteins (Brandtzaeg *et al.*, 1968) and all the protective factors of the colostrum. In this way the attachment of enteropathogenic bacteria to the intestinal epithelium may be prevented by Igs, or the lactoperoxidase system, IgM could bind complement for bactericidal activity, and IgG opsonize bacteria for phagocytosis; the Igs promoting the bacteriostatic activity of lactoferrin, and the lysozyme promoting complement binding by sIgA. Thus bacteria ingested during the period of suckling could be made innocuous. Although all these proteins could attach to potential pathogens immediately, the lactoperoxidase system would only be activated in the stomach by thiocyanate and the H_2O_2 produced by lactic acid bacteria, and lactoperoxidase is resistant to acid and proteolysis. Of all these antibacterial systems, only the lactoperoxidase system does not require specific antibodies and can therefore be regarded as a natural antibiotic.

In vivo Hilpert *et al.* (1977) showed that bovine Igs, mainly IgG_1 fed to babies, inactivated a toxin and could be detected in the faeces. In the faeces of calves all 3 classes of Igs, freed of hydrolysed fragments by chromatography, were detected after feeding of colostrum (Reiter, 1978). Logan *et al.* (1974) infected calves with enteropathogenic strain of *E. coli*. When fed saved whole colostrum, all the calves survived without diarrhoea, while the IgA fraction isolated from colostrum was found to be least effective, compared with IgM and IgG, in preventing diarrhoea, haemoconcentration, hyperkelaemia and uraemia. It appears also that IgG is the most active Ig in preventing attachment to the epithelium of the GI (Rutter *et al.*, 1976) although more work is required in this field.

Artificial feeding of the human newborn may be relatively successful in our sophisticated society, not least because of the nutritional and digestive resilience of the newborn, but also because of the high standard of hygiene. Feeding of processed milks under primitive hygiene conditions in underdeveloped societies is quite indefensible. Mata and his collaborators (see Mata and Urrutia, 1977) have conclusively demonstrated that breast feeding protects the human infant under the most appalling hygienic conditions; gastrointestinal disorders were of very low occurrence amongst Indian babies as long as they were exclusively suckled, but became frequent after weaning.

When breast feeding is not possible, such as in the case of preterm babies, human milk appears to be the first choice, either from its own mother or from a milk bank. In both cases it is common practice to drip feed through the nose and aspirate the saliva. The latter practice may be detrimental when we consider that saliva contains the same antibacterial factors as milk.

Milk collected for a milk bank is either fed raw after careful selection according to the best hygienic standards, or is heat treated. In both cases, the milk has been frozen at some stage which is bound to destroy the leukocytes—although it is still arguable whether the presence of leukocytes, particularly from another mother, is desirable.

Since the boiling of human milk has largely been abandoned, the milk is submitted to pasteurization, $\sim 63°C$ for 30 min. However, this time–temperature combination was adopted to kill *Mycobacterium tuberculosis* which is not a problem today. It is very likely that much lower time/temperature combinations would suffice to kill or at least heat shock the contaminating bacterial flora. Thus a higher proportion of the protective proteins could be preserved for the benefit of the baby.

In conclusion, colostrum and milk appear to be capable of suppressing potential pathogens in the neonate and thus promote a desirable balanced flora in the GI tract. It is therefore, of considerable interest that bovine colostrum and milk contain antibodies specific for pathogens and potential pathogens *but not* against the commensal and desirable bacterial flora—e.g. *Bacteroides* and *Lactobacillus* (Sharpe *et al.*, 1971). Such selective inhibitory action also applies to lactoferrin and the lactoperoxidase system. It is likley that human colostrum and milk fulfils the same role.

REFERENCES

Adinolfi, M., Glynn, A. H., Lindsa, M. P. and Milne, C. M. (1966). Seriological properties of A antibodies to *Escherichia coli* present in human colostrum. *Immunology* **10**, 517–526.

Aisen, P. and Liebman, A. (1968). The stability constant of the Fe^{++} conalbumin complexes. *Biochemical and Biophysical Research Communications* **30**, 407–413.

Allweiss, B., Dostal, J., Carey, K. E., Edwards, T. F. and Freter, R. (1977). The role of chemotaxis in the ecology of bacterial pathogens of mucosal surfaces. *Nature (London)* **266**, 448–450.

Aune, T. M. and Thomas, E. L. (1977). Accumulation of hypothiocyanite ion during peroxidase-catalyzed oxidation of thiocyanate. *European Journal of Biochemistry* **80**, 209–214.

Ballamy, J. E. C. and Nielson, N. O. (1974). Immuno-mediated emigration of neutrophiles into the lumen of the small intestine. *Infection and Immunity* **9**, 615–619.

Bishop, J. G., Schonbacher, F. L., Ferguson, L. C. and Smith, K. L. *In vitro* growth inhibition of mastitis causing coliform bacteria by bovine apolactoferrin and reversal of inhibition by citrate. *Infection and Immunity* **14**, 911–918.

Björck, L., Rosén, C.-G., Marshall, V. E. and Reiter, B. (1975). Antibacterial activity of the lactoperoxidase system in milk against pseudomonads and other Gram negative bacteria. *Applied Microbiology* **30**, 199–204.

Boulos, P. B., Dave, M., Whitfield, P. F. and Hobsley, M. (1977). Thiocyanate as a marker of saliva in gastric juice? *Gut* **18**, A496.

Brandtzeag, P., Fjellanger, I. and Gjeroldsen, S. T. (1968). Adsorption of immunoglobulins onto oral bacteria *in vivo*. *Journal of Bacteriology* **96**, 242–249.

Braun, O. H. (1976). Über die infektionsverhütende Wirkung der Muttermilch und deren moglichen Ursachen. *Klinische Paediatrics* **188**, 297–310.

Brock, J. H., Arzebe, F., Lampreave, F. and Piñero, A. (1976). The effect of trypsin and bovine transferrin and lactoferrin. *Biochimica et Biophysica Acta* **111**, 222–233.

Brock, J. H., Piñero. A. and Lampreave, F. (1978). The effect of trypsin and chymotrypsin on the antibacterial activity of complement, antibody and lactoferrin and transferrin in bovine colostrum. *Annales de Recherches Veterinaire* **9**, 287–294.

Bullen, J. J., Rogers, H. J. and Leigh, L. (1972). Iron binding proteins in milk and resistance to *Escherichia coli* in infants. *British Medical Journal* **1**, 69–75.

Bullen, J. J., Rogers, H. J. and Griffith, E. (1978). Role of iron in bacterial infection. *Current Topics in Microbiology, Immunology* **80**, 1–36.

Campbell, B. and Petersen, W. E. (1963). Immune milk—a historical survey. *Dairy Science Abstracts* **25**, 345–358.

Campbell, B., Sarwar, M. and Petersen, W. E. (1957). Diathelic immunization—a maternal-offspring relationship involving milk antibodies. *Science* **125**, 932–933.

Cañas-Rodriguez, A. and Smith, H. W. (1966). The indentification of the antimicrobial factors of the stomach contents of suckling rabbits. *Biochemical Journal* **100**, 79082.

Chaicumpa, W. and Rowley, D. (1972). Experimental cholera in infant mice: Protective effect of antibody. *Journal of Infectious Diseases* **125**, 480–485.

Documenta Geigy (1973). Scientific tables. 7th edn. p. 543–649. Geigy, Basle.

Dolby, J. M., Honour, P. and Valman, H. B. (1977a). Bacteriostasis of *Escherichia coli* by milk. I. Colonization of breast fed infants by milk resistant organisms. *Journal of Hygiene, Cambridge* **78**, 85–93.

Dolby, J. M., Stephens, S. and Honour, P. (1977b). Bacteriostasis of *Escherichia coli* by milk. II. Effect of bicarbonate and transferrin on the activity of infant feeds. *Journal of Hygiene, Cambridge* **78**, 235–242.

Donaldson, D. M., Ellsworth, B. and Matheson, A. (1974). Separation and purification of β-lysin from normal serum. *Journal of Immunology* **92**, 896–901.

Dowden, R. M., Brunner, J. R. and Philpott, D. E. (1967). Studies on milk globule membranes. *Biochimica et Biophysica Acta* **135**, 1–10.

Edelson, P. J. and Cohn, Z. A. (1973). Peroxidase-mediated mammalian cell toxicity. *Journal of Experimental Medicine* **138**, 318–323.

Evans, D. E. and Evans, D. J. Jr (1978). New surface-associated heat labile colonization factor antigen (CFA II) produced by entero toxigenic *Escherichia coli* of sero groups O_6 and O_8. *Infection and Immunity* **21**, 238–647.

Evans, D. G., Silver, R. P., Evans, D. J. Jr, Chase, D. G. and Gorbach, S. L. (1975). Plasmid controlled colonization factor associated with virulence in *Escherichia coli* enteropathogenic for humans. *Infection and Immunity* **12**, 656–667.

Evans, T. J., Ryley, H. C., Neale, L. M., Dodge, J. A. and Lewarne, V. M. (1978). Effect of storage and heat on anti microbial proteins in human milk. *Archives of Disease in Childhood* **53**, 239–241.

Eyres, R., Elliott, R. B., Howie, R. N. and Farmer, K. (1978). Low temperature pasteurization of human milk. *New Zealand Medical Journal* **87**, 135–138.

Falchuk, K. R., Perrotto, J. L. and Isselbacher, K. J. (1975). Serum lysozyme in Crohns disease and ulcerative colitis. *New England Journal of Medicine* **292**, 395–397.

Fleming, A. (1922). On a remarkable bacteriolytic element found in tissues and secretions. *Proceedings of the Royal Society B Sciences (London) 93,* 306–317.

Fodov, J. (1887). Die Fähigkeit des Blutes Bakterien zu vernichten. *Deutsche Medizinische Wochenschrift* **13**, 745–747.

Ford, J. E. (1974). Some observations on the possible nutritional signficance of vitamin B_{12} —and folate-binding proteins in milk. *British Journal of Nutrition* **31**, 243–257.

Ford, J. E., Law, B. A., Marshall, V. M. E. and Reiter, B. (1977). Influence of the heat treatment of human milk on some of its protective constituents. *Journal of Pediatrics* **90**, 29–35.

Giannella, R. A., Broitman, S. H. and Zamcheck, N. (1973). Influence of gastric acidity on bacterial and parasitic enteric infections. *Annales Internal Medicine* **78**, 271–276.

Gladstone, G. P. and Walton, E. (1971). The effect of iron and haematin on the killing of staphylococci by rabbit polymorphs. *British Journal of Experimental Pathology* **52**, 452–464.

Goldblum, R. M., Ahlstedt, S., Carlsson, B., Hanson, L. Å., Jodal, U., Lidin-Janson, G. and Sohl, A. (1975). Antibody-forming cells in human colostrum after oral immunization. *Nature (London)* **257**, 797–799.

Goldman, A. S. and Smith, C. W. (1973). Host resistance factors in human milk. *Journal of Pediatrics* **83**, 1082–1090.

Gothefors, L. and Marklund, S. (1975). Lactoperoxidase activity in human milk and in saliva of newborn infants. *Infection and Immunity* **11**, 1201–1215.

Green, D. E. and Pauli, R. (1943). The anti-bacterial action of the xanthine oxidase system. *Proceedings of the Society for Experimental Biology and Medicine (New York)* **54**, 148–150.

Griffith, E. and Humphrey, J. (1977). Bacteriostatic effect of human milk and bovine colostrum on *Escherichia coli*: the importance of bicarbonate. *Infection and Immunity* **15**, 396–401.

Groves, M. L. (1971). Minor milk proteins and enzymes. *In* "Milk Proteins" (Ed. H. A. McKenzie), *Chemistry and Molecular Biology,* Vol. 2. 396. Academic Press, London, New York.

Gullberg, P. (1973). Possible influence of vitamin B_{12}-binding protein in milk on the intestinal flora in breastfed infants. I. B_{12}-binding protein in human and bovine milk. *Scandinavian Journal of Gastroenterology* **8,** 479–503.

Gullberg, P. (1974). Possible influence of vitamin B_{12}-binding protein in milk on the intestinal flora of breastfed infants. II. Contents of unsaturated B_{12}-binding protein in meconium and faeces from breastfed and bottle fed infants. *Scandinavian Journal of Gastroenterology* **9,** 287–292.

Györgi, P. (1971). Biochemical aspects of human milk. *American Journal of Clinical Nutrition* **24,** 970–975.

Haber, F. and Weiss, J. (1934). The catalytic decomposition of hydrogen peroxide by iron salts. *Proceedings of the Royal Society, London* A **147,** 332–351.

Hanneberg, B. and Finne, P. (1974). Lysozymes in faeces from infants and children. *Acta Paediatrica Scandinavica* **63,** 588–594.

Hanson, L. Å. and Winberg, J. (1972). Breast milk and defence against infection in the newborn. *Archives of Disease in Childhood* **47,** 845–848.

Heddle, R. J., Knop, J., Steele, E. J. and Rowley, D. (1975). The effect of lysozyme on the complement action of different antibody classes. *Immunology* **28,** 1061–1066.

Henderson, S. G. (1942). The gastro intestinal tract of the healthy newborn infant. *American Journal of Roentgenology* **48,** 302–335.

Hill, I. R. and Porter, P. (1974). Studies of bactericidal activity to *Escherichia coli* of porcine serum and colostral immunoglobulins and the role of lysozyme with secretory IgA. *Immunology* **26,** 1239–1250.

Hilpert, H., Gerber, H., Amster, H., Pahud, J. J., Ballabriga, A., Arcalis, L., Farriaux, F., Peyer, de E. and Nussle, D. (1977). Bovine immunoglobulins, their possible utilization in industrially prepared infant milk formulae. *In* "Food and Immunology" (Eds. L. Hambraeus, L. Å. Hanson and H. McFarlane), 182, 196. Almquist and Wiksell International, Stockholm.

Hogg, D. McC. and Jago, G. R. (1970a) The antibacterial action of lactoperoxidase. The nature of the bacterial inhibitor. *Biochemical Journal* **117,** 779–790.

Hogg, D. McC. and Jago, G. R. (1970b) The oxidation of reduced nicotinamide nucleotides by hydrogen peroxide in the presence of lactoperoxidase and thiocyanate, iodide or bromide. *Biochemical Journal* **117,** 791–797.

Hoogendorn, H., Piessens, J. P., Scholtens, W. and Stoddard, L. A. (1977). Hypothiocyanate ion: the inhibitor formed by the system lactoperoxidase-thiocyanate hydrogen peroxide. I. Identification of the inhibiting compound. *Caries Research* **11,** 77–84.

Jacket, P. S., Aber, V. R. and Lowrie, A. B. (1978). Virulence of *Mycobacterium tuberculosis* and susceptibility to peroxidative killing systems. *Journal of General Microbiology* **107,** 273–278.

Johnston, R. B. Jr, Keele, B. B., Misra, H. P., Lehmeyer, J. C., Webb, L. S., Bachner, R. L. and Rajapopalan, K. V. (1975). The role of super oxide anion generation in phagocytic bactericidal activity. Studies with normal and chronic granulomatous disease leucocytes. *Journal of Clinical Investigation* **55,** 1357–1372.

Johnston, R. B. Jr, Godzik, C. A. and Cohn, Z. A. (1978). Increased superoxide anion production by immunologically activated and chemically elicited macrophages. *Journal of Experimental Medicine* **148,** 115–127.

Jones, G. W. (1977). The attachment of bacteria to the surfaces of animal cells. *In* "Microbial Interactions" (Ed. J. L. Reissig), 139–176. Chapman and Hall, London.

Kaplan, S. S., Quie, P. C. and Basford, R. E. (1975). Effect of iron on leucocyte function: Inactivation of H_2O_2 by iron. *Infection and Immunity* **12**, 303–308.

Kiermeier, F. and Kayser, C. (1960). Zur Kenntnis der Lactoperoxidase Aktivität in Kuhmilch und Abhängigkeit von biologischen Einflüssen. *Zeitschrift für Lebensmittel-Untersuchung und Forschung* **112**, 481–498.

Klebanoff, S. J. (1967). Iodination of bacteria: a bacteriocidal mechanism. *Journal of Experimental Medicine* **126**, 1063–1078.

Klebanoff, S. J. (1974). Role of superoxide anion in the myeloperoxidase-mediated antimicrobial system. *Journal of Biological Chemistry* **249**, 3724–3728.

Klebanoff, S. J. and Smith, D. C. (1970). Peroxidase-mediated activity of rat uterine fluid. *Gynecological Investigations* **1**, 21–30.

Klebanoff, S. J., Clem, W. H. and Luebke, R. G. (1966). The peroxidase-thiocyanate-hydrogen peroxide antimicrobial system. *Biochemica Biophysica Acta* **117**, 63–72.

Korhonen, H. (1973). Untersuchungen zur Bakterizidie der Milch und Immunisierung der bovimen Milchdrüse, p. 88. PhD Dissertation, Helsinki.

Krause, R. M. (1958) Studies on bacteriophages of haemolytic streptococci: II. Antigens released from the streptococcal cell walls by phage-associated lysin. *Journal of Experimental Medicine* **108**, 803–821.

Krawezuk, J., Sawicki, Z. and Krawczynski, J. (1978). Diagnostic value of lysozyme activity, estimation in the feces of infants with acute diarrhoea. *Journal of Clincal, Chemical, and Clinical Biochemistry* **16**, 343–347.

Krinsky, N. I. (1974). Singlet excited oxygen as a mediator of the anti-bacterial action of leucocytes. *Science (Washington DC)* **186**, 363–365.

Law, B. A. and Reiter, B. (1977). The isolation and bacteriostatic properties of lactoferrin from bovine milk whey. *Journal of Dairy Research* **44**, 595–597.

Logan, E. F., Stenhouse, A. and Ormrod, D. J. (1974) The role of colostral immunoglobulins in intestinal immunity to enteric coli bacillosis in the calf. *Research in Veterinary Science* **3**, 290–301.

Logothetopulos, J. H. and Myant, N. B. (1956). Concentration of radio-iodide and ^{35}S-labelled thiocyanante by the stomach of the hamster. *Journal of Physiology* **133**, 213–219.

McCelland, D. B. L. and Furth, R. von. (1975). In vitro synthesis of lysozyme by human and mouse tissues and leucocytes. *Immunology* **28**, 1099–1114.

McCelland, D. B. L., McGrath, J. and Samson, R. R. (1978) Antimicrobial factors in human milk. *Acta Paediatrica Scandinavica Supplement* **271**, 1–20.

Maffei, H. V. L. and Nóbrega, F. J. (1975). Gastric pH and microflora of normal and diarrhoeic infants. *Gut* **16**, 719–726.

Magnusson, K. E., Stendahl, O., Stjernström, I. and Edebo, L. (1978). The effect of colostrum and colostral antibody sIgA and phagocytosis of *Escherichia coli* O' 86. *Acta Pathologica et Microbiologica Scandinavica* Section B **86**, 113–120.

Marshall, V. M. (1978) *In vitro* and *in vivo* studies on the effect of the lactoperoxidase–thiocyanate–hydrogen peroxide system on *Escherichia coli*. PhD Thesis, Reading University.

Marshall, V. M. and Reiter, B. (1976). The effect of the lactoperoxidase/thiocyanate/hydrogen peroxidase system on the metabolism of *Escherichia coli*. *Proceedings of Society for General Microbiology* **3**, 109.

Mason, S. (1962). Some aspects of gastric function in the newborn. *Archives of Disease in Childhood* **37**, 387–391.

Masson, P. L. (1970). "La Lactoferrine". Arscia, Bruxelles. Librarie Maloine, Paris.

Masson, P. L., Heremans, J. F., Prignot, J. and Wauters, G. (1966). Immuno-histochemical localization and bacteriostatic properties of an iron-binding protein from bronchial mucus. *Thorax* **21**, 538–544.

Mata, L. J. and Urrutia, J. J. (1977). Infections and infectious diseases in a malnourished population: a long-term prospective field study. *In* "Food and Immunology" (Eds L. Hambraeus, L. Å. Hanson and H. McFarlane), 42–57. Almquist and Wiksell International, Stockholm.

Michael, J. G., Ringenbock, R. and Hottenstein, S. (1971). The anti-microbial activity of human colostral antibody. *Journal of Infectious Diseases* **124**, 445–448.

Morrison, M. and Allen, P. Z. (1963). The identification and isolation of lactoperoxidase from salivary gland. *Biochemical and Biophysical Research Communications* **13**, 490–494.

Morrison, M. H. and Steele, W. F. (1968). Lactoperoxidase, the peroxidase in the salivary gland. *In* "Biology of the Mouth". (Ed. P. H. Parson), 89–110. American Society for the Advancement of Science.

Morrison, M. H., Hamilton, B. and Stotz, E. (1957). The isolation and purification of lactoperoxidase by ion exchange chromatography. *Journal of Biological Chemistry* **228**, 767–776.

Nakamura, O. (1923). Über Lysozymwirkungen. *Zeitschrift für Immunitätsforschung Experimentelle und Klinische Immunologie* **38**, 425–447.

Nathan, C. F., Brukner, L. H., Silverstein, S. C. and Cohn, Z. A. (1979a). Extracellular cytolysis by activated macrophages and granulocytes. I. Pharmacologic triggering of effector cells and release of hydrogen peroxide. *Journal of Experimental Medicine* **149**, 84–99.

Nathan, C. F., Nogueira, N., Juangbhanich, C., Ellis, J. and Cohn, Z. (1979b). Activation of macrophages *in vivo* and *in vitro*: Correlation between peroxide release and killing of *Tryponsoma cruzi*. *Journal of Experimental Medicine* **149**, 1056–1068.

Oram, J. D. and Reiter, B. (1965). Phage associated lysins affecting Group N and D streptococci. *Journal of General Microbiology* **40**, 57–70.

Oram, J. D. and Reiter, B. (1966). Inhibitory substances present in milk and secretion of the dry udder, p. 93. Report of National Institute for Research in Dairying.

Oram, J. D. and Reiter, B. (1968). Inhibition of bacteria by lactoferrin and other iron-chelating agents. *Biochemical et Biophysica Acta* **170**, 351–365.

Ørskov, I., Ørskov, F., Sojka, W. J. and Leach, J. N. (1961). Simultaneous occurrence of E. *coli* B and L antigens in strains from diseased swine. Influence of cultivation temperature on two new *E. coli* K antigens K_{87} and K_{88}. *Acta Pathologica et Microbiologica Scandinavia* **79**, 142–152.

Ørskov, I., Ørskov, F., Smith, H. W. and Sojka, W. J. (1975). The establishment of K_{99}, a thermo labile, transmissible *Escherichia coli* antigen, previously called 'KC$_0$', possessed by calf and lamb enteropathogenic strains. *Acta Pathological et Microbiologica Scandinavia* **B83**, 31–36.

Osserman, E. F., Confield, R. F. and Beychok, S. (1974). "Lysozyme". Proceedings of a conference, New York, 1972. Academic Press, New York.

Osugi, T. (1977). Development of peroxidase-mediated antibacterial activity in embryonic salivary glands of the mouse. *Archives of Oral Biology* **22**, 237–241.

Paape, M. J. and Guidry, A. J. (1977). Effect of fat and casein in intracellular killing by milk leucocytes. *Proceedings of the Society of Experimental Biology and Medicine* **155**, 588–593.

Padgett, G. A. and Hirsch, J. E. (1967). Lysozyme: its absence in tears and leucocytes of cattle. *Australian Journal of Experimental Biology and Medical Science* **45**, 569–571.

Paxson, C. L. and Cress, C. C. (1979). Survival of human milk leucocytes. *Journal of Pediatrics* **94**, 61–64.

Peaker, M. and Linzell, J. L. (1975). Citrate in milk: a harbinger of lactogenesis. *Nature (London)* **253,** 464–465.

Peterson, R. G. and Hartsell, E. (1955). The lysozyme spectrum of the Gram negative bacteria. *Journal of Infectious Diseases* **96,** 75–81.

Pitt, (1974). Necrotizing enterocolitis, Report, 68th Roth Conference on pediatric Research, p. 53–56.

Pitt, J. ,Barlow, B. and Heird, W. C. (1977). Protection against experimental necrotizing enterocolitis by maternal milk. I. Role of milk leucocytes. *Pediatric Research* **11,** 906–909.

Raptopoulou-Gigi, M., Marwick, K. and McClelland, D. B. L. (1977). Antimicrobial proteins in sterilized human milk. *British Medical Journal* **1,** 12–14.

Reiter, B. (1967). Relationship of the agglutinins of the milk fat globule to the cold agglutinins of the erythrocytes. Annual Report, National Institute for Research in Dairying, p. 89.

Reiter, B. (1976). Bacterial inhibitors in milk and other biological secretions with special reference to the complement–antibody, transferrin–lactoferrin and lactoperoxidase–thiocyanate–hydrogen peroxide system. *In* "Inhibition and inactivation of vegetative microbes" (Eds F. A. Skinner and W. B. Hugo), p. 31–60. Academic Press.

Reiter, B. (1978a). Review of the Progress of Dairy Science: antimicrobial systems in milk. *Journal of Dairy Research* **45,** 131–147.

Reiter, B. (1978b). Reveiw of non specific antimicrobial factors in colostrum. *Annales de Recherches Veterinaires, Paris* **9,** 205–224.

Reiter, B. (1979). The lactoperoxidase–thiocyanate–hydrogen peroxide system. *In* "Oxygen free radicals and tissue damage". CIBA Foundation Symposium No. 65 (new series).

Reiter, B. and Bramley, A. J. (1975). Defence mechanisms of the udder and their relevance to mastitis control. *In* "Proceedings of Seminar on mastitis control" (Eds F. H. Dodd, T. K. Griffien and R. G. Kingwill), 210–215. International Dairy Federation.

Reiter, B. and Brock, J. H. (1975). Inhibition of *Escherichia coli* by bovine colostrum and post colostral milk. I. Complement-mediated bactericidal activity of antibodies to a serum susceptible strain of *E. coli* of the serotype 0111. *Immunology* **28,** 71–82.

Reiter, B. and Brown, P. (1976). Inhibition of the haemagglutination of red blood cells by K_{88} and K_{99} adhesin using milk fat and fat globule membrane. *Proceedings of the Society for General Microbiology* **3,** 109.

Reiter, B. and Gibbons, R. A. (1964). Some further aspects of the lactoperoxidase–thiocyanate–hydrogen peroxide inhibitory system with special reference to the behaviour of spermatoza in cervical mucus. Annual Report, National Institute for Research in Dairying, p. 87.

Reiter, B. and Marshall, V. M. E. (1975/76). The *in vivo* antibacterial activity of the lactoperoxidase–thiocyanate–hydrogen peroxide system in milk. Academic Report, National Institute for Research in Dairying, p. 90.

Reiter, B. and Oram, J. D. (1962). Inhibition of a streptococcal bacteriophage by suramin. *Nature (London)* **193,** 651–652.

Reiter, B. and Oram, J. D. (1967). Bacterial inhibitors in milk and other biological fluids. *Nature (London)* **216,** 328–330.

Reiter, B., Pickering, A., Oram, J. D. and Pope, G. S. (1963). Peroxidase-thyocyanate inhibition of streptococci in raw milk. *Journal of General Microbiology* **33,** xii.

Reiter, B., Pickering, A. and Oram, J. D. (1964). An inhibitory system—lactoperoxidase/thiocyanate–hydrogen peroxide—in raw milk. *In* "Microbial Inhibitors in Food" (Ed. N. Molin), p. 297–305. 4th International Symposium on Food Microbiology Almqvist and Wiksell, Uppsala.

Reiter, B., Björck, L., Marshall, V. M., Longman, A. G. and Cousins, C. M. (1973/74).

Preservative effect of the lactoperoxidase–thiocyanate–hydrogen-peroxide system in milk. Annual Report, National Institute for Research in Dairying, p. 98.

Reiter, B., Brock, J. H. and Steel, E. D. (1975). Inhibition of *Escherichia coli* by bovine colostrum and post colostral milk. II. The bacteriostatic effect of lactoferrin—one a serum susceptible and serum resistant strain of *E. coli*. *Immunology* **28**, 83–95.

Reiter, B., Marshall, V. E., Björck, L. and Rosén, C.-G. (1976). Non specific bactericidal activity of the lactoperoxidase–thiocyanate–hydrogen peroxide system of milk against *Escherichia coli* and some Gram negative pathogens. *Infection and Immunity* **13**, 800–807.

Reiter, B., Marshall, V. M. and Philips, S. M. (1980). The lactoperoxidase, thiocyanate–hydrogen peroxide system. I. The antibiotic activity in the calf abomasum. *Research in Veterinary Science* **28**, 116–122.

Robinson, J. E., Harvey, B. A. and Soothill, J. F. (1978). Phagocytosis and killing of bacteria and yeasts by human milk cells after opsonization in aqueous phase of milk. *British Medical Journal* **1**, 1443–1445.

Rogers, H. J. (1976). Ferric iron and the antibacterial effects of horse serum 7S antibodies to *Escherichia coli* 0111. *Immunology* **30**, 425–433.

Rogers, H. J. and Synge, C. (1978). Bacteriostatic effect of human milk on *Escherichia coli*: the role if IgA. *Immunology* **34**, 19–28.

Ruddell, W. J. J., Blendis, L. M. and Walters, C. L. (1977). Nitrite and thiocyanate in the fasting and secreting stomach and in saliva. *Gut* **18**, 73–77.

Russel, M. W. and Reiter, B. (1975). Phagocytic deficiency of bovine milk leucocytes: an effect of casein. *Journal of the Reticuloendothelial Society* **18**, 1–13.

Russel, M. W., Brooker, B. E. and Reiter, B. (1976). Inhibition of the bacteriocidal activity of bovine polymorphonuclear leucocytes and related systems by casein. *Research in Veterinary Sciences* **20**, 30–35.

Russel, M. W., Brooker, B. E. and Reiter, B. (1977). Electron microscopic observations of the interaction of casein micelles and milk fat globules with bovine polymorphonuclear leucocytes during the phagocytosis of staphylococci in milk. *Journal of Comparative Pathology* **87**, 43–52.

Rutter, J. M., Jones, G. W., Brown, G. T. H., Burrows, M. R. and Luther, P. D. (1976). Antibacterial activity of colostrum and milk associated with protection of piglets against enteric disease caused by K_{88}-positive *Escherichia coli*. *Infection and Immunity* **13**, 667–676.

Salajka, E., Cernohovs, J. and Sarmanova, Z. (1975). Association of the colonization of the intestine by pathogenic strains of haemolytic *E. coli* in weaned piglets with withdrawal of antibody contained in the dam's milk. *Documenta Veterinaria Brno* **8**, 43–55.

Samson, R. R., Mirtle, C. and McClelland, D. L. (1979). Secretory IgA does not enhance the bacteriostatic effects of iron-binding or vitamin B_{12}-binding proteins in human colostrum. *Immunology* **38**, 367–373.

Schindler, J. S. and Bardsley, W. G. (1975). Steady state kinetics of lactoperoxidase with ABTS as a chromogen. *Biochemical and Biophysical Research Communications* **67**, 1307–1312.

Schindler, J. S., Childs, R. E. and Bardsley, W. G. (1976). Peroxidase from human cervical mucus. The isolation and characterization. *European Journal of Biochemistry* **65**, 325–331.

Sellwood, R., Gibbons, R. A., Jones, G. W. and Rutter, J. M. (1975). Adhesion of enteropathogenic *Escherichia coli* to pig intestinal brush borders: the existence of two pig phenotypes. *Journal of Medical Microbiology* **8**, 405–411.

Selsted, M. E. and Martinez, R. J. (1978). Lysozyme; Primary bactericidin in human plasma sserum active against *Bacillus subtilis*. *Infection and Immunity* **220**, 7782–791.

Sharpe, M. E., Latham, M. J. and Reiter, B. (1975). The immune response of the host animal to bacteria in rumen and caecum. *In* "Digestion and metabolism in the ruminant"

(Eds I. W. McDonald and A. C. Warner), 193–204. The University of New England Publishing Unit.

Spik, G., Sheron, A., Montreuil, J. and Dolby, J. M. (1978). Bacteriostasis of a milk sensitive strain of *Escherichia coli* by immunoglobulins and iron-binding proteins in association. *Immunology* **35**, 663–671.

Stelmaszyńska, T. and Zgliczyński, B. (1971). Studies on hog intestine mucosa peroxidase. *European Journal of Biochemistry* **119**, 56–61.

Stephens, S., Harkness, R. A. and Cockle, S. M. (1979). Lactoperoxidase activity in guinea pig milk and saliva: correlation in milk of lactoperoxidase with bactericidal activity against *Escherichia coli*. *British Journal of Pathology* **60**, 252–258.

Stjernstrom, I., Magnusson, K. E., Stendahl, O. and Tagesson, C. (1977). Liability to hydrophobic and charge interaction of smooth *Salmonella typhimurium* 395 MS sensitized with Anti-MS Immunoglobulin G and complement. *Infection and Immunity* **18**, 261–265.

Thomson, J. and Morell, D. B. (1967). The structure, location and distribution of salivary gland peroxidase. *Journal of Biochemistry* **62**, 483–486.

Vakil, J. R., Chandan, R. C., Parry, R. M. and Shahani, K. M. (1969). Susceptibility of several microorganisms to milk lysozyme. *Journal of Dairy Science* **52**, 1192–1197.

Wardlaw, A. C. (1962). The complement-dependent bacteriolytic activity of normal human serum. I. The effect of pH and ionic strength and the role of lysozyme. *Journal of Experimental Medicine* **115**, 1231–1249.

Weidel, W. (1951). Über die Zell-membran von *E. coli* B. I. Präperierung der Membranen. Analytische Daten. Morphologie und Verhalten der Membranen gegen über den Bakteiophagen der T-Serie. *Zeitschrift für Naturforschung* **126**, 421–425.

Wilkinson, P. C. (1972). Characterisation of chemotactic activity of casein for neutrophil leucocytes and macrophages. *Experientia* **28**, 1051–1052.

Wood, J. L. (1975). Biochemistry. *In* "Chemistry and Biochemistry of Thiocyanic Acid and its Derivatives" (Ed. A. A. Newman), 156–221. Academic Press, London, New York.

Wright, R. C. and Tramer, J. (1958). Factors influencing the activity of cheese starters. The role of peroxidase. *Journal of Dairy Research* **25**, 104–118.

DISCUSSION

Wood   With regard to the maturity of lactation, you said that you had had some milk from mothers who had been delivered preterm, and that lactoperoxidase was not to be found there. This seems to be very interesting and might be well worth looking at on a larger scale. I think that immature breast milk is higher in protein content than is mature breast milk. By "immature" I mean where the baby is delivered before 40 weeks. I should be surprised if the milk were found to be deficient in some other protective mechanism. It is worth going into, I think.

Reiter   I do not know about the other proteins but it was a surprise to us to find this deficiency in lactoperoxidase. You must remember that in the case of any of the protective proteins that we talked about, lactoperoxidase is the only one that increases after parturition. In the cow it reaches a maximum in five days and then decreases slowly. In human milk I think it is three days. Incidentally, in regard to

Dr Bullen's work, I quite agree that the lactoferrin has a place. But his animals (guinea-pigs) dosed with haematin, were killed at three days; after three days the bactericidal activity of the guinea-pig milk can be reversed by a reducing agent, indicating that the lactoperoxidase system is active. The organism might multiply up to 40 times. I should like very much to follow that up, particularly since haematin reacts with H_2O_2. For each factor to be investigated a different animal is needed. With the guinea-pig we definitely want to consider both lactoferrin and lactoperoxidase. It is interesting to note that the calf is born without lactoperoxidase in the saliva. The baby is born with lactoperoxidase in the saliva. If the baby suckles it will contribute lactoperoxidase to the milk which is relatively low in human milk.

Walker-Smith Could I comment on gastric pH? There is a difference between gastric pH of breast fed babies and bottle fed babies. Maffei and Nóbreya (1975) showed that gastric pH in normal breast fed babies was higher than in normal bottle fed infants. Thus there is a relative gastric hypo-acidity in breast fed babies as compared to bottle fed babies. It is interesting to speculate whether nature has made it safer for the "good things" in breast milk which may be sensitive to low pH to reach the small intestine intact.

Reiter Did you say that the gastric pH was higher?

Walker-Smith Yes, in breast fed babies. Although they have more acid stools, they secrete less gastric acid.

Soothill I was interested that we found milk polymorphs working better than you did. Could this be a species difference? Ours was human. If yours was bovine, the difference might arise from the difference in casein concentration or fat globule formation. Could this be another example of the superiority of human milk?

Reiter It was bovine. You see, when we used polymorphs isolated from the blood we got normal bactericidal activity as with other species, but when we took bovine polymorphs and suspended them in milk and measured, after 2, 4 and 6 h, ingestion and bactericidal activity, intracellular killing progressively decreased.

Tyrrell If I may make a contribution on a slightly different subject, Dr Matthews in our laboratory demonstrated that normal human milk contains a nonantibody, antiviral substance. It is rather peculiar in that it seems to impair the entry of viruses into cells, thus you must have to have both the cell and the virus and this inhibitor present in the system at the same time in order to demonstrate its effect, but it works on a very wide range of viruses. It was found to be inactivated in the process of producing powdered milk or drying. It is present in cows' milk and a number of other species besides humans. I think we would like to know two things. One is exactly what it is, and the other is whether it really helps the baby at all. It does appear to be associated with the glycoproteins—its activity is associated with the polysaccharides, and may even be found in IgA rich fractions apparently in the glycosylated part of the molecule rather than in the antigen binding sites. This is another system which may have an effect on the overall experience of an animal fed naturally, but I do not know of anybody who has proved that there is a beneficial effect. Do you?

Reiter I have seen the abstract and was very much intrigued by it. I can only say, the more the merrier! Do those viruses attach to erythrocytes?

Tyrrell Some of the susceptible viruses attach to erythrocytes, others do not.

Reiter But of course they would have to enter some mammalian membrane at some stage, and I just wondered whether preparation of fat globule membranes were looked at. They can be produced easily.

Tyrrell Something very similar is found on other biologically important sites too; for example, I recently had a conversation with an American colleague (Dr S. Baron) who seems to have stumbled on something rather similar in normal tissue cultures being produced by the cells. He was looking for an inhibitor, which he thought might be interferon, and he turned up a substance which has very similar properties to what we found in milk. So they may not be unique at all.

Reiter Dr Harrison (Bath University) let me have some fractions of glycopeptide fractions isolated from fat globule membranes. He had the same idea, independently, to use the fat globular membrane as a model for the intestinal membrane. The glycopeptide inhibited haemagglutination by *E. coli*, but haemagglutination is much less specific than the attachment to FGM or brush border.

Kuitunen Can you comment on Prof. Ballabriga's attempts to vaccinate cows and in that way develop better cows' milk for babies?

Reiter I do not know about the Spanish work, but I know that Dr Hilbert (Nestlés) has vaccinated cows and isolated immunoglobulins. They did two trials: one in Spain and one in France, when they fed these bovine immunoglobulins to babies with diarrhoea. I do not know what has happened since. A few millilitres of human colostrum does just as well, if you can get hold of it.

Walker-Smith Could I ask the general body of opinion whether people think *E. coli* enteritis is now common enough to justify the production of such a milk? If such a milk were to be produced, it would be more applicable to the developing world, but it would be practical to have a milk with such antibodies in a country like this nowadays?

Reiter We cannot rear piglets with bovine powdered milk, 25% die; we cannot even rear calves easily, the hygienic conditions are of course different. I would definitely not advocate the replacement of breast milk, but we are thinking about a cheap whey powder (containing lactoperoxidase) for postweaning feeding, when the real trouble starts.

Marshall Do you think that this milk which is going to protect all these infants in the developing world will be able to overcome the problem of the consumption of massive amounts of bacteria from the contaminated water supply?

Reiter This is a nasty one, because of course we cannot. If we make a powder and it is made up with contaminated water, this is dangerous. We have two trials going on in Keyna and Mexico in which we suppress bacterial contamination in the milk by the lactoperoxidase system so that the milk arrives in a fit state at 30°C, travelling for 6 h from the collection centre. But this is a question of the challenge dose.

Marshall This has been shown recently in Gambia. The water for domestic consumption contained from 2.6×10^2 to 4.0×10^{10} ml^{-1} (Rowland *et al.*, 1977). Thus a lot of bacteria are being fed to infants and you will need a great deal of antibody to cope with them.

Reiter Can you explain to me also why they throw away the colostrum? Is it taboo in The Gambia.

Marshall I do not know.

Soothill I think we shall be very cautious in recommending sending any sort of milk powder for infant feeding to developing countries. But if areas where this is less potentially damaging, is there any serious evidence that those far more readily available antibodies, IgG antibodies from blood, would not work just as well or nearly as well as IgG antibodies from the milk of the animal?

Reiter That has been tried, of course, particularly IgM, in calves, but there was a great difficulty because of problems of virus infections. Blood from the slaughterhouse was diluted with distilled water, precipitating the IgM which was fed to calves to prevent diarrhoea. I am not thinking of replacing breast feeding— that would be a crime. But postweaning food is something worthwhile considering.

Walker-Smith Harking back to Bill Marshall's point, it is clear in the developing world that if breast fed infants at the same time are also receiving enormous amounts of bacteria in their weaning food that they may develop gastroenteritis. Thus, it is hardly likely that an artificial milk with antibodies would be better than breast feeding, which does not prevent gastroenteritis in such circumstances. However, if the weaning food were replaced by a food supplement such as this and could be provided in a manner such that it would not be bacterially contaminated, this should be a practical proposition. Although we are convinced that breast feeding is best, we must remember that severe dehydrating gastroenteritis can occur in breast fed babies who are also having a heavily bacterially contaminated weaning food in addition.

REFERENCES

Maffei, H. V. L. and Nóbrega, F. J. (1975). Gastric pH and microflora of normal and diarrhoeic infants. *Gut* **16**, 719–726.

Rowland, M. G. M. and McCollum, J. P. K. (1977). *Transactions of the Royal Society of Tropical Medicine and Hygiene* **71**, 199–203.

Advances in Immunization for Protection of the Fetus and Newborn against Infection

J. W. G. SMITH

National Institute for Biological Standards and Control,
Hampstead, London, UK

The newborn baby may suffer the effects of infection acquired *in utero*, during labour, or shortly after birth and may also be harmed indirectly from maternal or placental infection (Banatvala, 1977; Fox, 1977; Gamsu, 1977). The newborn baby can be immunized, usually passively with immunoglobulin given shortly after birth, but the possibilities are greater of providing indirect protection by means of immunity transferred from the mother, who may be immunized either actively with vaccines or, sometimes, passively with immunoglobulin, and these procedures may additionally protect the fetus and newborn by preventing maternal infection. Protection of the baby by vaccination of those who care for the mother or baby will not be considered here, although there are circumstances where this could be of value, for example, the vaccination of medical and nursing staff against rubella, or the administration of live poliomyelitis vaccine to interfere with transmission of enteroviruses in nurseries.

197

Numerous microbial pathogens, including protozoa, mycoplasmas, bacteria, chlamydias and viruses, both wild and vaccine strains, have been shown capable of harming the fetus and newborn baby, and these effects have been well reviewed in recent years (Dudgeon, 1976; Alberman and Peckham, 1977; Tobin et al., 1977; Hurley et al., 1978; Waterson, 1979). Whilst all human pathogens are presumably capable of attacking the newborn baby, who is susceptible to relatively low grade pathogens, a high proportion of neonatal infections are caused by a more restricted range of organisms, such as Escherichia coli, pseudomonads, staphylococci (Pryse-Davies and Hurley, 1979). This may imply the possibility of using vaccines against some of these pathogens but, apart from certain important exceptions, in practice the incidence of serious neonatal infections due to most individual pathogens is so low that the use of vaccines is unlikely to be worthwhile. The range of pathogens that may harm the fetus when the pregnant mother is infected is probably much smaller, but there is still much to be learnt, particularly in the case of maternal infections which are infrequent or difficult to diagnose, or in which the risk of damage to the fetus is low or the effects on the baby subtle and not revealed until later in life (Brown and Karunas, 1972; Siegal, 1973). The application of immunization procedures to protect the fetus and newborn baby depends not only on the availability of vaccines but also on epidemiological knowledge, of the risks presented by particular pathogens and of the safety and effectiveness of corresponding vaccines when given to the newborn, older age groups or to the pregnant woman. If, for example, the possibility that influenza gives rise to fetal abnormality or malignancy were to be verified (Fedrick and Alberman, 1972; Hakulinen et al., 1973), active immunization of pregnant mothers could be of value. Conversely, a demonstrated risk to the fetus from a vaccination procedure would act as a contra-indication to maternal immunization and as an encouragement to inducing the particular immunity before the age of child bearing was reached. Such decisions are dependent on epidemiological studies to evaluate the risks involved, and are mentioned in order to emphasize the need for such work, difficult though it may be.

Immunization already has an established place in the prevention of congenital defects and infections of the newborn. BCG vaccination, for example, is used to protect babies born into infected families (DHSS, 1972). Active and passive immunization against rubella was introduced solely for preventing congenital defects, although the optimal policy for the use of live rubella vaccine is still debated, as is the value of immunoglobulin for nonimmune mothers (Peckham and Marshall, 1979). Vaccinia immunoglobulin for the passive immunization of babies born of mothers affected by vaccinia virus has also been available for a number of years. Numerically, the most valuable immunization procedure for protection of the newborn may be the use of tetanus toxoid in pregnant women to prevent tetanus neonatorum. It has been estimated that more than 50 000 people die in the world each year from tetanus, and a high proportion are newborn babies in the developing countries (Bytchenko, 1966). Immunization of the pregnant mother with two spaced doses of adsorbed toxoid will prevent this disease and attempts are being made to develop vaccines which will be effective in a single dose (Kielmann and Vohra, 1977; D'Sa *et al.*, 1978). These established procedures will not be referred to further, attention being instead confined in this brief review to certain infections in which recent progress suggests that practical benefits may become available in the relatively short-term future.

CYTOMEGALOVIRUS

Human cytomegalovirus (CMV) usually causes subclinical infection but, as with other herpesviruses, infection is common, and about 70% of young adults possess serum antibodies to the virus and may remain symptom-free carriers for life. Infection first acquired in early pregnancy is often transmitted to the fetus (Stern and Tucker, 1973) and in a proportion of cases leads to permanent defects, notably mental retardation (Alberman and Peckham, 1977). However, reactivation of latent infection in pregnancy has by no means been excluded as a cause of fetal damage (Stagno *et al.*, 1977). As many as 1·0% of babies may be congenitally infected and one in ten of these suffer symptoms (Hanshaw *et al.*, 1973); the infection is an important cause of congenital defect and a successful vaccine could be of great value.

Two attenuated live vaccines are under investigation. The AD169 strain, attenuated by H. Stern and S. D. Elek (Elek·and Stern, 1974) by repeated passage in a variety of cells, has been shown to be immunogenic when given subcutaneously to healthy volunteers, and relatively free from immediate side-effects, apart from local soreness and, occasionally, fever. The Towne strain, attenuated by S. A. Plotkin by passage 125 times in WI-38 human diploid fibroblasts, is also under study, and when given subcutaneously has caused seroconversion in 14 seronegative subjects (Just *et al.*, 1975; Plotkin *et al.*, 1976). Neither strain appears to be recoverable from vaccinees, in contrast to the 4–5% of naturally infected persons who are found to excrete virus in the urine or other secretions. Early evidence suggests that antibodies decline after vaccination, so that the duration of serological immunity is uncertain. Clinical studies are in progress to evaluate these strains in renal transplant patients who, when infected from blood transfusion, are believed to have a higher rate of graft rejection than those who remain uninfected.

There are important difficulties in the way of utilizing herpesvirus vaccines, quite apart from question of the degree of protection and the duration of immunity they may induce. Differences in the antigenic properties and DNA chemistry of strains have been reported, so that the protective antigens could also differ (Huang *et al.*, 1976). Infected persons usually carry latent virus for life, and there is the possibility that carriage of vaccine strains could be harmful. Since the role of reactivated latent virus in causing congenital defect is uncertain, the safety of vaccine virus in this respect would require very careful evaluation. Herpesviruses, such as the Epstein-Barr virus and herpes simplex type II virus in man, and certain animal herpesviruses, are associated with cancer and the possibility of vaccine virus causing such a complication has to be considered. Nevertheless, an attenuated, immunogenic herpes vaccine virus should be safer than the wild virus, and the prevention of congenital defect from CMV is now at least a possibility.

HEPATITIS A

Infection with hepatitis A virus is the commonest cause of jaundice in pregnancy (Haemmerli, 1966), but the fetus *in utero* does not appear to be affected, although birth may be premature. Infection in late pregnancy or the puerperium may be transmitted to the baby during or after birth.

Passive Immunization

Normal human immunoglobulin is protective against hepatitis A if given before or within one or two weeks of exposure (Krugman, 1963; Public Health Laboratory Service, 1968), and its use in pregnant women who are travelling to areas of high endemicity could therefore have some influence in reducing prematurity from this cause, as well as neonatal hepatitis. There is no evidence that passive immunization is of benefit when given to the patient after the onset of jaundice. However, in the event of jaundice in late pregnancy or the puerperium, the use of normal human immunoglobulin for the baby would seem to be advisable, although there appear to be no specific reports of its value in these circumstances.

Active Immunization

Formalin inactivated vaccine prepared from the liver of infected marmosets has been developed and shown to be protective in eight of these animals when given in eight injections spaced over 14 weeks (Provost and Hilleman, 1978). The vaccine is liable to come to clinical trial in the next year or two. It is of potential value for travellers to areas where the infection is common, and used in this way could indirectly benefit the neonate.

HEPATITIS B

Although not established as a cause of congenital defect, hepatitis B virus can infect the newborn, mainly from mothers who themselves acquire the infection in late pregnancy or the puerperium, and such infants may have persisting antigenaemia. Of 27 infants infected when their mothers had acute hepatitis in pregnancy, 13 were found to be carriers, but of 21 babies of mothers who were asymptomatic carriers only one developed antigenaemia (Schweitzer et al., 1973). Hepatitis B infection in early pregnancy appears not to be associated with a risk to the fetus, possibly because protective antibody is also transferred; the viral antigen for which this antibody is specific is not certain, but it is probably the HBe antigen (Tobin et al., 1977).

Passive Immunization

Human antihepatitis B immunoglobulin is available, prepared from donors with antibody to hepatitis B surface antigen (HBsAg). When given to exposed adults it can certainly delay the onset of symptoms and viraemia in exposed subjects, and is probably protective (Seeff et al., 1975), but in one study follow-up for over six months revealed that hepatitis could develop after this time; however, re-exposure could not be excluded and proteases in the immunoglobulin may have impaired its activity in vivo (Grady and Lee, 1975; Prince, 1978). At present, antihepatitis B immunoglobulin is regarded as of protective value and therefore worth giving to exposed subjects, but a sound estimate of its effectiveness has yet to be made. If not available, normal immunoglobulin may be of some use, but its effect may not be great in circumstances of heavy exposure, as may be the case in the fetus and newborn (Prince, 1978).

In preventing neonatal infection hepatitis B immunoglobulin could be given (a) to mothers who, on screening, are found to be carriers, as their babies are at risk from transplacental transfer, ingestion of blood and secretions at birth, and from the milk. The risk to such infants appears to be low, except possibly in certain racial groups, such as those of Chinese origin living in Taiwan and Japan (Cossart, 1978; Derso et al., 1978). Infants born of maternal carriers whose blood is positive both for HBe antigen and when tested for DNA polymerase appear to be at greater risk than those whose mothers are negative in these tests (Beasley et al., 1977). The protective value to the fetus or newborn baby of giving immunoglobulin to the pregnant mother in such cases has not been established and could not at present be advised; (b) to mothers who have acute HBsAg-positive hepatitis during the third trimester. The effect of passive maternal immunization in this event is open to study; (c) to infants born of mothers who either develop infection in late pregnancy or puerperium, or are carriers of HBsAg, especially if HBe antigen and RNA polymerase positive. There is clinical trial evidence that spouses can be protected in this way and the use of specific immunoglobulin for the baby has therefore been recommended (US Advisory Committee, 1977; Prince, 1978). Continued protection of babies of HBeAg-positive mothers may require repeated injections of anti-HBsAg immunoglobulin.

Active Immunization

In 1971 S. Krugman and colleagues showed that heated serum from a hepatitis B carrier induced a degree of protection in volunteers (Krugman *et al.*, 1971). More recently, experimental vaccine has been prepared by concentrating hepatitis surface antigen from the blood of carriers and inactivating at 60°C for 10 h. Such a vaccine has proved protective in a small number of experimental chimpanzees, but its safety is uncertain; there has apparently been one incident of such material transmitting infection to a chimpanzee. French workers have studied a vaccine prepared by purifying HBsAg by affinity chromatography and treating with formalin. This vaccine was immunogenic in five chimpanzees, and 96 human volunteers who worked in a renal unit were vaccinated with two injections. Forty six of the volunteers were studied serologically five months later and 35 had had an antibody response, although natural exposure could not be excluded as a cause in a proportion of these subjects. Comparison with nonvaccinated subjects suggested that protection against antigenaemia was induced for this five month period (Maupas *et al.*, 1976). Other workers are attempting to purify the protective hepatitis B polypeptides and a subunit vaccine, prepared by means of caesium chloride centrifugation followed by formalin inactivation, has proved immunogenic in chimpanzees (Purcell and Gerin, 1975). The synthesis of these antigens is also a future possibility (see review by Zuckerman, 1977).

The most promising approach to a hepatitis B vaccine is the production of HBsAg in *Escherichia coli* by means of genetic engineering. The core antigen has been expressed in this way using as starting material DNA isolated from Dane particles (Burrell *et al.*, 1979). The nucleotide sequence of the gene coding for HBsAg has recently been established (Valenzuela *et al.*, 1979) and there seems to be no reason why the antigen should not be expressed in a suitable micro-organism in the near future. Although the main use of such a vaccine would be outside the field of fetal and neonatal protection it could be of definite value in this respect when used in women who are known, or liable, to be exposed to infection.

RESPIRATORY SYNCYTIAL VIRUS

Respiratory syncytial virus (RSV) is an important and common pathogen in the first year of life (Martin *et al.*, 1978). Its most serious respiratory manifestations—bronchitis, bronchiolitis and pneumonia—are most frequently seen in the first six months of life. The infection is occasionally fatal and has been incriminated as a cause of cot death. It may also give rise to longterm respiratory sequelae (Downham *et al.*, 1975; Hall *et al.*, 1979). In a UK survey of cases of RSV infection admitted to hospital, 0·96% were in the first month of life and 17·7% in babies one to three months old (Report, 1978). Of 23 neonatal infections reported in a study from the USA, severe illness occurred mostly in the fourth week of life, symptoms of infection in the first three weeks usually being milder. Four of the 23 cases were fatal, three of these being over three weeks of age (Hall *et al.*, 1979). The main value of vaccines would therefore apply after the neonatal period, but if immunization could be accomplished early, it could have benefits in the first month of life. In any event, to protect against the main effects of the virus an effective vaccine requires to be capable of immunizing successfully the very young infant. Passive immunity derived from the mother may be responsible for the relative sparing of infants in the first three weeks of life, but such a limited effect does not encourage the possibility that vaccination of older girls and women would indirectly provide much protection for the young baby (Glazen *et al.*, 1978; Hall *et al.*, 1979).

Reinfection of children is common (Henderson *et al.*, 1979) and when it occurred one year after the first infection the resulting illness was not significantly less severe clinically than first infections, although third episodes were milder, an effect which appeared to be independent of the inverse association between age and severity. A single dose of live vaccine may not, therefore, be capable of inducing a high level of immunity nor one of long duration; however, even a short period of immunity could be valuable in protecting babies during their early months of life when the infection is most dangerous.

Active Immunization

Attempts to develop vaccine have been made for some years. An inactivated preparation was subjected to clinical trial in 1966, but vaccinated infants who subsequently became infected in an outbreak 9 months later tended to have a more severe illness than controls (Kapikian *et al.*, 1969). The cause is not known, but serum antibody, in the absence of other parameters of immunity, may have been responsible for a hypersensitivity to the virus. A similar state of affairs was resolved in the case of measles by means of live vaccines, and since live, attenuated vaccines have proved so successful in immunizing against virus infections recent attention has been directed to the preparation of live RSV vaccines. Chanock and his coworkers, using passage in calf kidney and bovine fetal kidney tissue culture and 5-fluorouridine as a mutagen, have developed a number of temperature sensitive (*ts*) mutants incapable of growth at 39°C. The first mutant vaccine studied was a cold-adapted strain which in infants and children was immunogenic in 26 of 39 tested, but caused mild respiratory illness in three infants aged 6–12 months, one of whom developed bronchitis. A *ts* mutant vaccine was tested in 32 infants and children aged 6 months to 6 years. The vaccine was infective but caused rhinitis in seven children, one of whom developed otitis media, possibly as a secondary consequence of the vaccine-induced upper respiratory infection (Parrott *et al.*, 1975). Virus recovered from vaccinated children included a proportion which had undergone partial reversion of the *ts* property (Hodes *et al.*, 1974). Further strains are under investigation by this group, potential candidate vaccine strains being studied in primates (Belshe *et al.*, 1978), and *ts* mutants are also being studied in the laboratory in the UK (Gimenez and Pringle, 1978).

Preliminary studies have also been reported of a live RSV vaccine given subcutaneously. The strain was passaged in WI-38 cells but there appears to be no evidence that it is attenuated. When given to children 7–23 months of age, 19 of 22 showed an antibody response and did not develop clinical RSV illness (Buynak *et al.*, 1978). Immunization by the introduction of virulent or attenuated virus by an unusual route has a long history, centuries in the case of variolation, and this RSV vaccine may prove to be a modern example.

The possibility of using a live, attenuated RS vaccine in infants is thus being actively studied, despite the difficulties of establishing a suitable vaccine strain, the background of adverse effects from killed vaccine, and the likely difficulty of inducing an immunity in the young, immunologically immature baby.

VARICELLA-ZOSTER

Maternal varicella in early pregnancy may be transmitted to the fetus, giving rise to such defects as atrophic limbs, cortical atrophy, micro-ophthalmia, cataract and skin lesions, but since adult infection is uncommon, varicella is a rare cause of congenital defect. However a small proportion of medical students and nurses are found nowadays to lack varicella antibodies and this proportion could become greater in developed countries. The virus may also attack the newborn of sero-negative mothers who develop the infection shortly before or after giving birth, infection being acquired by the fetus via the placenta or by direct exposure after birth. Neonatal varicella is serious and is associated with a case fatality ratio of at least 10% (Meyers, 1974), and the rate may be higher when the infection develops more than 4 days after birth, possibly because in such cases the baby is unlikely to have had any passive maternal antibody (Gershon, 1975).

Passive Immunization

Evidence has accumulated that varicella-zoster immune globulin, from the blood of donors convalescent from zoster, is capable of preventing infection in exposed subjects when given before or within 3 days of exposure. When given up to a week after exposure a degree of attenuation of the infection is possible (Balfour and Groth, 1979). It could therefore be of value to protect susceptible pregnant women in contact with varicella, although it might be difficult to be certain in individual cases that the woman is susceptible to the infection. Varicella-zoster immunoglobulin is in short supply and its use in pregnancy might at present be considered to have a lower priority than, for example, its use in exposed leukaemic children, in whom it is life saving. Specific immune globulin has also been advised in the USA for neonates whose mothers develop varicella at or near delivery. Although a prophylactic effect in the newborn has not specifically been established, the procedure is undoubtedly of great potential value in preventing this uncommon but serious neonatal infection and represents a significant advance.

Active Immunization

If, as has happened with other infectious diseases, an increasing proportion of women reach child bearing years without having had chickenpox, vaccination of girls against this disease might become necessary in order to prevent its serious effects on the fetus and the newborn. A live attenuated vaccine, the OKA strain, has been developed by Takahashi in Japan by passage in human embryonic lung cells, guinea-pig embryo cells and WI-38 human diploid cells. It has been subjected to clinical trial in normal adults and in children, including leukaemic and immunocompromised patients (Asano and Takahashi, 1977). Results so far reported suggest that the vaccine is safe, immunogenic and protective, even in the highly susceptible groups. M. Just, in Switzerland, has used a vaccine, derived from the Japanese strain, on an experimental basis in sero-negative medical students, again with apparent success. There is now interest in the UK in studying the use of this vaccine in immunocompromised children. Should this early promise be sustained, its application would require careful appraisal. General vaccination of infants, for example, might have drawbacks, since partial uptake, by inducing a degree of herd immunity, could increase the proportion of susceptible young women in the population.

GROUP B HAEMOLYTIC STREPTOCOCCI

The association of group B streptococci with infection of the newborn was not appreciated as being other than a rarity until 1964 (Eickhoff et al., 1964). In the USA it has now been reported as the main cause of menigitis in the first two months of life, and has been estimated to affect approximately one baby in 500, of whom about half die, and many of those who survive suffer disablement (Franciosi et al., 1973; Horn et al., 1974) Infection appears to be less common in the UK than in the USA.

Early onset disease presents within the first 5 days of life, usually in the form of respiratory infection and septicaemia. In these cases, labour is often difficult and the Streptococcus is probably acquired by the neonate during birth from the maternal vagina, which is frequently colonized asymptomatically. Alternatively, infection may be acquired by exposure after birth, giving rise to late onset disease, usually meningitis. The source of infection in these cases is less certain; transmission by those who handle the baby may be important.

Of the five recognized serotypes of group B streptococci, type III causes most neonatal infections in the USA, where it is associated with nearly 90% of meningitis and 50% of septicaemia cases (Wilkinson, 1978). In the UK about 57% of meningitis cases and 38% of other neonatal systemic infections are due to type III (Parker, 1979). A successful vaccine against type III infection, if used to immunize the pregnant mother, might be capable of inducing passive protection in the baby, and incorporation in the vaccine of polysaccharide antigens protective against types Ia and Ib should extend coverage to about 90% of infections in the UK.

Evidence that vaccination of the mother could protect the neonate by means of passively transferred antibody depends on the following observations. (a) Few maternal vaginal carriers of group B streptococci have seriously infected babies, especially in the case of late onset disease, suggesting that passive maternal antibody may be protective. (b) Mothers with affected babies tend to have lower group B type III polysaccharide antibody levels in their serum than those whose babies are unaffected (Baker and Kasper, 1976). (c) Anticapsular type-specific antibody is protective in mice infected with type I strains (Baker, 1977) and bactericidal against type III strains (Balitimore et al., 1977). (d) Successful polysaccharide vaccines have been developed from the protective capsular antigens of *Haemophilus influenzae, Neisseria meningitis* and *Streptococcus pneumoniae*. Although such a vaccine has not yet been developed for the prevention of group B streptococcal disease, there is much interest in the possibility, particularly in the USA (Baker, 1977).

DISCUSSION

The potential scope for the use of immunization for preventing congenital defect and neonatal infection is, in practice, probably limited. Defects are common and affect about 1:37 babies, but the proportion caused by maternal infection is unknown and may be small. Of the multitude of infectious agents capable of attacking the human adult, only a few have been implicated as responsible for a significant number of congenital defects. In these instances, however, immunization may have an important role, and promising developments in relation to CMV and varicella, for example, have been referred to. But the specific preventive tool of immunization is unlikely to find wide application in controlling those cases due to one of a large range of infrequent causative agents, although its potential can properly be evaluated only in the light of greater knowledge of the specific causes of congenital defect.

In the case of neonatal infections, the role of immunization is similarly limited by the wide variety of microbes that can attack the baby, any individual species or antigenic variety being itself a rare cause of harm. Additionally, chemoprophylaxis can often be used to prevent these infections, especially in at-risk cases, such as the debilitated or premature baby born after a prolonged and difficult labour who may be at risk from the attack of almost any pathogen. However, the identity of the responsible pathogen(s) can usually be determined more readily than is the case with congenital defect. As a result the range of organisms and the frequency with which they affect the newborn is becoming better established, so that the possibility of using active or passive immunization for control of the more common or more dangerous ones is open to consideration, for example, herpes simplex viruses, hepatitis viruses, varicella, and group B streptococci. *Escherichia coli* is common among the pathogens responsible for severe infection of the newborn and recent studies suggest that, among the numerous antigenic types of *E. coli*, strains possessing the K1 capsular polysaccharide antigen are particularly important (Sarff *et al.*, 1975). Whilst it may be difficult to vaccinate the newborn baby against this antigen, as polysaccharides are often poorly immunogenic in those under the age of one year, maternal immunization is possible. A greater use of passive immunization of the neonate can also be envisaged, using immunoglobulin known to contain antibody against specific pathogens, especially viruses, for which chemoprophylaxis is at present unavailable, or bacterial species which are often antibiotic resistant, such as *Pseudomonas* spp. It might become practicable to prepare, in quantities sufficient for clinical use, monoclonal human antibody against a number of the pathogens causing infection of the newborn. However, the possibility of using immunization against more than a few of the neonatal pathogens does not seem great, although its scope might well increase as information accumulates on the importance of specific pathogens in causing intra-uterine and neonatal damage.

REFERENCES

Alberman, E. and Peckham, C. (1977). Long-term effects following infections in pregnancy. *In* "Infections and Pregnancy" (Ed. C. R. Coid), 489–514. Academic Press, London, New York.

Asano, Y. and Takahashi, M. (1977). Clinical and serologic testing of a live varicella vaccine and two-year follow-up for immunology of the vaccinated children. *Pediatrics* **60**, 810–814.

Baker, C. J. (1977). Summary of workshop on perinatal infections due to group B streptocci. *Journal of Infectious Diseases* **136**, 137–152.

Baker, C. J. and Kasper, D. L. (1976). Correlation of maternal antibody deficiency with susceptibility to neonatal group B streptococcal infection. *New England Journal of Medicine*, **294**, 753–756.

Balfour, H. H. and Groth, K. E. (1979). Zoster immune plasma prophylaxis of varicella: a follow-up report. *Journal of Pediatrics* **94**, 743–746.

Baltimore, R. C., Kasper, D. L., Baker, C. J. and Goroff, D. K. (1977). Antigenic specificity of opsonophagocytic antibodies in rabbit antisera to group B streptococci. *Journal of Immunology* **118**, 673–678.

Banstuda, J. E. (1977). Health of mother, fetus and neonate following maternal viral infections during prenancy. *In* "Infections and Pregnancy" (Ed. C. R. Coid), 437–488. Academic Press, London, New York.

Beasley, R. P., Trepo, C. and Stevens, C. E. (1977). The e antigen and vertical transmission of hepatitis B surface antigen. *American Journal of Epidemiology* **105**, 94–98.

Belshe, R. B., Richardson, L. S., London, W. T., Sly, D. L. Camargo, E., Prevar, D. A. and Chanock, R. M. (1978). Evaluation of five temperature-sensitive mutants of respiratory syncytial virus in primates. II Genetic analysis of virus recovered during infection. *Journal of Medical Virology* **3**, 101–110.

Brown, G. C. and Karunas, K. S. (1972). Relationship of congenital anomalies and maternal infection with selected enteroviruses. *Journal of Epidemiology* **93**, 207 217.

Burrell, C. J., Mackay, P., Greenaway, P. J., Hopschneider, P. H. and Murray, K. (1979). Expression in *Escherichia coli.* of hepatitis B virus DNA sequences cloned in plasmid pBR 322. *Nature* **279**, 43–47.

Buynak, E. B., Weibel, R. E., McLean, A. A. and Hilleman, M. R. (1978). Live respiratory syncytial virus vaccine administered parenterally. *Proceedings of the Society for Experimental Biology and Medicine* **157**, 636–642.

Bytchenko, B. (1966). Geographical distribution of tetanus in the world 1951–60. A review of the problem. *Bulletin of the World Health Organisation* **34**, 71–104.

Cossart, Y. E. (1978). Transmission of hepatitis B from mother to infant. *Medical Journal of Australia* **2**, 550–551.

DHSS (1972). Immunisation against infectious diseases. HMSO.

Derso. A., Boxall, E. H., Tarlow, M. J. and Flewett, T. M. (1978). Transmission of HBsAg from mother to infant in four ethnic groups. *British Medical Journal* **1**, 949–952.

Downham, M. A. P. S., Gardner, P. S., McQuillin, J. and Ferris, J. A. J. (1975). The role of respiratory viruses in childhood mortality. *British Medical Journal* **1**, 235–239.

D'Sa, J. A., Dastur, F. D., Awatramani, V. P., Dixit, S. K. and Nair, K. G. (1978). Tetanus immunisation with one dose vaccine—preliminary data. *Journal of the Association of Physicians of India* **26**, 891–894.

Dudgeon, J. A. (1976). Infective causes of human malformations. *British Medical Bulletin* **23**, 77–83.

Eickhoff, T. C., Klein, J. O., Daley, A., Ingall, D. and Finland, M. (1964). Neonatal sepsis and other infections due to group B beta-haemolytic streptococci. *New England Journal of Medicine* **271**, 1221–1228.

Elek, S. D. and Stern, H. (1974). Development of a vaccine against mental retardation caused by cytomegalovirus infection *in utero*. *Lancet* **i**, 1–5.

Fedrick, J. and Alberman, E. D. (1972). Reported influenza in pregnancy and subsequent cancer in the child. *British Medical Journal* **2**, 485–488.

Fox, H. (1977). Infections of the placenta. *In* "Infections and Pregnancy" (Ed. C. R. Coid, 251–288. Academic Press, London, New York.

Franciosi, R. A., Knostman, J. D. and Zimmerman, R. A. (1973). Group B streptococcal neonatal and infant infections. *Journal of Pediatrics* **82**, 707–718.

Gamsu, H. (1977). Health of mother, fetus and neonate following bacterial, fungal and protozoal infections during pregnancy. *In* "Infections and Pregnancy", (Ed. C. R. Coid), 344 436. Academic Press, London, New York.

Gershon, A. A. (1975). Varicella in mother and infant: problems old and new. *In* "Infections of the Fetus and the New-Born Infant", (Eds S. Krugman and A. A. Gershon), Vol. 3, 79–96. New York.

Gimenez, H. B. and Pringle C. R. (1978). Seven complementation groups of respiratory syncytial virus temperature-sensitive mutants. *Journal of Virology* 27, 459–464.

Glazen, W. P., Paredes, A. and Taber, L. M. (1978). Pathogenesis of respiratory syncytial (RS) virus bronchiolitis in infants. *Pediatric Research* 12, 492–498.

Grady, G. F. and Lee, V. A. (1975). Hepatitis B immune globulin—Prevention of hepatitis from accidental exposure among medical personnel. *New England Journal of Medicine* 293, 1067–1072.

Haemmerli, U. P. (1966). Jaundice during pregnancy with special emphasis on recurrent jaundice during pregnancy and its differential diagnosis. *Acta Medica Scandinavica* Suppl. 144.

Hakulinen, T., Hovi, L., Karkinen-Jääskeläinen, M., Penttinen, K. & Saxén, L. (1973). Relation between influenza during pregnancy and childhood leukaemia. *British Medical Journal* 4, 265–267.

Hall, C. B., Kopelman, A. E., Douglas, R. G., Geiman, J. M., Meagher, M. P. and McQuillan, J. (1979). Neonatal respiratory syncytial virus infection. *New England Journal of Medicine* 300, 393–396.

Hanshaw, J. B., Schultz, F. W., Melish, M. M. and Dudgeon, J. A. (1973). Congenital cytomegalovirus infection. *In* "Intrauterine Infections", (Eds K. M. Elliott and J. Knight), 23–32. Ciba Foundation Symposium No. 10 (new series) Elsevier, Amsterdam.

Henderson, F. W., Collier, A. M., Clyde, W. A. and Denny, F. W. (1979). Respiratory syncytial virus infections, reinfections and immunity. A prospective longitudinal stray in young children. *New England Journal of Medicine* 300, 530–534.

Hodes, D. S., Kim, H. W., Parrott, R. H., Camargo, E. and Chanock, R. M. (1974). Genetic alteration in a temperature-sensitive mutant of respiratory syncytial virus after replication *in vivo*. *Proceedings of the Society for Experimental Biology and Medicine* 145, 1158–1164.

Horn, K. A., Zimmerman, R. A., Knostman, J. D. and Meter, W. T. (1974). Neurological sequelae of group B streptococcal neonatal infections. *Pediatrics* 53, 501–504.

Huang, E. S., Kilpatrick, B. A., Huang, Y.-T. and Pagano, J. S. (1976). Detection of human cytomegalovirus and analysis of str variation. *Yale Journal of Biology and Medicine* 49, 29–43.

Hurley, R., de Louvois, J. and Drasar, F. (1979). Perinatal and neonatal infections. Proceedings of a Symposium, 9 June, 1978. *Journal of Antimicrobiol Chemotherapy* 5, Suppl. A.

Just, M., Buergin-Wolff, A., Emoedi, G. and Hernandez, R. (1975). Immunisation trials with live attenuated cytomegalovirus Towne 125. *Infection* 3, 111–114.

Kapikian, A. Z., Mitchell, R. H., Chanock, R. M., Shvedoff, R. A. and Steward, C. E. (1979). An epidemiological study of altered clinical reactivity to respiratory syncytial (RS) virus infection in children previously vaccinated with an inactivated RS virus vaccine. *American Journal of Epidemiology* 89, 405–421.

Kielmann, A. A. and Vohra, S. R. (1977). Control of tetanus neonatorium in rural communities—immunisation effects of high-dose calcium phosphate-adsorbed tetanus toxoid. *Indian Journal of Medical Research* 66, 906–916.

Krugman, S. (1963). The clinical use of gamma globulin. *New England Journal of Medicine* 269, 195–201.

Krugman, S., Giles, J. P. and Hammond, J. (1971). Viral hepatitis type B (MS-2 strain). Studies on active immunisation. *Journal of the American Medical Association* 217, 41–45.

Martin, A. J., Gardner, P. S. and McQuillen, J. (1978). Epidemiology of respiratory virus infection among pediatric inpatients over a six-year period in North East England. *Lancet* ii, 1035–1038.

Maupas, P., Goudeau, A., Coursaget, P., Drucker, J. and Bagnos, P. (1976). Immunisation against hepatitis B in man. *Lancet* i, 1367–1370.

Meyers, J. D. (1974). Congenital varicella in term infants: risk reconsidered. *Journal of Infectious Diseases* 129, 215–217.

Parker, M. T. (1979). Infections with group B streptococci. *Journal of Antimicrobial Chemotherapy* 5, Suppl. A, 27–37.

Parrott, R. H., Kim, H. W., Brandt, C. D. and Chanock, R. M. (1975). Potential of attenuated respiratory syncytial virus vaccine for infants and children. *In* "Developments in Biological Standardisation" (Ed. F. T. Perkins), Vol. 28, 389–398. Karger, Basel.

Peckham, C. and Marshall, W. C. (1979). Rubella and other virus infections in pregnancy. *Journal of Antimicrobial Chemotherapy* 5, Suppl. A, 71–80.

Plotkin, S. A., Farquhar, J. and Hornberger, E. (1976). Clinical trials of immunisation with the Towne 125 strain of human cytomegalovirus. *Journal of Infectious Diseases* 134, 470–475.

Prince, A. M. (1978). Use of hepatitis B immune globulin; reassessment needed. *The New England Journal of Medicine* 299, 198–199.

Provost, P. J. and Hilleman, M. R. (1978). An inactivated hepatitis A virus vaccine prepared from infected marmoset liver. *Proceedings of the Society for Experimental Biology and Medicine* 159, 201–203.

Pryse-Davies, J. and Hurley, R. (1979). Infections and perinatal mortality. *Journal of Antimicrobial Chemotherapy* 5, Suppl. A, 59–70.

Public Health Laboratory Service Report. (1968). Assessment of British gammaglobulin in preventing infectious hepatitis. *British Medical Journal* 3, 451–454.

Purcell, R. H. and Gerin, J. L. (1975). Hepatitis B subunit vaccine: a preliminary report of safety and efficacy tests in chimpanzees. *American Journal of the Medical Sciences* 270, 395–399.

Report. (1978). Respiratory syncytial virus infection; admissions to hospital in industrial, urban and rural areas. Report to the Medical Research Council Sub-committee on Respiratory Syncytial Virus Vaccines. *British Medical Journal* 2, 796–798.

Sarff, L. D., McCracken, G. H., Schiffer, M. S., Glode, M. P., Robbins, J. B., Ørskov, I. and Ørskov, F. (1975). Epidemiology of *Escherichia coli* K1 in healthy and diseased new-born. *Lancet* i, 1099–1104.

Schweitzer, I. L., Mosley, J. W. and Ashcavai, M. (1973). Factors influencing neonatal infection by hepatitis B viruses. *Gastroenterology* 65, 277–283.

Seeff, L. B., Zimmerman, H. J., Wright, E. C., Schiff, E. R., Kiernan, T., Leevy, C. M., Tamburro, C. H. and Ishak, K. G. (1975). Hepatic disease in asymptomatic parenteral narcotic drug abusers: a veterans administration collaborative study. *American Journal of Medical Science* 270, 41–47.

Siegal, M. (1973). Congenital malformations following chickenpox, measles, mumps and hepatitis. Results of a cohort study. *Journal of the American Medical Association* 226, 1521–1524.

Stagno, S., Reynolds, D. W., Huang, E-S., Thames, S. D., Smith, R. J. and Alford, C. A. (1977). Congenital cytomegalovirus infection: occurrence in an immune population. *New England Journal of Medicine* 296, 1254–1258.

Stern, H. and Tucker, S. M. (1973). Prospective study of cytomegalovirus infection in pregnancy. *British Medical Journal* 11, 268–270.

Tobin, J. O'H., Jones, D. M. and Fleck, D. G. (1977). Aetiology, Diagnosis, Prevention and Control of Infections Affecting Pregnancy in Humans. *In* "Infections and

Pregnancy" (Ed. C. R. Coid), 1–52. Academic Press, London, New York.

US Advisory Committee. (1977). Immune globulins for protection against viral hepatitis. *Morbidity and Mortality Weekly Report*. US Department of Health, Education and Welfare **26,** 425–442.

Valenzuela, P., Gray, P., Quiroga, M., Zaldivar, J., Goodman, J. M. and Rutter, W. J. (1979). Neucleotide sequence of the gene coding for the major protein of hepatitis B virus surface antigen. *Nature* **280,** 815–819.

Waterson, A. P. (1979). Virus infections (other than rubella) during pregnancy. *British Medical Journal* **3,** 564–566.

Wilkinson, H. W. (1978). Analysis of group B streptococcal types associated with disease in human infants and adults. *Journal of Clinical Microbiology* **7,** 176–179.

Zuckerman, A. J. (1977). Hepatitis B vaccines, *Nature* **267,** 578–579.

DISCUSSION

Wood I certainly realize the importance of your last comments about the real difficulties in applying immunological protection to more infants in view of the comparative rarity of the problems caused by the infections you have mentioned. But I would like to persuade you to think of this in a slightly different context. Our objective is to further reduce perinatal morbidity and perinatal mortality to the point where there is almost no avoidable perinatal loss or morbidity because we are now a society with a policy of restriction of family size, small families with a lot invested in individual children. There is a case for trying very hard to make sure that all that is preventable is prevented. The cost of handicap is now very high, not only in a personal but also in a financial sense. The cost of a handicapped infant to society is measurable in hundreds of thousands of pounds.

Lambert To add to what Joe Smith said, we will have more and more changes in the future in existing policies of immunization because of the effects of those policies themselves. The current example is measles; we have a perfectly well defined measles immunization policy which is, however, not accepted in a wholehearted way. There therefore is no statistical possibility of the eradication of measles in the foreseeable future. The only certain epidemiological result is an increasing average age of acquiring measles in the children who get it, with the result that we are already seeing a considerable amount of writing from the USA about epidemics of measles in adolescents and young adults. They licensed in 1963 and we licensed in 1968 so they are some way ahead of us, but we are about to see an appreciable number of women of child bearing age now who are nonimmune to measles. We know extraordinarily little about measles in pregnancy and measles in the neonate simply because nearly every woman so far has had measles antibody.

So I think we shall have to think a lot about the future measles immunization programme in the next decade in relation to possible neonatal measles. The same may apply to other common banal pathogens. One sees a surprising number of nurses from the West Indies, young girls of 18, 20, 22, who get varicella, and in one of our geriatric units there was recently an outbreak among the staff of West Indian birth originating in an elderly patient with zoster which actually caused the ward to be closed because all the girls got chickenpox.

Stern   I would agree with Prof. Wood that we must look at this in absolute terms. For example, in the case of CMV although the number of congenital defects due to this virus may be small in proportion to the total number of congenital defects in the population, yet we can calculate that CMV infection produces as many as 200–300 severely mentally retarded babies every year. This is enough to fill a whole hospital every year, so the financial implications are very considerable.

Chairman   You could supplement that and say it is a relatively large proportion that is preventable with present knowledge and that was the denominator that Prof. Wood was asking us to use.

Dewdney   If we are extending our discussion to the slightly older child, I suppose the most cost effective vaccine we could produce is that to control dental caries. As you are raising the streptococcal question in your talk, I wonder, Dr Smith, if you could comment on progress with that vaccine.

Smith   There are two groups working on it in the UK; Cohen at Downe and Lehner at Guy's. *Streptococcus mutans*, extraordinarily enough, seems to be the major cause of dental caries. It produces an aminoglycan which forms plaque, localizing the organism onto the tooth enamel. It ferments sugar in the diet to produce acid which erodes the tooth. Cohen's group, Bowen in particular, have vaccinated monkeys with killed *Streptococcus mutans*. They then put the animals on a cariogenic diet which consists of bananas plus sweets and Mars bars and things of that sort which produces dental caries in a period of 3–18 months or so. They have shown a significant measure of protection. These are difficult studies to do because of the need to follow these animals for up to three years to get results. Lehner's group has come up with similar evidence using a different monkey species.

I think there are a lot of difficulties to be overcome. There are a number of serological types of *Streptococcus mutans*. There are also other organisms which can cause dental caries. It would be advisable to purify a streptococcal vaccine and use only the effective antigen and progress is being made on this. There is also the association of streptococci with rheumatic heart disease to consider. Nevertheless there is enormous interest in a vaccine against caries, a very costly disease.

Soothill   I think that we really should take some note of what happens in the human. The immunodeficient human has better teeth than the control. The difference is probably due to diet. But there is no clinical pointer to immunodeficiency, that immunological mechanisms play any part in caries though they do in gum disease and aphthous ulcers.

Smith   I think that Lehner's group and others have shown that the crevicular fluid does contain antibacterial factors including phagocytes, complement, lysozyme and immunoglobulin and have produced evidence that this fluid has an antibacterial effect. Presumably, this is why the vaccine works.

Soothill But does it work in human caries? The clinical impression suggests not.

Marshall The evidence that influenza is more severe in the pregnant woman than a nonpregnant woman is debatable. The effect on the fetus depends on which epidemic you study. I would like to raise the following question. In the event of a severe outbreak of influenza in a community and assuming that the appropriate vaccine is available, would a policy of vaccinating pregnant women, either with killed or live vaccine, be worth considering?

Smith I think, as you rightly state, that the evidence that influenza in pregnancy does any harm is very small. I think there are two or three studies which have shown a positive effect, one from Finland, I believe, and a few from this country, mainly relating to the H2N2 epidemic. Even so, these were very small effects needing a large population to show them up. On the other hand, vaccine has not been used in pregnancy on a sufficient scale to demonstrate that it has no harmful effects. About 3 or 4% of those vaccinated do get a febrile response. Conceivably that could be associated with greater risk of stillbirth, so the equation might be finely balanced.

Marshall Has live influenza vaccine been given to pregnant women?

Smith Not as far as I know.

Cooper I have a different impression from that of John Soothill about dental problems in immunodeficient patients. In our experience, the incidence of dental caries and gingival diseases is higher in patients with immunodeficiency. Even if one selects isolated IgA deficiency, that is the case. The difficulty is in determining whether the immunodeficiency is directly related with the increase in tooth and gum diseases. Immunodeficient children frequently breathe through their mouth, receive a lot of sugar laden medications, and are often fed around the clock because of their frequent infections, especially of the ears and upper respiratory tract. These secondary factors could contribute to their dental problems.

Soothill I said they have a high incidence of gingival disease but not dental caries.

Cooper Caries included.

Hayward I wondered if you were being unduly pessimistic at the end. Is it not possible to reduce dramatically the incidence of umbilical tetanus infections by immunizing the mother before birth, which would be a major public health achievement? Secondly, as far as immunization against dental caries is concerned, it is extremely difficult to persuade anyone to accept immunization. Is it not easier to use fluoride in toothpaste?

Smith The first one, tetanus. I think probably the best example of immunization in preventing illness in the newborn is tetanus immunization. It is responsible for well over 50000 deaths each year, mostly in developing countries as neonatal tetanus. This can be prevented by two spaced injections of a good adsorbed toxoid. There is a lot of work going on to prepare a vaccine which will work in pregnant women in one dose. That certainly is a very cost effective means. As far as dental caries is concerned, I think the sort of question you raised ought to go into the debate. You may, for example, suggest that chlorhexidine in toothpaste can have an effect in diminishing the numbers of *Streptococcus mutans*, but it turns out that there is no real strong evidence that chlorhexidine prevents dental caries. Fluoride in water will certainly have an effect, but I do not think that it will eliminate it. You still get dental caries in areas where there is fluoride. Regular dental hygiene is another obvious way. But, again, children may have dental care every six months and still get caries. This is why the dentists with whom I have discussed this seem to think that if there was a vaccine that would be accepted as safe it could be very valuable, particularly in Britain where we get a lot of dental caries.

Denman Could I return to the question of the efficacy and safety of vaccinating against viruses such as herpes simplex and cytomegalovirus? It is fairly well accepted now that the major form of immunity which controls the growth and dissemination of these agents, is cell mediated immunity. You have alluded to the fact that people have looked sequentially at lymphocyte transformation in individuals who have been immunized with vaccines of this sort. It does seem on this evidence that a cell mediated immune response is evoked. But my question really relates to the possibility that this test may be inadequate in terms of predicting the longterm development of cell mediated immunity and also in predicting the possible ill effects of such vaccines in those individuals who might have some inability to handle such viruses or vaccines because of defects in their own cell mediated immunity responses. Indeed, they may have defects of the sort which have been postulated to predispose to severe infections by this group of viruses, for example, to severe recurrent herpetic cold sores. Do you believe that it is sufficient to look short-term at lymphocyte transformation as a means of satisfying oneself that one is likely to have established longterm cell mediated immunity? Should one be looking, or have people looked, longterm at other more longlasting markers of cell mediated immune responses such as cytoxic responses and interferon production when cells from immunized individuals are challenged with virus *in vitro*? The reason I stress this point is, first the fact that lymphocyte transformation is often a very fleeting response after immunization both in animals and in man in whom persisting virus infections have been established. Secondly, there is some debate as to whether lymphocyte transformation *in vitro* necessarily reflects the establishment of true cell mediated immunity. One wonders whether we should be using such screening procedures after immunization to try and get a better idea of what would be predictive tests for individuals at risk of the longterm complications you so nicely listed.

Smith To my knowledge, I do not think that it has been greatly studied in people who have had herpes vaccines. I think that cytotoxicity has in varicella vaccinees and that there is a cytotoxic effect. I think that in the CMV studies lymphoblast transformation was used because it was perhaps easier to do and larger numbers could be studied. I think that the ultimate proof of efficacy comes from clinical trial with long follow up to find the duration of immunity. Takahashi is trying varicella vaccine in people with a variety of immunological defects, and one of the aspects of his study is to try to determine the parameters which must be present in these subjects for the vaccine to work. The extraordinary thing is that it is apparently working in leukaemic children, producing protection, but the numbers are not very large.

Stern Dr Denman was talking about the transience of lymphocyte transformation. Was he referring to herpesviruses, which establish longterm latent infection? In the CMV vaccination studies that we have been doing on renal transplant patients, there is a very striking response in the lymphocyte transformation test-usually within about three weeks, which then settles down to a base level after a further two to three weeks. This base level has been maintained now for at least nine months. There is no evidence of any other fall-off. But if we are talking about preventing congenital infection, the most important consideration is persistence of antibody in the mother. In our volunteers, antibodies have been maintained after vaccination now for almost five years, which is encouraging for possible longterm persistence of antibody. When there is reactivation of CMV infection in a pregnant woman, this can sometimes result in interuterine infection. Although we do not perhaps have enough data, what data we do have at the moment suggests that, although the fetus becomes infected, it is not damaged. Perhaps if maternal antibody crosses the placenta at about the same time as the virus, the severity of fetal infection is ameliorated. The only thing that matters is persistence of antibody in the mother.

Turano What do you think about vaccination in the case of respiratory syncytial virus? We had quite a severe outbreak in Naples. At the same time we isolated a strain of virus from the newborn which was not harmful at all. The babies from which we isolated the virus recovered without after effects. In Naples, on the other hand, they died. There is a debate now as to the efficacy of the vaccine. What do you think about that, from your information?

Smith An outbreak of RS virus in a nursery has recently been reported. There were 23 cases in neonates, with four deaths. The greatest severity was in the fourth week of life. In the first three weeks of life the illness was mild. One of the babies who died was about three weeks old but there were some other contributory factors. The other three deaths were in the fourth week of life. RS virus as a pathogen appears to extend into the neonatal period, therefore it is legitimate to consider it here. An implication is that there is some passive immunity but it is not very effective, and seems to last for only about three weeks. There is obviously great interest in producing a vaccine which will give protection when it is most required in the second to the sixth month of life. Chanock's group in the USA has studied so far four vaccines in children. The first, a killed RSV vaccine, was used in about 1967 and the vaccinated children, when exposed subsequently had a more severe infection. Since then he has concentrated on live vaccines. He has tried, secondly, a cold adapted strain which was immunogenic in children aged from three to six years, but I think it caused an unacceptable degree of illness in them. More recently he has gone on to temperature sensitive mutants, and has developed two vaccine strains, TS1 and TS2, both of which appear to be immunogenic in chimpanzees, although he has rejected the TS1 because it causes rhinorrhoea. When used in young children it was found that one of the subjects got an otitis media. He thought that perhaps the rhinorrhoea had precipitated a bacterial infection leading to otitis media. The TS2 mutant appears not to cause rhinorrhoea in chimpanzees and he is now extending this into clinical trial, with children aged from 3 to 6 years. If it proves effective he is intending to bring the age down. This vaccine is given intranasally, I believe. Its restrictive temperature is 39°C, so that the virus will probably not grow in the lungs. I do not think that he has yet any evidence of protection in young children. There is a group in the UK, Pringle and colleagues in Glasgow, who have established that the RS virus has seven complementation groups. He is trying to develop vaccine strains where there is a lesion on perhaps more than one of the complementation groups. There are also parallel studies in regard to RS vaccines in calves.

Sir Ashley   I should like to make a small point in support of what Dr Denman said about the use of tests to designate cell mediated immunity. He mentioned lymphocyte transformation. I think we are in danger of being too glib when we say "This is all right, therefore there is cell mediated immunity". One sees quite misleading papers saying that cell mediated immunity is normal in this or that group of persons because their lymphocytes were transformed in a particular way. But even if one shows transformation all one is really saying, misleadingly, is "This car will go because I have shown that petrol will go through the carburettor".

Damage to the Fetus and Newborn from Prophylactic Procedures

W. C. MARSHALL

The Hospital for Sick Children,
Great Ormond Street, London WC1, UK

The assessment of the benefits of immunization requires accurate information on both the incidence of the infection as well as adverse reactions to the immunoprophylactic agent. Unfortunately there is a tendency for adverse reactions to come into prominence only when the incidence of the disease declines to very low levels.

Those agents which may be a hazard to the fetus and newborn can be determined by an examination of the circumstances in which vaccines are used in any particular community. They may be used as an elective procedure in a comprehensive immunization programme, for foreign travel or during exposure or possible exposure to outbreaks or importation of a nonendemic infectious disease. In all these circumstances a pregnant woman or one who may become pregnant in the immediate future may require immunization. In some circumstances immunization of the newborn may be necessary. From a practical point of view it seems prudent to make the general statement that all live vaccines are contra-indicated during pregnancy or just before conception. Inactivated vaccines, on the other hand, and preparations used for passive immunoprophylaxis are not generally hazardous. Chemoprophylaxis during pregnancy for the prevention of malaria with currently available drugs is not hazardous. If new vaccines are introduced evaluation of side effects would have to include possible effects on the fetus.

The problems of live vaccines in pregnancy has been brought into prominence by the introduction of rubella vaccines. In the UK only the following vaccines are likely to be given in pregnancy—vaccinia, yellow fever, rubella and oral polio vaccine; mumps and measles vaccines on the other hand are very unlikely to be used in adults and it is too early to comment on live influenza vaccines.

Vaccinia: There is no doubt that vaccinia virus can infect the fetus. But the number of documented infections is suprisingly small in view of the millions of doses of smallpox vaccine that have been used. Levine and his colleagues in an extensive review in 1974 reported only 20 cases, (Levine *et al.*, 1974). The majority resulted from primary vaccination. However there were two instances of where revaccination was performed but 19 and 21 years had elapsed since the previous vaccination. An unexpected risk to the pregnant woman occurred when infection was acquired from a recently vaccinated offspring. The survival rate was very low but the infant described by Waddington *et al.* (1964) survived and is of particular interest because attempts to revaccinate this boy in later infancy were unsuccessful.

In a study by Rahjvajn *et al.* (1973), 101 women were successfully vaccinated in the first trimester but virus were not isolated from the products of conception obtained from therapeutic abortions performed for reasons other than the vaccination; but the majority of these were not primary vaccinations. Several prospective studies totalling 8599 pregnancies with 11 104 controls revealed no cases of fetal vaccinia but there was some evidence of increased fetal wastage following vaccination in the first trimester in the series reported by MacArthur (1952) and by Bieniarz and Dabrowski (1956).

Within the past year attention has been drawn to the risks of vaccination in pregnancy in the UK and a report from Australia of vaccination of a woman at eight weeks gestation which resulted in the birth of a 500 gm infected infant of 24 weeks who survived only 1 hour (Anon., 1979a).

Yellow fever: Millions of doses of the 17D strain of vaccine have been used in the field without reports of ill effects (Saenz, 1971). More specifically, Smith *et al.* (1938) stated that there were no adverse effects among the pregnant women who were included in 59 000 individuals in the Brazilian vaccine trials. Nevertheless, adminstration of this vaccine should be avoided if possible or at least deferred until after the first trimester.

Poliovirus vaccine: The Sabin type vaccine has been tested in pregnant women at all stages of pregnancy without ill effects, (Prem, *et al.*, 1960). Several infants with a variety of types of congenital malformation born to women who had received oral

TABLE I.

Characteristics of 9 patients with Rubella vaccine-like virus isolated from therapeutic abortion specimens.*

Prevaccination rubella immunity status	Time of vaccination in relation to conception (weeks)		Gestation at abortion (weeks)	Interval between vaccination and abortion (weeks)	Tissue(s) positive for rubella virus
	Before	After			
Susceptible		2	6	4	Undifferentiated products of conception
Susceptible		3	8	5	Decidua
Susceptible		9	14	4	Placenta
Susceptible	7		13	20	Fetal eye
Susceptible		7	13	6	Products of conception, fetal bone marrow
Susceptible	2		7	9	Products of conception
Unknown	2		14	16	Placenta, fetal eye
Unknown		11	13	2	Placenta, fetal kidney
Unknown		1	11	10	Placenta, decidua

* Data from Center for Disease Control: Rubella Surveillance, July 1973–Dec. 1975.

polio vaccine have been investigated virologically but no evidence of intrauterine infection found. However, the theoretical risks of this vaccine can be readily overcome by the use of killed polio vaccine.

Rubella: The attenuated strains of rubella currently used in vaccines can infect the fetus (Table I). But the risk would seem to be confined to vaccination of the sero negative women (Vaheri *et al.*, 1972; Modlin *et al.*, 1976). Vaccination of the pregnant woman therefore remains a cause for concern and it is a frequent practice to terminate the pregnancy in cases of inadvertent vaccination. Twenty to fifty pregnancies have been terminated per annum in the UK since the introduction of rubella vaccines. However, a number of the terminations may have not been required if the prevaccination rubella immune status had been known. This situation could have been avoided if the recommendation that women of child bearing age should have rubella serology performed before considering vaccination (sero-positive individuals will not require vaccine) had been carried out. This policy should continue unchanged at the present time (Anon., 1979).

Although the fetus can be infected the role of the virus in the causation of damage is not known. The Center for Disease Control in the USA has information on the infants born to 65 rubella susceptible women who received vaccine when pregnant or within three months of conception (Preblud *et al.*, 1978). Two infants, now aged 18 and 22 months, had laboratory evidence of congenital infection and these and the remainder are stated to be alive without signs of damage. It was concluded that the maximum theoretical risk of congenital malformations would be less than 5·5%, a risk lower than the chance occurance of congenital malformations. But since defects, such as deafness, may not become evident for several months or even years after birth in congenital rubella, the duration of obser-vation is critical in the evaluation of risks, and these infants may not have been observed for long enough to state that there has been no evidence of damage. Such information is encouraging but is based almost on experience in the USA where the rubella vaccine prepared in human diploid cells (RA27/3) has not been widely used. There are known to be some differences in the immune responses between RA27/3 vaccine and the Cendehill and HPV77/DE5 vaccines. Thus all rubella vaccines in current use have not yet been fully evaluated for this risk.

Mumps and Measles: At the present neither of these live vaccines are likely to be administered to adults hence the pregnant woman is not subject to largely unknown risks. Yamauchi *et al.*, (1974) recovered mumps vaccine virus from the placenta in two of three susceptible women who volunteered to receive vaccine prior to termination of their pregnancies. Therefore it must be assumed that this virus could infect the fetus.

The epidemiology of measles is undergoing an important change in the USA with reports of epidemic measles in young adults (Krause *et al.*, 1979), This may have arisen from a lack of exposure to natural infection in childhood or due to failure of measles vaccine. Because of the risks of measles in young adults consideration may be given to using measles vaccine in this age group. No information is available on the risks of attenuated measles virus to the fetus. A risk must be considered to exist and extreme caution should be exercised if measles vaccines were to be administered to adolescent or adult women who may be pregnant.

BCG vaccine: This vaccine does not appear to be harmful to the fetus but it would be prudent to avoid vaccination during pregnancy unless their is an immediate excessive risk of unavoidable exposure to infective tuberculosis (Anon., 1979 c).

New live vaccines: Live influenza virus vaccines should be avoided but such a recommendation is based on the general statement concerning all live vaccines in pregnancy. Trials with live cytomegalovirus vaccines have already commenced and this vaccine will introduce another potential hazard. It will be necessary to pay special attention to the susceptible pregnant woman in the trials of the vaccine.

Passive immunoprophylactics: Substances used today are all of human origin and there is no evidence that they are harmful to the fetus if administered during pregnancy.

Live vaccines in the neonatal period: The major hazard is confined to congenital combined immunodeficiency states. Vaccinia virus and BCG vaccines pose the greatest threat to these infants and the practical problem is the recognition of the disorder. This could be suspected or made if there is a family history of a similar disorder but such a diagnosis will not be achieved in the first affected child of a family because the infant will not have lived long enough to exhibit clinical manifestations of the immunodeficiency disorder.

Yellow fever vaccine is not advised in infants under one year of age because of a stated increased risk of neurological complications.

Environmental agents are only one of the many factors known to cause fetal damage and theoretically they are the most easily controlled. Should the need to immunize a pregnant woman or newborn infant arise careful attention to the composition of the material used is important.

REFERENCES

Anon. (1979 a). Adverse reactions to smallpox vaccination. *Weekly Epidemiological Record* **54**, 276.

Anon. (1979 b) Rubella: who needs a blood test? *Lancet* **i**, 1329–1331.

Anon. (1979c). BCG vaccines, ACIP Recommendations. *Morbidy and Mortality Weekly Report*. Center for Disease Control **29**, 241–244.

Bieniarz, J. and Dabrowski, Z. (1956). Influence of anti-smallpox vaccination on the course of pregnancy. *Polski Tygodnik Lekarski* **2**, 2183–2188.

Krause, P. J., Cherry, J. D., Deseda-Tous, J., Champion, J. G., Strassburgh, M., Sullivan, C., Spencer, M. J., Bryson, Y. J., Welliver, R. C. and Boyer, K. M. (1979). Epidemic Measles in Young Adults. *Annals of Internal Medicine* **90**, 873–876.

Levine, M. M., Edsall, G. and Bruce-Chwatt, L. J. (1974). Live vaccine in pregnancy–risks and recommendations. *Lancet* **ii**, 34–38.

MacArthur, P. (1952). Congenital Vaccinia and Vaccinia Gravidarum. *Lancet* **ii**, 1104–1106.

Modlin, J. F., Herrman, K., Brandling-Bennett, A. D., Eddins, D. L. and Hayden, G. (1976). Risk of Congenital Abnormality after inadvertent rubella vaccination of pregnant women. *New England Journal of Medicine* **294**, 272–274.

Preblud, S. R., Nieburg, P. I. and Hinman, A. R. (1978). Rubella Vaccination and Pregnancy. *British Medical Journal* **2**, 960–961.

Rahjvajn, B., Krznar, B., Stiljkovic, C., Orescanin, M. and Smerdel, S. (1973). Vaccination against smallpox in early pregnancy. *Acta Medica Jugoslavica* **27**, 351–357.

Saenz, A. C. (1970). Yellow fever Vaccines: Achievements, Problems, Needs. *In* "International Conference on Application against Viral, Rickettsial and Bacterial Diseases of Man. Washington D.C., December, 1970", 31–34. PAHO Washington.

Smith, H. H., Penna, H. A. and Paoliello, A. (1938). Yellow fever vaccination with cultured virus (17D) without immune serum. *American Journal of Tropical Medicine* **18**, 437–463.

Vaheri, A., Vesikari, T., Oker-Blom, N., Seppala, M., Parkman, P. D., Veronelli, J. and Robbins, F. C. (1972). Isolation of attenuated rubella vaccine virus from human products of conception and uterine cervix. *New England Journal of Medicine* **286**, 1071–1074.

Waddington, E., Bray, P. T., Evans, A. D. and Richard, I. D. G. (1964). Cutaneous complications of mass vaccination against smallpox in South Wales 1962. *Transactions of The St John's Hospital Dermatological Society* **50**, 22–42.

Yamauchi, T. Wilson, C. and St Geme, J. W. (1974). Transmission of live, attenuated mumps virus to the human placenta. *New England Journal of Medicine* **290**, 710–712.

DISCUSSION

Soothill   I think one point needs clarifying. Bill Marshall has said that, if the polio vaccine is given after 6 weeks, there is no difference between the conversion rate if the child is breast fed or bottle fed. That does not show information about the individual. If there were only a relatively small number of the mothers producing high titres of antipolio antibodies in their milk you would not get a statistical effect, but you might well have an important failure of protection in certain individuals. If the first half of the colostrum story is correct, I think we ought to go on worrying about the second half of the story in terms of each individual, as opposed to the group as a whole. Am I wrong?

Chairman   Perhaps I can take that question on board a little. I think that what Bill has suggested is a slight oversimplification. The failure to get good takes with polio vaccine in the tropics is not merely due to immunoglobulins in the colostrum, or even merely to interference in the gut because of the endemicity of other enteroviruses. It is still a bit of a mystery as to what it is that goes wrong in the tropics. It may well not be a simple immunological problem at all; there may be some other, what we choose to call nonspecific, factors involved.

Soothill   Is there clear evidence that either specific or nonspecific factors in human milk can interfere with the immunization procedure in some individuals at any stage of lactation?

Marshall   De Forrest 1973 has shown no difference in antibody responses to three doses of oral polio vaccine in breast and bottle fed infants, vaccinated at 2, 3 and 6 months of age. Antibody levels are highest in colostrum therefore immunization may not be effective in the newborn, but colostrum seems to be only one factor to be considered in the tropics (Plotkin *et al.*, 1966).

Walker   There has been some experience with using high titre antibodies directed against hepatitis B virus in mothers who are infected during the latter part of pregnancy, when there is a high risk of neonatal hepatitis. Using that information, I wondered if the use of hyperimmune γ globulin directed against chickenpox might be as effective when mothers develop chickenpox during the latter part of pregnancy and have infants who have a very high mortality. Has that been looked at at all, or is there any prospective study that is under way in respect to that?

Marshall   The CDC are releasing zoster immunoglobulin (ZIG) in the USA for this reason. In the UK you can only get ZIG from the Central Public Health Laboratory, Colindale, by providing pre and postvaccination serum samples. So this information should become available.

Walker Is there any information to suggest that this is effective in preventing high mortality?

Smith I do not think there is evidence that ZIG given to the mother will protect the neonate.

Hayward But is it not the problem that the children who are most severely affected by chickenpox are the ones whose mothers developed chickenpox extremely late, and you may therefore not be able to give the baby antibody in time? I think that this poses enormous logistic problems.

As to the other question with which you ended, there is a certain amount of information on what happened to children who received immunoglobulin injections after birth. After a year their IgG levels were somewhat lower (O'Brien and Kempe, 1963). There are, of course, a lot of other children who receive vast amounts of immunoglobulin from very early on in the form of blood transfusions, and someone else may know what happens to them.

Reeves With regard to the failure of certain vaccines to take in the Third World population, how important do you feel malnutrition may be as a factor here? A lot of work has been done on the effects of malnutrition on different aspects of the immune response. To what degree may this be a limiting factor in the success of any major immunization programme in the Third World?

Marshall I think it may be a limiting factor. Certainly the information that is available is very scanty. The major problem in immunization in tropical countries is having potent vaccines. Whilst one could go to East or West Africa, and conduct a vaccine trial with almost 100% efficacy in almost any group, the moment the vaccine is issued to clinics, you get trouble with storage. The major limiting factor in tropical countries, allowing for malnutrition, is still the availability of potent vaccines.

Faulk There is an impressive amount of information that has been generated over the past ten years on the role of nutrition in immune responses and many people around this table have contributed to this growing fund of knowledge. In brief, a malnourished child has a type of acquired immunodeficiency in which there is a relative hypofunction of T cells. This is measured by a lack of response to skin testing, by a deficiency of T cell rosettes, and by a relatively intact B cell function. The pattern of diseases in those children does, in a way, reflect their form of acquired immunodeficiency. For instance, measles is a very serious disease in malnourished populations, as is tuberculosis. On the other hand, those diseases which depend primarily on B cell function do not seem to be particularly outstanding. So I would think that the answer to your question is yes, in that it is one part of the host response to certain infectious organisms, particularly if the response is primarily T cell dependent.

Hayward I think it is worth citing some superb data by Mehta and others from southern India in which they immunized over a thousand babies in the newborn period with BCG and followed up to see what happened. If I remember rightly, the rate of becoming PPD skin test positive was somewhat low amongst all of them, but they found that the immunized infants, in comparing immunized with nonimmunized infants, were little different and it made little difference to the number who ultimately developed pulmonary tuberculosis. But there was a very dramatic fall in the incidence of tuberculous meningitis amongst the immunized who came from relatively rich families, whereas the immunized who came from poor families who were by implication malnourished did not have a reduced incidence of tuberculous meningitis.

Marshall Presumably you can overcome any artificially induced immunity by a large enough dose of the infecting agent, as in the case of a massive inhalation of tubercle bacilli by a child who has been vaccinated with BCG.

Hayward The other important thing is that for immunization to work well you must be reasonably fed at the time you are receiving the antigen stimulus.

Marshall Could I raise a question concerning newborn vaccination with BCG and smallpox? One of the major causes of deaths from smallpox vaccine in the USA when it was a routine procedure, was progressive vaccinia in infants with presumably combined immunodeficiency (Nef *et al.*, 1967). Likewise, most cases of disseminated BCG infection would appear to be in children who had congenital immunodeficiency disorders. How you avoid this is very difficult. A family history is helpful but the newborn infant has not lived long enough to give any clinical suspicion of a congenital immunodeficiency disorder.

Hayward I quite agree, and the cost of screening for immunodeficiency disorders would be much too high. The societies in which we are in a position either to test for or treat severe congenital immunodeficiency are on the whole rather well off, newborn tuberculosis is rare and smallpox is exceptional. So I do not think this is likely to be a big problem in the future.

Reeves I still think we should take this whole question of malnutrition very seriously because in framing a policy for any particular eradication programme, we may find that where you have a malnourished population who have a T cell defect, vaccines being given in order to enhance cell mediated responses to, for instance, budding viruses are not going to be particularly successful. Whereas if you are trying to achieve a significant antibody response, that may be entirely satisfactory.

Marshall Please do not think I was dismissing malnutrition as unimportant, it is the most important disease in the world, but the vaccine stability is also important.

Denman I was intrigued by your observations about the mother immunized with vaccinia during pregnancy and the fetus contracted generalized vaccinia. When tested later on, the child was unresponsive to skin testing. Do you think there is any general possibility that viruses can specifically delete those cells which are programmed to respond to a specific virus infection? That has been shown with respect to rubella virus, for example, there is an old paper showing that a child with a congenital rubella syndrome eventually developed full immunological competence, but was unable to respond to rubella either in the form of skin testing or lymphocyte transformation or development of antibody. I wonder whether there is a general issue and attenuated agents given during pregnancy could conceivably cause specific tolerance if they could pass the placenta and react with specifically reactive clones and cells.

Marshall Vaccination in the case you cite was at 24 week gestation. Would the elimination of clones be very difficult at this stage? But these cases are very rare; there are two or three examples of infants who lacked detectable antibody. But has antibody been sought by all available methods? Some children with congenital rubella have no CF antibody, and skin testing is difficult; I do not know of a good skin test antigen for rubella.

Chairman I think it is fair to say that the usual story applies: most infants with congenital rubella are making lots of antibody.

REFERENCES

De Forest, A., Parker, B., Parker, M. S., Diliberti, J. H., Taylor Yates, H., Sibinga, M. S. and Smith, D. S. (1973). *Journal of Pediatrics* **83,** 93–95.

Nef, J. M., Lane, J. M., Perj, J. H., Moore, R., Millar, J. D. and Henderson, D. A. (1967). *New England Journal of Medicine* **276,** 125–132.

O'Brian, D. and Kempe, C. H. (1963). *Pediatrics* **32,** 4–9.

Future Prospects for the Protection of the Fetus and Newborn

A. C. ALLISON

International Laboratory for Research on Animal
Diseases, P.O. Box 30709, Nairobi, Kenya.

Anyone who attempts to predict the course of biological science for a long time ahead is injudicious. The history of the subject shows that it is full of surprises. Who, in 1940, would have predicted the tremendous power of antibiotics for controlling bacterial infections and who, in 1950, would have predicted the spectacular developments of molecular biology that were to take place in the following decade? Instead of looking into the crystal ball I shall review some recent and not-so-recent studies that may help to explain the cellular basis of the high susceptibility of newborns to infections. I shall also describe some recent major technical developments which should facilitate diagnosis of infections in the fetus and newborn. Some of them have therapeutic potential as well.

CELLULAR BASIS OF SUSCEPTIBILITY OF THE NEWBORN TO INFECTIONS

A general feature of most virus infections in humans and experimental animals is the increased resistance to disease which develops in the course of growth and maturation of the host (Sigel, 1952). The changes are particularly dramatic in the neonatal period. In the absence of antibody acquired passively from the mother, herpesvirus and other virus infections are often very severe in the neonatal period, becoming steadily milder during infancy and early childhood. Adults are more susceptible to virus infections than are children, for example having a higher probability of developing paralysis when exposed to polio virus, mononucleosis when infected with EB virus and complications after infection with childhood exanthems. In old age infections become still more severe, presumably owing to failure of host defence mechanisms (Makinodan *et al.*, 1971).

When analysing the cellular basis of the susceptibility of newborns to infections, several cell types must be considered. These include: B lymphocytes making antibodies; T lymphocytes helping antibody formation, developing specific cytotoxicity or releasing mediators; polymorphonuclear leukocytes, which are especially important in controlling pyogenic bacterial infections; macrophages, which play a major role in defence against viruses and intracellular bacteria and parasites; and the recently described natural killer cells, which appear also to be important in resistance to infectious diseases. The ontogeny of these systems in the fetus and newborn is a large subject, which cannot be reviewed fully here. I shall confine my remarks to a few well-studied topics in which I had a personal interest. Most of the experimental work has been performed on mice, because of the availability of inbred strains and well characterized immunoglobulin subclasses and histocompatibility systems. There appear to be analogies between the responses of newborn mice and humans to infections, which is encouraging since we all want to apply our experimental results to man; but these analogies should not be pressed. This is especially true of fetal infections because of the marked differences between rodent and human placentas.

T LYMPHOCYTES AND IMMUNOLOGICAL TOLERANCE

One of the explanations which has been advanced for the severity of virus infections in the fetus and newborn has been that infections during this period induce tolerance whereas later infections elicit immune responses (Burnet, 1960). It is now clear that this is only partly true. Rubella and other infections of the human fetus *do* result in specific antibody formation. Even the classical example, lymphocytic choriomeningitis infection of mice, now appears more complex than was originally thought. Since this is an interesting model, I shall discuss it briefly.

Lymphocytic choriomeningitis (LCM) virus, using several strains of virus and of mice, produces a severe and often lethal infection (Lehmann-Grubbe, 1973). In mice deprived of T lymphocytes the virus replicates in the brain and other tissues but the animals do not suffer harmful effects, so an immunopathological reaction involving T lymphocytes is thought to be responsible for the pathogenesis of the disease.

Virus readily passes from infected mothers to their fetuses, and when a mouse is infected in fetal or early postnatal life it becomes a chronic carrier of the virus but does not develop choriomeningitis. This suggests that T lymphocytes become unresponsive to viral antigens. However, the carrier mice do make antibodies and develop an immune complex glomerulonephritis (Oldstone and Dixon, 1969). Hence tolerance is not induced in B lymphocytes, which respond to neonatal infection by making antibodies to LCM viral antigens.

Likewise, when mice are injected with native foreign serum proteins, tolerance is readily induced in the population of specific helper T lymphocytes but not in the antibody-forming B lymphocyte population. The same is true of autoantigens, which explains many puzzling features of self-tolerance and autoimmunity (Allison, 1977). A similar selective tolerance of T lymphocytes may occur in virus infections of humans. For example in Africa and some Mediterranean countries there is widespread exposure of young persons to hepatitis B virus. More than 5% of these become persistent carriers of the virus in the absence of demonstrable liver disease. One interpretation is that early exposure to the virus induces selective tolerance of T lymphocytes, which are required for recovery from infection but also damage the liver by an immunopathological reaction. Persistent virus infection with little disease is also seen in immunosuppressed renal transplant patients, whereas medical or nursing staff infected with the same virus develop hepatitis.

Another well studied example is the susceptibility of newborn mice and hamsters to the oncogenic effects of some viruses. Polyoma virus is a widespread infection of wild mice and colonies of laboratory mice unless special precautions are taken to eliminate it. Under natural conditions virus infection does not lead to tumour development because newborns are passively protected by antibodies acquired from their mothers. They later become infected horizontally—i.e, not from their mothers—when their immune system is mature enough to control tumour development. When a newborn mouse is infected with polyoma virus in the absence of antibodies many tumours develop, whereas if the infection is delayed for even a few weeks, the virus multiplies efficiently in many organs but no tumours are seen. The tumour cells have a virus specific antigen that elicits resistance to transplantation. The importance of T lymphocytes is shown by the fact that polyoma virus infection of adult mice deprived of T lymphocytes (thymectomized and treated with antilymphocytic serum, or nude mice) results in the formation of tumours, and this process can be prevented by transfer of immune T lymphocytes (see Allison, 1974; Allison et al., 1974). The question arises whether polyoma virus infection of newborn mice induces tolerance in T lymphocytes or just a delay in mounting cell mediated immune responses. The latter is true. If mice are infected as newborns and their lymphoid cells are taken six weeks later, they can prevent the appearance of polyoma tumours in immunosuppressed recipients (Allison, 1970). Thus in some circumstances virus infections of newborn induce selective tolerance of T lymphocytes while in others the T lymphocyte response is delayed when compared with the rapid response mounted in adults.

The latter is important in oncogenesis, and could also be decisive in those virus infections where cell mediated immunity plays a major role in recovery, such as pox virus and herpesvirus infections.

NATURAL KILLER CELLS

Another cell type that has attracted interest recently is the natural killer (NK) cell, a lymphoid cell that is cytotoxic without previous immunization. Activity of NK cells shows marked differences in various strains of mice, and is evidently under genetic control. Activity of NK cells is also related to age: it is low in the fetus and newborn, increases sharply after birth to reach a maximum at about 6–8 weeks of age in the case of mice, and thereafter declines so that it is quite low in old age. The properties of NK cells have recently been reviewed (Santoli and Koprowski, 1979). Activity of NK cells in experimental animals or using human cells in culture can be increased by interferon (Gidlund et al., 1978; Trinchieri and Santoli, 1978) and decreased by corticosteroids (Cudkowicz and Hochman, 1979).

When human lymphocytes are stimulated in a mixed lymphocyte reaction or by pokeweed mitogen, they produce a distinct type of interferon (type II or immune interferon). It is reasonable to suppose that production of immune interferon and activation of natural killer cells might play a role in immunity to infectious diseases. Evidence that this is the case comes from studies of children with what appear to be selective deficiencies of immune interferon production and NK activity. These investigations have been made by Dr J.-L. Virelizier who was for three years in my laboratory at the Clinical Research Centre and has for the last three years been working in an excellent clinical immunology laboratory in the Hôpital des Enfants Malades, Paris.

The first case was a 5-year-old girl unable to recover from Epstein-Barr virus (EBV) infection (Virelizier et al., 1978). She had a chronic disease with fever, lymphoid hyperplasia, interstitial pneumonitis, thrombocytopenia and polyclonal hypergammaglobulinaemia. Evidence for persistent EBV infection included very high titres of antibodies (IgM and IgG) to viral capsid antigen and early antigen, the presence of cells containing EBV-associated nuclear antigen in lymph nodes and blood, and the establishment of spontaneous permanent lymphoblastoid cell lines from both sources over a period of a year. Following exacerbation of the polyclonal proliferation of immunoblasts the patient died 19 months after the onset of the disease. Despite thorough investigation the only defect in cellular or humoral immunity that could be detected was a selective failure to sectrete immune interferon when peripheral blood mononuclear cells were stimulated in culture. Another case with a similar syndrome has been observed by Virelizier (unpublished data).

A congenital or acquired defect of immune interferon secretion might be expected to result in impaired NK activity. This hypothesis was tested by Virelizier *et al.* (1979) by parallel examination of immune interferon secretion in a mixed leukocyte reaction and NK activity against a human erythroblastic cell line (K562) of peripheral blood leukocytes from children with various immunological disorders. Four patients showed a combined defect of these two types of immune function. The patients showed increased suseptibility to virus infections, one patient having chronic BCG and toxoplasma infections. In contrast to the four patients described, other patients suffering from recognized deficiencies of B or T lymphocytes gave either normal results or showed dissociated defects in the NK and immune interferon secretion assays. These results are consistent with an important role of endogenous interferon in the *in vivo* control of NK activity and resistance to infection. The low NK activity in newborn babies is presumably one factor predisposing them to infection.

It is tempting to extend this generalization further, and to suppose that the relative resistance of children as compared with adults to virus infections (poliomyelitis, exanthemata, EB virus etc.) may be related to higher and more readily increased NK activity in children. The still greater susceptibility of old persons to zoster and other infections may be related to the decline in NK activity with age.

INTERFERON

Interferon activates NK cells, and may therefore increase immunity to viral and bacterial infections and tumours. Interferon can also act on cells in which virus is replicating, inhibiting that process. For some time the prospect of using interferon in severe chronic virus infections has been discussed, and new potent preparations of human interferon from several different sources are available (from cultures of human fibroblasts, leukocytes and lymphoblastoid cell lines). These have been used in human patients with chronic hepatitis B virus infections and malignancies, without serious complications and apparently with benefit.

The use of potent, purified preparations of human interferon in newborns with uncontrolled virus infections should be tried. It must be borne in mind that Gresser *et al.* (1975, 1978) have found that repeated administration of interferon to mice in the neonatal period is followed by hepatitis and, later glomerulonephritis; so there are potential complications associated with the use of interferon in human newborns. However, in life threatening virus infections the use of interferon would be justified, and, with luck, might greatly improve the chances of recovery.

Whether interferon given to the mother can protect the fetus against virus infection is another interesting question which should be analysed experimentally in monkeys (where the placenta is less different from the human than is the rodent placenta).

Since interferon can limit cell proliferation there is another potential complication to the fetus, but this is probably less hazardous than damage due to virus infections.

IMMATURITY OF MACROPHAGE FUNCTION AS A FACTOR IN THE SUSCEPTIBILITY OF NEWBORNS TO VIRUS INFECTIONS

When herpes simplex virus or several other viruses are injected into newborn mice or other experimental animals by any route, a lethal infection is produced. Mice a few weeks old became resistant to most viruses inoculated by most routes, whereas intracerebral injection of virus into mice of this age or even adults results in a lethal encephalitis. This has led to the concept that the central nervous system remains sensitive to virus infections while in young animals a barrier develops in other organs of the body preventing the spread of viruses to the central nervous system.

A role of macrophages in age related restriction of herpesvirus (HSV-1) replication was suggested by Johnson (1969). Studying viral antigens by immunofluorescence, he showed that macrophages are the level at which infections are arrested in adult mice. When peritoneal cells from suckling mice were infected in culture the virus spread to form clumps of fluorescent cells. Peritoneal cells from adult mice did not support the complete replication of virus, although Stevens and Cook (1971) subsequently showed that herpes simplex virus undergoes an abortive infection in these cells. In our laboratory further studies were undertaken. Administration of silica particles or anti-macrophage serum, which depletes macrophages, made weanling mice more susceptible to infection (Zisman et al., 1970). Infectious center assays showed that HSV-1 replicates efficiently in cultures of peritoneal cells from newborn but not adult mice. Transfer of peritoneal cells from adult to newborn mice increases the resistance of the latter to HSV-1 infection (Hirsch et al., 1970). Focal necrotizing hepatitis produced by HSV-2 in mice in another model in which the role of macrophages in age related resistance has been studied. After intraperitoneal inoculation of the virus numerous focal areas of necrosis develop in the livers of mice aged up to 4 weeks (Mogenson et al., 1974). In older mice there are a few small lesions (Mogenson, 1977). Again HSV-2 replicates in cultures of peritoneal cells from 3-week-old, but not 8-week-old mice. Silica treatment increased the number of foci in adult mice and transfer of peritoneal cells from 8-week-old to 3-week-old mice decreased the number of foci to nearly as few as seen in adult mice.

The human correlate of these animal model infections is neonatal infection with

HSV (see Nahmias *et al.*, 1975). The infection is usually acquired during passage through the birth canal and hence is most often caused by HSV-2, the genital strain of the virus. The infection is characterized by widespread dissemination of the virus with lesions in many organs, including the central nervous system and liver. It is often fatal. The number of cases in premature infants is disproportionately high.

POSSIBLE USE OF HIGHLY SPECIFIC ANTIBODIES PRODUCED BY THE HYBRIDOMA TECHNIQUE

Antibodies have been widely used for diagnostic purposes and to prevent diseases, for example, γ-globulin replacement therapy in patients with hypogammaglobulinaemia, passive protection with antitoxins and antivenins and administration of immune serum to susceptible persons exposed to viruses. However, antibodies conventionally produced by immunizing animals or occurring in convalescent humans have limitations. They are mixtures of molecules with different immunological specificities and properties such as capacity to activate complement or bind to receptors or leukocytes. Their supply of often limited and no two batches are alike.

It was therefore a great advance when Köhler and Milstein (1965) announced that they could fuse an antibody-forming cell with a tumour cell and obtain cloned cell lines (hybridomas) that could be propagated indefinitely in culture and in mice and would continue to produce large amounts of the same antibody. Thus the capacity to make specific antibody, which in normal cells of the B lymphocyte lineage is limited to a finite number of cell divisions, is immortalized. Hybridomas, with many different specificities have already been produced, and their preparation is now becoming an industry. Some antiviral antibodies secreted by hybridomas have group specificity, others individual specificity. Some neutralize virus but many do not. The hybridomas can be sent from one laboratory to others, ensuring a uniform supply of potent antibodies. This is important for reproducibility, and it is safe to predict that in five years many diagnostic antibodies will come from hybridomas. The same is true of antibodies used for radioimmunoassay of hormones and other biological products.

What could be done for infections of the fetus and newborn? Monoclonal antibodies could be prepared against infectious agents to which the fetus and newborn are susceptible. Small amounts of viral or bacterial antigens could be recognized quickly using new techniques (enzyme linked assays and others) for rapid diagnosis. Monoclonal antibodies could also be used to determine the class of antibodies formed in an infant, which can indicate whether it was infected as a fetus. In our laboratory we have developed small immuno-absorbent columns (4 μl). Pipette tips are packed with commercially available sepharose linked to protein

A. Hybridoma antibodies passed through the column and bound to the protein A and after washing can be used to absorb antigens added to the column. The antigens can be eluted if required. Monoclonal antibodies against human IgM or IgG subclasses could be used to determine the class specificity of antimicrobial antibodies.

These few remarks give some indication of the potential of the monoclonal antibody technique for diagnosis. There is no reason why monoclonal antibodies should not also be used for prophylaxis and therapy. Most of the monoclonal antibodies so far available are murine, but why should these not be injected into humans (horse serum has been widely used)? B lymphocyte cell lines transformed by EB virus release some antibodies of defined specificity (Steinitz *et al.*, 1977; Zuranski *et al.*, 1978), but the yield is low. Higher yields are expected by fusing human antibody-forming cells with human myeloma cells in culture, and there are unpublished reports that this has been successful. It therefore seems likely that human monoclonal antibodies will be available in a few years. These could be purified, treated so as to inactivate any potential oncogenic viruses or nucleic acids and used as a new generation of magic bullets to seek out and neutralize or opsonize or phagocytosis viruses or bacteria in the newborn. The right subclass of monoclonal antibody could be chosen to ensure attachment to receptors on leukocytes.

TRANSFUSIONS IN INFECTIONS OF THE NEWBORN

The case fatality rate of early onset group B streptococcal septicaemia remains high despite early antibiotic therapy. There is evidence that trasfusions of whole blood to the patients increases the likelihood of survival (Courtney *et al.*, 1979). In a group of 49 infants whole blood or exchange transfusions was associated with a significant improvement in survival, regardless of other variables (more than two-thirds of cases survived). Whether this was due to replacement of factors in the newborn required for opsonization or of leukocytes that are not functioning properly in the neonatal period, remains to be established. If the former is the case, purified factors might be used, and their preparation will be discussed in the next section. If leukocytes are required the use of the cell separator and replacement therapy (which has been of such value is reducing infections in patients with malignant disease after aggressive chemotherapy) might be successful in the neonatal period. It would be effective against viruses as well as bacteria, since leukocytes facilitate neutralization. Perhaps replacement therapy should be routine.

WAYS OF PRODUCING AND PURIFYING FACTORS

A second major technical advance in recent years is the cloning of DNA coding for proteins in *Escherichia coli*. Already insulin and other proteins have been produced in the bacteria, and it is conceivable that the same could be done with complement components or other factors required to protect the newborn from infection. The purification of proteins from bacterial secretions or fresh serum would be possible by immuno-absorbent systems (see above) or substrate absorption systems. This type of technology is now being developed but may be of major importance in a few years. The paediatricians and infectious disease specialists should tell their laboratory colleagues what components they want (complement components, interferon and so on) and it is likely that ways will be found to produce the required material in quantity at tolerable expense. This is why meetings such as the Beecham Colloquia are useful—they provide an opportunity for clinicians, laboratory investigators and crystal ball gazers to come together and exchange views. I have covered a few possibilities that might have application to infections of the newborn. The next five years will reveal whether any of these come to pass or whether other, unexpected developments make a major impact.

REFERENCES

Allison, A. C. (1970). On the absence of tolerance in virus oncogenesis. *In* "Proceedings of the IV Quadrennial International Conference on Cancer" (Ed. L. Sèveri), p. 653.

Allison, A. C. (1974). Interactions of antibodies, complement components and various cell types in immunity against viruses and pyogenic bacteria. *Transplant Reviews* **19**, 3–55.

Allison, A. C. (1977). Autoimmune Diseases: Concepts of Pathogenesis and Control. *In* "Autoimmunity: Genetic, Immunologic, Virologic, and Clinical Aspects" (Ed. N. Talal), 91–139. Academic Press, New York.

Allison, A. C., Monga, J. N. and Hammond, V. (1974). Increased susceptibility to virus oncogenesis in congenitally thymus-deprived nude mice. *Nature, London* **252**, 766–767.

Burnet, F. M. (1960). "Principles of animal virology", 2nd edn, 246–258. Academic Press, New York.

Courtney, S. E., Hall, R. T. and Harris, D. J. (1979). Effect of blood transfusions in early-onset group B streptococcal septicaemia. *Lancet* **ii**, 462–463.

Cudkowicz, G. and Hochman, P. S. (1979). Do natural killer cells engage in regulated reactions against self to ensure homeostasis? *Transplant Reviews* **44**, 13–41.

Gidlund, M., Orn, A., Wigzell, H., Seyik, H. and Gresser, I. (1978). Enhanced NK cell activity in mice injected with interferon and interferon inducers. *Nature, London* **273**, 759.

Gresser, I., Morel-Maroger, L., Verroust, P., Rivière, Y. and Guillan, J. C. (1978). Anti-interferon globulin inhibits the development of glomerulonephritis in mice infected with lymphocytic choriomeningitis virus. *Proceedings of the National Academy of Science, USA* **75**, 3413–3416.

Gresser, I., Tovey, M. G., Maury, C. and Chouroulinkov, I. (1975). Lethality of interferon preparations for newborn mice. *Nature, London* **258**, 76–78.

Gresser, I., Tovey, M. G., Maury, C. and Bandu, M. T. (1976). Role of interferon in the pathogenesis of virus diseases in mice as demonstrated with the use of anti-interferon serum. 11 Studies with herpes simplex, Moloney sarcoma, vesicular stomatitis, Newcastle disease, and influenza viruses. *Journal of Experimental Medicine* **144**, 1316.

Hirsch, M. S., Zisman, B. and Allison, A. C. (1970). Macrophages and age-dependent resistance to herpes simplex virus in mice. *Journal of Immunology* **104,** 1160–1165.

Johnson, R. T. (1969). The pathogenesis of herpes virus encephalitis II. A cellular basis for the development of resistance with age. *Journal of Experimental Medicine* **120,** 359–374.

Köhler, G. and Milstein, G. (1975). Continuous culture of fused cells secreting antibody of predefined specificity. *Nature* **256,** 495–7.

Lehmann-Grubbe, F. (1973). "Lymphocytic choriomeningitis virus and other arena-viruses" p. 339. Springer-Verlag, Berlin.

Makinodan, T. E., Perkins, E. H. and Chen, M. G. (1971). Immunologic activity of the aged. *Advances in Gerontology Research* **3,** 171–198.

Mogenson, S. G. (1977). Role of macrophages in hepatitis induced by herpes simplex virus types 1 and 2 in mice. *Infection and Immunity* **17,** 268–273.

Mogenson, S. C., Teisner, C. B. and Andersen, H. K. (1974). Focal necrotic hepatitis in mice as a biological marker for differentiation of *Herpes virus hominis* type 1 and type 2. *Journal of General Virology* **25,** 151–155.

Nahmias, A. J., Visintine, A. M., Reimer, C. B., Del Bueno, I., Shore, S. L. and Starr, S. E. (1975). Herpes simplex virus infection of the fetus and newborn. *Progress in Clinical Biological Research* **3,** 63–67.

Oldstone, M. B. A. and Dixon, F. J. (1969). Pathogenesis of chronic disease associated with persistent lymphocytic choriomeningitis viral infection. I. Relationship of antibody production to disease in neonatally infected mice. *Journal of Experimental Medicine* **129,** 483–505.

Santoli, D. and Koprowski, H. (1979). Mechanism of activation of human natural killer cells against tumour and virus-infected cells. *Immunological Reviews* **94,** 125–163.

Sigel, M. M. (1952). Influence of age on susceptibility to virus infections with particular reference to laboratory animals. *Annual Review of Microbiology* **6,** 247–280.

Steinitz, M., Klein, G., Koskinies, S. and Hakel, O. (1977). EB virus induced B-lymphocyte cell lines producing specific antibody. *Nature, London* **269,** 420–422.

Stevens, J. G. and Cook, M. C. (1971). Restriction of herpes simplex virus by macrophages. An analysis of the cell–virus interaction. *Journal of Experimental Medicine* **133,** 19–38.

Trinchieri, G. and Santoli, D. (1978). Antiviral activity induced by culturing lymphocytes with tumour-derived or virus transformed cells. Enhancement of human NK cell activity by interferon and antagnostic inhibition of susceptibility of target cells to lysis. *Journal of Experimental Medicine* **147,** 1314–1333.

Virelizier, J. L., Lenoir, G. and Griscelli, G. (1978). Persistent Epstein-Barr virus infection in a child with hypergammaglobulinaemia and immunoblastic proliferation associated with a selective defect in immune interferon secretion. *Lancet* **ii,** 231–234.

Virelizier, J.-L., Lipinski, M., Tursz, T. and Griscelli, C. (1979). Defects of immune interferon secretions and natural killer activity in patients with immunological disorders. *Lancet* **ii,** 696–697.

Zisman, B., Hirsch, M. S. and Allison, A. C. (1970). Selective effects of anti-macrophage serum, silica and anti-lymphocyte serum on pathogenesis of herpes virus infections of young adult mice. *Journal of Immunology* **104,** 1155–1159.

Zuranski, V. R. Jr, Haber, E. and Black, P. H. (1978). Production of antibody to tetanus toxoid by tantinous lymphoblastoid cell lines. *Science* **199,** 1439–1441.

DISCUSSION

Adinolfi   I have not clearly understood if you said that the interferon deficiency in the children you mentioned is genetically controlled. Did you say that there are mice with a genetic deficiency of interferon? If so, what types of infection or tumour develop in these mice?

Allison I said that there are differences in interferon production and natural killer activity in different strains of mice. For example, A mice are low producers of interferon under standard conditions and they also have low natural killer activity. They are much more susceptible to certain infections, e.g., malaria and herpes virus infections, than other strains of mice. As to the children with progressive disease, two of these occurred in one family, so it is likely that there was an inherited defect. The others were found in children with severe recurrent infections, including progressive mononucleosis in which the tissues became infiltrated with mononuclear cells and the patients eventually died.

Wood You really have given us quite a challenging task in connection with leukocyte function. I was thinking of how one would deal with a group B streptococcal infection where you perceive a child is sick and have about six hours to get something done. With leukocyte infusions in small babies one is impressed with how nonlaudable pus becomes laudable pus within a couple of hours and the effect fades again after another 12 or 24 h as the leukocytes are used up. One of the the problems one can see is whether this treatment would produce iso-immunization which would have longterm problems for a child.

Allison I think that the longterm risk of iso-immunization is slight. The situation is desperate and one wants to cure the child.

Wood I have another comment. I would like to test the immunological temperature, in a sense. Micheal Denman was talking about the delayed hypersensitivity component of immunity to virus infections, and whether the use of a dialysable transfer factor has any possibilities in the newborn or in the pregnancy.

Allison In the case of transfer factor, the world is divided into the believers and the nonbelievers. I am in the latter category.

Denman Can we return to your thoughts about monoclonal antibodies, particularly in respect to therapy? Could you first outline whether you believe that there are occasions where the ability to give monoclonal antibody of high specificity would help eliminate specific agents? And in that context, how do you envisage dealing with the problem whether antibodies may enhance infections or may block other mediators? How does one sort out that situation even if you do have monoclonal antibodies available?

Allison What I had in mind was, in serious infections, to give an antibody of IgG subclass which would interact with leukocytes. In the human this is IgG 1 and IgG 3. Preliminary experiments could be done in mice but it seems likely that this passive immunity would benefit the child. As regards viruses, Dr Smith mentioned on the first day that some monoclonal antibodies do not neutralize while others do. In the case of influenza virus, for example, we know that only antibodies against the variant specific determinants of the haemagglutinin neutralize. Antibodies against other determinants on the haemagglutinin or other surface proteins do not neutralize. You would have to make sure that the antibodies were neutralizing. Probably interaction with leukocytes is important in neutralization so one would choose sub-classes which interact with leukocytes. I think that this is perfectly feasible.

Wood I think that it is a most attractive idea. If I understand you correctly, the technique achieves a large output of material?

Allison It produces a large amount of very specific material. In other words, you are dealing with one antibody which is directed against a particular determinant.

Adinolfi I would like to ask about the maturation of macrophages in the newborn. Do you agree there is a dichotomy in maturation of the function of the macrophages? It has been suggested that phagocyte activity is normal in the newborn but the function of macrophages as helper cells is incomplete during perinatal life.

Allison We have done some work on this in mice. Newborn mice have macrophages which are deficient in terms of virucidal capacity. Intraperitonal inoculation of certain viruses produces damaging effects in newborns; but if you take peritoneal cells from older animals and put them into the peritoneum of newborns they will resist the infection, particularly in the presence of very small amounts of antibody. Deficient function of mononuclear cells (macrophage and natural killer cells) is certainly one of the features of newborn mice and probably humans.

Bullen Just one point about giving polymorphs to babies. We have produced antipolymorph sera in New Zealand white rabbits and it has no effect on polymorphs from Sandy Lop rabbits. If you infuse a lot of polymorphs into babies, you might induce antipolymorph antibodies which might have bad effects.

Allison This is a potential complication but you are dealing with a child who will probably die if you do not intervene. I think the element of risk is justified.

Hayward We screen probably most of our neonates for severe infection at some time or other, and the problem is to know in which ones to intervene. We find it logistically extremely difficult to give polymorph infusions despite the fact that we have donors available, cell separators etc., simply because by the time you can get this arranged either the child is on antibiotics and you think it is going to get better, or the child is moribund. I think that there are enormous logistical problems which far outweigh the worries as to whether anti-white-cell antibodies are likely to be made.

Denman Could we ask Dr Allison a little more about the mouse strains and patients with NK cell deficiency and interferon deficiency? On *a priori* grounds one would assume that there might be common stem cells, both for cells of the monocyte–macrophage series, granulocytes and NK cells, in terms of bone marrow differentiation. How satisfied are you Dr Allison, that there is not a more generalized defect in an earlier stage in bone marrow differentiation which could also involve other progeny and not exclusively NK cells?

Allison In the children we have been discussing, B and T lymphocyte counts and performance tests have been normal, and there is no evidence for any defect in monocytes or polymorphs. The only defect found in these children is a defect in interferon production by T lymphocytes, either in mixed lymphocyte reactions or when they are stimulated by pokeweed mitogen, an interferon inducer in human lymphocytes. In contrast, the proliferative responses of the lymphocytes are normal. One does not know whether the failure to produce interferon is related to the absence of demonstrable natural killer cell activity in these patients, but the fact is that these patients had a selective defect in that aspect of the system, and they had progressive infections.

Marshall Could somebody comment on the immunosuppressive aspect of antimicrobials. In desperate situations antibiotics are used empirically, if we select the wrong antibiotic could there be adverse effects because of immunosuppression.

Allison I was going to bring this up the other day in regard to the effect of antibiotics on polymorph function. A lot of work has been done on the effect of anti-biotics on lymphocyte functions, particularly by Forsgren in Sweden. Several antibiotics have suppressive effects, both on human lymphocyte reactions *in vitro* in relation to the usual proliferative responses to mitogens and mixed lymphocyte cultures, antibody promotion *in vitro*, and in large doses are immunosuppressive in experimental animals *in vivo*. Whether they are suppressive in therapeutic doses in man is uncertain.

Marshall So if you are measuring the immune responses in ill infants, this is one factor that you would obviously have to take into account in evaluating the results?

Allison Yes. The children with progressive mononucleosis or toxoplasma infection I mentioned were not being treated at the time; obviously that would have complicated the issue. They were looked at over a period of several months and tested repeatedly.

Cooper I should like to return to the fascinating information about immunodeficient patients who do not make interferon. I know of no biologic precedent for this informative experiment of nature. As I recall, interferon is of two molecular forms. One is produced by responding immunocompetent cells and one is produced by any virus infected cell. Do these children not make either, or just the former type?

Allison It is the immune interferon that we are talking about, which is produced by the reactive cells.

Cooper They could, then, presumably make other kinds of interferon, if their cells were infected with EBV?

Allison They presumably could, but EBV multiplies selectively in B lymphocytes and nasopharyngeal cells.

Reeves I should like to refer to the point about possible adverse effects of antibacterial agents on lymphocyte function, which is obviously a very important one. I wonder how much of the data relates to *in vitro* effects in terms of inhibition of lymphocyte stimulation and how much concerns *in vivo* phenomena. It is well known that there is a multitude of agents which can completely flatten *in vitro* lymphocyte responsiveness. A therapeutic dose of two tablets of soluble aspirin can blot out reactivity *in vitro*, yet most of us do not seem to suffer from serious infection when we take such therapy.

Allison Observations were made of the effect of the antibiotics on *in vitro* responses of human lymphocytes and *in vivo* immune responses were tested in experimental animals. In both cases suppressive effects were seen. Whether these are important in patients nobody knows. I do not believe that in the very complicated situations in which antibiotics are used in young children one knows whether it is the effects of massive doses of antibiotics or other defects of the neonate which are being observed.

O'Grady People have looked fairly carefully at patients who have been treated with those agents which have produced most immunosuppression in experimental systems, such as chloramphenicol, trimethoprim and rifampicin, and there is to my knowledge no evidence of any interference with the way that the patients handle the infections.

Hayward When it comes to discussing the effect of the aminoglycosides, we have to bear in mind that almost all of us do our lymphocyte cultures in medium containing aminoglycosides—probably gentamicin nowadays but it used to be penicillin and streptomycin. We have used ampicillin and cloxacillin with equal effectiveness.

Wood I suppose it is possible that in some infections lymphocyte stimulation would already have started before we knew there was something to treat, and that our treatment might come some time after lymphocyte reactivity had been initiated. Or would that be a bonus in the sense that it might be harder to stop by antibiotics once it had got going? Perhaps you could also say if antibiotic depressed lymphocyte function is reversible.

Allison The effects which have been described are reversible, as far as I know, and the major effect is during the early period of transformation. That is the main message which comes out of the work of Forsgren in Sweden. I simply do not know whether it is important in practice. There is an interesting synergism of rifampicin with cell mediated immunity. Where you have depressed cell mediated immunity, as in lepromatous leprosy, rifampicin cannot eliminate the bacteria as in the T cell deficient animal.

Lambert It is interesting to see two completely different types of ideas arising out of Dr Allison's remarks. The problem is how to detect trouble at the very moment when normal colonization with an incredible number and variety of organisms is taking place. On the one hand, there is the idea of trying to detect and boost particular defects of host resistance. On the other, there is the idea of immunological rather than antibiotic "magic bullets" to intercept the specific pathogens, or the banal organsisms getting into the wrong place. On that latter theme—which relies on early diagnosis—I do not think that we need to be too gloomy. The Danish Serum Institute antipneumococcal serum, for example, contains antibody against 88 serotypes, of which only about two are cross-reactive. It does not seem too far fetched to build a capacity for early detection of a large number of antigens, either unusual ones, such as toxoplasmosis, or banal ones in the wrong place, and to use these as diagnostic markers.

Denman Could we ask you a little bit more specifically about that point? It is obviously very critical. Supposing you take the example of Brian Greenwood's demonstration, that you can diagnose meningococcal meningitis very rapidly by performing immuno-electrophoresis on the cerebrospinal fluid. If you took, say, very highly specific, very high affinity, antibody against the precise antigen in which you were interested using the sort of techniques you described, is there any evidence that you would get a reaction which could be detected that much more quickly—in say, fifteen minutes as opposed to the four to six hours it takes at present?

Lambert You can speed it up for the *Pneumococcus* and *Meningococcus* anyway.

Allison One could probably set up an Elisa test, or radio-immuno assay with one of these antibodies, which would reduce it to an hour or thereabouts. It is really a question of hours rather than days.

Chairman I should like to pick up what Dr Allison said earlier about detecting muramic acid and remind everybody that, of course, gas chromatography is now a standard method of identifying anaerobes by picking up the volatile fatty acids which they produce as metabolites. This can be done with clinical material and not only with material grown in culture. In our laboratory, Dr Sanderson has recently got it working on swabs of pus. If you take a little bit of fluid from pus, a purulent discharge, you can identify the organism in it. This is something which can be done in a matter of an hour or so. I do not think that we have got to the end of this. We have just shown that something in principle is possible. There are tantilizing bits of information in the literature like being able to detect squalene in the circulation of people with influenza. It is worth exploring the products of other bacteria and tissue fluids from patients with other serious generalized infections and see if we cannot use this type of physicochemical characterization. It does have the advantage that, although you have to know what you are looking for in the sense that you have to set up the gas chromatographic apparatus in order to look for a certain class of substances, nevertheless you do not need to put a specific reagent into it. You do not have to have a specific antibody against the partciular *Clostridium* in order to be able to do it.

Hayward   I still feel that we are missing the logistic problems. We probably see several flat babies in the emergency room every week and only a small proportion of those are going to suffer from identifiable infections which we might readily be able to treat. Now we have gas chromatographs, we have facilities for counter current immuno-electrophoresis and all these various things. It is difficult and expensive to get people to come in and do these tests where there is going to be a very low yield at two o'clock on a Sunday morning. It may well be easier, rather than preparing monoclonal antibody, to try and prepare immunoglobulin from healthy adults which has a reasonably high titre of antibody against a range of group B streptococci; there are several different antigenic varieties of group B streptococci, so if you have a monoclonal antibody which reacts with one then you have to know which group B streptococci you are dealing with or else you can try to select a monoclonal antibody which reacts with a shared carbohydrate, in which case we may be less confident about its use. I suspect that in the immediate future we may be making more use of selected human sera, rather than concentrating on highly specific reagents.

Chairman   I think the advantage of monoclonal antibodies is that if you do find out exactly what you want, then you can make it by monoclonal technology. I think Tony is a bit optimistic still about making human immunoglobulin types. But the point is that it would be possible, if you knew exactly what determinant you wanted, to make lots of it and to go on making exactly the same, whereas the problem with immunizing animals, or with material from human donors, is that you can never be quite sure whether the next batch will be the same as the last one.

Allison   And in tests like radio-immuno assay for hormones, I can predict that within three or four years all the reagents which will be used will be monoclonal, simply because of reproducibility from one institution to another. Eventually this must be true of diagnostic reagents. It is simply a matter of time before people get used to the idea. The problem is to know what agents you really want. It is up to a group such as yourselves to tell us what reagents you think would be particularly useful.

O'Grady   I should like to come back to the issue of muramic acid. Since bacteria contain a number of substances not present in mammalian tissue their identification is a very attractive way of making a diagnosis. We have made a number of rather half-hearted attempts to look for muramic acid in small quantities and it has turned out in our hands to be very difficult. I wonder if you could say a little more about where you have got to technologically. Do you have two days of difficult chemistry to clean up the material before you start?

Allison   I should say that this work which is going on at the moment by a young British man who is now in the USA. The whole thing can be done in a matter of an hour or two. The essential procedure is one step precipi- tation—conjugation to make a volatile product, and then gas chromatograph;

it could become quite standardized. It works in the low nanogram range and could probably be made more sensitive.

Soothill I feel that the implication of the monoclonal antibodies are really very exciting, but we are not really confining its therapeutic potential in the neonate to diagnosis. Will it be possible to make human material for therapeutic purposes? If so and if the speculations that the phagocyte function is poor in the neonate are correct, then that might limit the therapeutic effect of such antibody which really depends on phagocytes. In the past people have suggested putting nasty things on anticancer antibodies. Could we combine a chemotherapeutic with an antibody effect by adding anti-bacterial chemotherapeutic agents to the antibody and letting the antibody deliver them safely to the right place, and so bypass the dependence on complement and phagocytes?

Allison One might, but I must say that a lot of work has gone on in cancer with antibodies and I think that in general it has been very disappointing. So I personally am not an enthusiast, but I could be convinced if any good evidence along those lines were forthcoming.

Soothill But the antigenicity of the cancer is rather limiting. I am suggesting that the antigenicity of the bacteria might be greater.

Allison That could well be.

Chairman You have to think, too, of the micro-anatomy of the situation when your antibacterial conjugate arrives. Maybe it will get, say, a sulfphonamide on to the outside of the bacterium, but it is not going to do much good until it gets inside and starts inhibiting its metabolism. That is a little technical problem which has not been solved.

Sir Ashley I do not see that adding an antibody would make it home in at all. No antibody homes in to anything. It is a purely chance effect that it meets the bacterium somewhere in the tissue, and equally with the molecules of an antibiotic, I have never known an antibody which said, "By God! there's a bacterium", and homes in on it.

Soothill My point is that antibodies do not do anything to bacteria unless there is an intact complement and phagocyte system, and we are speculating that the complement in the phagocyte system of the neonate may not be very good. That may explain some of our special problems. Can we bypass the dependence of antibacterial function on good complement?

Dewdney We have been pretty speculative about prospects for therapy of the newborn. Do you not feel it is more likely in the foreseeable future that we shall develop much better chemotherapy? I say that because for perhaps the first time we are beginning to see what look to be very potent antiviral drugs of high selectivity for virus infected cells being evaluated in clinical trials in adults. I would have thought that those would contribute more significantly to the control of virus infection in the newborn than any of these exciting and very speculative immunological procedures.

I would also like to ask whether perhaps the newborn with defects of immunological function may not respond as well to these chemotherapeutic agents as the adult does?

Allison   In relation to the last point, that was what I was implying by the remarks about the reinforcement of chemotherapy by immunity in, for example, mycobacterial infections ,which is an example of this type of collaboration.

Since the title of the Colloquium is 'Immunological Aspects of Infection in the Foetus and Newborn", I confined my remarks to that. Like you, I think better chemotherapy, and in particular chemotherapy that does not interfere with the function of granulocytes and lymphocytes would be highly desirable. It may be that one could actually choose chemotherapeutic agents for the newborn as compared with the adults for this very reason.

Faulk   One of the major problems which we have not thoroughly discussed is that of the diagnosis of intra-uterine infections perhaps because these are usually diagnosed retrospectively. I wonder if prospective diagnoses could be made by measuring bacterial products by gas chromatography of maternal blood.

Allison   I have even wondered about amniotic fluid in some circumstances. But maternal blood certainly one could try.

Cole   Could I ask Prof. Soothill, when he said that there is evidence that phagocyte function is depressed in the newborn in group B streptococcal infection, has any trial of fresh frozen plasma adminstration been undertaken in this condition? Because as he pointed out, phagocyte function involves not just the phagocyte itself but the opsonin system, and it is much easier to give fresh frozen plasma than it is to give granulocytes.

Soothill   I do not know whether that has been done. It was Tony Allison, not I, who pointed out a number of aspects of his concern about the poverty of phagocyte function in the neonatal period. The data on humans are fairly scanty. Certainly the interaction of the humoral and the cellular phase of the process is very important, and there is a considerable role for plasma infusion in those, for instance, who have defective yeast opsonization.

Cole   Do we know whether the phagocytes of these newborns will engulf group B streptococcus? Because the tools now available such as chemolumines-cence can give a very quick answer on this, and I am surprised that the actual organism has not been used in the test, (i.e. group B streptococci of the various serotypes).

Soothill   I have not, and I do not know anyone else who has.

Hayward   There is quite a lot of data on this subject from Hill in Salt Lake City indicating the effectiveness, for instance, of exchange transfusion of plasma containing or not containing appropriate anti group B strep. antibodies, and so on, which I would refer you to. As far as the effect of the possible immaturity of the newborn polymorph is concerned, I think this is rather a debatable issue. Miller's data says that they migrate less well, but there is another paper which is open to interpretation that this is due to differences of nuclear size and an artefact of the leading front method of measuring mobility. His other data says that they have a less deformable surface membrane on the basis of aspiration into microtubes. I think we need data telling us whether the heterogeneity of neutrophil maturity in the newborn is partly responsible for the different functional results we obtain. A population of cells that contains a large number of immature cells as well as perhaps a quantitatively normal number of mature cells may respond differently *in vitro* from the way in which it responds *in vivo*, where the mature cells will localize.

Smith I am speculating, but there are probably a number of pregnancies which you know are going to give rise to a fetus which is abnormal in some way, or susceptible to infection. There is probably scope for screening tests to detect these before birth, as with rhesus incompatibility. Under those circumstances you might wish selectively to use immunization with available vaccines to offer protection before inducing labour or Caesarian section. I was thinking of infections like *Pneumococcus* spp., *Haemophilus influenzae* B, and *Neisseria meningitidis* where there are good effective vaccines and in which circulating passive antibody plays a major role in protection. I do not know whether this is realistic because it depends on the ability to forecast the susceptible baby.

Chairman When you say "forecast", are you thinking of something like the at risk registers where one just adds up the number of facts that you have of a quite general nature about the patient?

Smith Yes, I do not know how realistic that is in relation to the infection risk.

Chairman Before the child is born it is a bit difficult.

Marshall We have discussed polymorph function and opsonization and so forth, is there any evidence on these aspects of host defence to explain sex differences in mortality and morbidity in newborn infections?

Chairman I think we shall have to end the discussion at this point—particularly as for the first time, I think, a question has been thrown out which no one has sought to answer immediately. I think we have reached the end of our planned and unplanned agenda.

Index

Acute phase reaction, 47
Antibody, 94, *see also* Milk antibodies
  anti-idiotype, 112
  maternal, 74, 96, 97, 108, 113, 123, 131, 228
  monoclonal, 233, 237, 242
Antigen absorption, 85
Antimicrobials, immunosuppression by, 239, 240

B Cells, 8, 111, 116, 118, 120, 121, 143, 153, 223, 228
Bacterial toxins, 83
BCG Vaccination, 107, 198, 220, 221, 223, 231
Bordetella pertussis, 9
Bronchus-associated lymphoid tissue, 143

C3 Receptors, 8
Chickenpox *see* Varicella-zoster
Chlamydial infections, 72, 75
Chlorhexidine, 70, 214
Colostrum, 41, 96, 123, 124, 131, 145, 152, 162, 163, 182, 184, 195, 222
Complement, 14, 20–37, 64, 126, 130, 146
  components of, 21, 47–49, 97, 107
  genetic polymorphism of, 34
  levels in fetal serum, 27

levels in maternal serum, 31
  phylogeny of, 36
  synthesis, 25, 32
Coxsackie virus infection, 9
Cytomegalovirus, 3, 15, 78, 108, 118, 151, 153, *see also* Immunization

Diathelic immunization, 154, 183
Di George Syndrome, 119, 121

Enterochelin, 134
Enterocolitis necrotizing, 84
Enteromammary immune system, 140–142, 149–150
Enteroviruses, 4, 8, 75, 76
Epstein-Barr virus, 4, 8, 111, 228, 230
Escherichia coli, 70, 95, 124, 130, 131, 132, 134, 163, 179, 198
  antibodies to, in milk, 124, 139
  endotoxins of, 115, 118

Fc Receptor, 11, 56, 115, 116, 119
Fever, 10

Gastric barrier, 84, 91, 181, 193
Gastroenteritis, 71, 72, 195

Giardia lamblia, 101, 141
Glycocalyx, 87
Graft-versus-host disease, 94, 119, 121, 152
Granulocyte, *see* Polymorph

Haemachromatosis, 137
Hepatitis viruses, 4, 50, 84, 229, 231, *see also* Immunization
Herpes virus hominis, 3, 230, 233
Hexachlorophane, 70, 78
Hofbauer cells, 57, 65
Hybridoma technique, 233
Hypogammaglobulinaemia, 120, 162

IgA, 13, 51, 60, 87, 100, 104, 111, 112, 120, 125, 126, 130, 132, 135, 139, 140, 153
  secretory, 87, 93, 94, 97, 99, 102, 124, 130, 135, 139, 140, 183
IgD, 89
IgE, 89
IgG, 11, 15, 50, 56, 60, 64, 74, 96, 108, 111, 112, 117, 120, 126, 139, 140, 183, 223, 237
IgM, 13, 14, 87, 108, 111, 112, 117, 120, 126, 139, 140, 183
Immune complexes, 64, 65, 116, 117, 121
Immunization
  against cytomegalovirus, 199, 214–215
  against dental caries, 212
  against group B haemolytic streptococci, 75, 205–206
  against hepatitis A, 200
  against hepatitis B, 200–202
  against influenza, 213
  against measles, 211, 220
  against poliomyelitis, 197, 218–219, 222
  in pregnancy, 213, 218
  against respiratory syncytial virus, 202–204, 215
  against rubella, 2, 198, 219, 220
  against smallpox, 218
  against tetanus, 213
  against tuberculosis, 111, *see also* BCG
  against varicella-zoster, 204–205
  against yellow fever, 218, 221
Immunodeficiency, 33, 47, 79, 80, 100, 107, 121, 152, 154, 213, 221, 224
  immunological tolerance, 228

Influenza, 213
Interferon, 3, 231
  immune, 230–231, 239

Lactobacilli, 126, 131
Lactoferrin, 41, 51, 60, 97, 99, 124, 125, 130, 132, 146, 156, 160–164, 193
Lamina propria, 86, 87, 153, 154
Large intestine, bacterial flora of, 126, 135
Leukocyte transfusion, 234, 237
Listeria monocytogenes, 71, 72
Lymphocytic choriomeningitis, 9, 117, 228
Lymphocytes, maternal, 62, 112
Lysozyme, 37–40, 51, 84, 93, 97, 130, 132, 146, 156–160

Major histocompatibility complex, 55
Malaria, 5–6, 15, 54
Mammary gland, 135, 146, 151
Measles, 211, 220
Milk
  antibacterial factors in, 155
  antistaphylococcal factor in, 97
  antiviral substance in, 193
  bacterial contamination of, 194–195
  cellular immune response of, 144–146
  fat globules in, 179–181
  fatty acids in, 178
  hydrogen peroxide in, 168, 176
  iron binding proteins of, 125, 130
  lactoperoxidase system, 156, 164–167, 174, 177, 183, 192–193
  leukocytes in, 175–177
  mucosal growth factor of, 102–103
  passive protection by, 95
  thiocyanate in, 167
  vitamin B12 binding protein in, 179
  xantheoxidase in, 178
Milk antibodies, 96, 125, 140, 144, 146, 156, 162
  following vaccination, 144
Mucins, intestinal, 90
Mumps virus, 5, 220

Natural killer cells, 228, 230
Neutrophil, *see* Polymorph

Panencephalitis
  measles, 2
  rubella, 2
Peyer's patches, 86, 89, 104, 143, 151, 153, 154
Peristalsis, 90, 92
Pinocytosis, 84, 87
Placenta
  chorioamnionitis, 53
  Fc receptors, 56–57, 60, 64–66
  fetal stem vessels, 54, 57, 64
  intervillous spaces, 54, 56, 64
  mesenchymal stroma, 54, 56, 57
  transferrin receptors, 55, 60–64
  trophoblasts, 11, 54, 55
Placentitis, 10, 12, 13
Poliovirus, 5, 76, 77, 218–219, 228
Polymorphonuclear leukocytes, 73, 78, 81, 107, 228
Polyoma virus infection, 229
Properdin, 21, 24
Prostaglandins, 104
Pseudomonas infections, 71

Rifampicin, 6
Rotavirus, 17, 72
Rubella, 2, 3, 108, 117, 228, *see also* Immunization
  vaccine damage from, 219–220

Salmonella infections, 134, 135, 137
Systemic lupus erythematosus (SLE), 66
Small intestine
  bacterial adherence to, 84, 88
  bacterial penetration of, 84
  cell mediated immunity, 89
  nonimmunological defences of, 90–93
  secretory immunity, 89
Staphylococcal infections, 70, 71, 79
Streptococcal group B infections, 70, 71, 72, 77, 80, 108, *see also* Immunization
Sudden infant death syndrome, 101–102
Suppressor cells, 109, 116, 118, 119, 121, *see also* T Cells
Syphilis, 108

T Cells, 9, 55, 64, 108–110, 115, 116, 118, 120, 121, 143, 152, 223, 228
Tetanus, 231
Thalassaemia, 136
Toxoplasmosis, 5, 50, 108, 231, 239
Transfer factor, 237
Transferrin, 56, 60, 63, 124, 136, 156, 162
Trophoblast, *see* Placenta
Tuberculosis, 6, 224

Vaccines, 2, 74, 150, 198, 217, 218, 219, 222
Vaccination, *see* Immunization
Vaccinia virus, 107, 218
Varicella-zoster, 4, 108, 222–223, *see also* Immunization
  congenital syndrome of, 3
Vibrio cholerae, 126, 131

Yersinia enterocolitica infections, 136

Zoster immune globulin, 204, 222, 223